T0244233

THE RICH FLEE AND THE POOR TAKE THE BUS

THE RICH FLEE AND THE POOR TAKE THE BUS

How Our

Unequal Society

Fails Us during

Outbreaks

TROY TASSIER

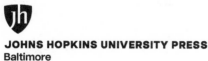

JOHNS HOPKINS UNIVERSITY PRESS
Baltimore

Johns Hopkins University Press

2715 North Charles Street

Baltimore, Maryland 21218

www.press.jhu.edu

Library of Congress Cataloging-in-Publication Data

Names: Tassier, Troy, author.

Title: The rich flee and the poor take the bus : how our unequal society
   fails us during outbreaks / Troy Tassier.

Description: Baltimore, Maryland : Johns Hopkins University Press,
   [2024] | Includes bibliographical references and index.

Identifiers: LCCN 2023013410 | ISBN 9781421448220 (alk. paper) |
   ISBN 9781421448237 (ebook)

Subjects: MESH: Epidemics—economics | Epidemics—epidemiology |
   Socioeconomic Disparities in Health | Social Determinants of Health |
   Risk Factors

Classification: LCC RA649 | NLM WA 105 | DDC 614.4/9—dc23/eng
   /20230726

LC record available at https://lccn.loc.gov/2023013410

A catalog record for this book is available from the British Library.

*Special discounts are available for bulk purchases of this book. For
more information, please contact Special Sales at specialsales@jh.edu.*

To Mary Beth, Katherine, and Nick

CONTENTS

PREFACE

At first the deaths mounted slowly. Then, in late summer, they exploded across the city. By August 1625, there were upward of 4,000 people dying per week in a city with a population of only 300,000. Anyone who could afford to escape the plague distanced themselves from the crowded conditions of London. Newly crowned King Charles prohibited Londoners from entering Whitehall Palace. Parliament adjourned to Oxford. Others who had enough wealth, or a lucky opportunity, escaped to the countryside.

Thomas Dekker, a playwright and pamphleteer, wrote *A Rod for Run-awayes* in protest of those who fled London: "We are warranted by holy Scriptures to flie from *Persecution,* from the *Plague,* and from the *Sword* that pursues us: but you flye to save your selves, and in that flight undoe others."[1] In part, Dekker was objecting to the wealthy carrying the plague to those who lived in the countryside. He demonstrated this harm in the illustration that adorns the cover of his pamphlet. He reserved his strongest words, however, for the financial "undoe-ing" of the poor who were left behind in the city.

When the wealthy left London, shops closed. Churches and charities did not receive alms. The price of bread and grain soared. The economy collapsed. Dekker's "rod" of punishment was raised against the rich for their financial abandonment of the poor as much as the contagion that they created in the countryside. He chastised the wealthy for not providing financial support for those who could not afford to flee to physical safety and for those who faced starvation. Eventually, King Charles intervened by levying a tax

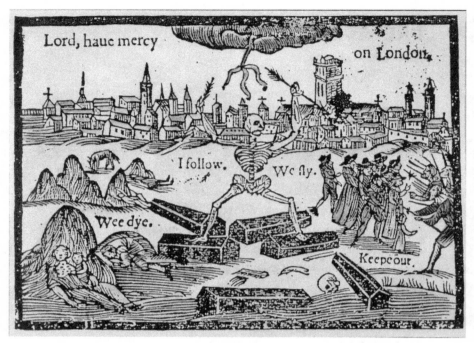

Plague in 1625. Cover image of Thomas Dekker's pamphlet
A Rod for Run-awayes. New York Public Library/Science Source

on those who fled, which he used to feed those who had
been left behind.[2]

In Dekker's description of the plague in 1625, we see
that the movements and behaviors of people—and the financial circumstances of individuals—determined who was
safe and who was sick, who was financially secure and who
was destitute. In London, the actions and interactions of
people, their collective social norms, and their individual beliefs, along with the king's policies, all helped to determine
the path of the plague and its economic consequences. Economics, epidemics, and society were intricately intertwined
in 1625.

They are intertwined today as well.

An old adage in epidemiology claims, "If you've seen one epidemic, you've seen one epidemic." Just like each individual human being is unique, so is each epidemic. Yet, there are regularities to human behavior. And there are regularities to epidemics and how societies and individuals behave in response to them.

While the details change over the years, one result is the same: today and in the past, the most physical and financial harm from epidemics falls upon the people who are least privileged and most marginalized. It is society's responsibility to protect such people when epidemics arrive. We often failed to live up to this responsibility in the past. We failed again with our response to COVID-19.

To avoid this failure in the future, we must understand why this history repeats. Inequality, discrimination, racism, and a lack of financial security all magnify the harm done to vulnerable groups during epidemics. The linkages between these issues and epidemics are not always direct nor simple. They involve a tangled web of interactions among individuals across communities and society. These interactions are the pathways that allow epidemics to spread. But there are other factors, too. Selfish decisions by individuals and firms can create epidemic harm for others just as they did in Dekker's time. Lack of access to high-quality health care leaves some individuals without preventative care, even before an epidemic, while others are without critical care after being infected. Still other people are forced to balance at the margins of poverty, left to choose between epidemic safety and financial survival. Many of the most marginalized face all of these issues simultaneously. By more clearly understanding how each of these issues are interconnected, we can better protect marginalized groups when an epidemic arrives.

We cannot wait until the next epidemic strikes to address these issues. Universal access to high-quality health care, living wages for all workers, lower levels of socioeconomic inequality, and more robust public health funding would prepare us for an epidemic in the future. These improvements would also create a more just society in the present. This book demonstrates why achieving these goals is important. I hope that it will inspire the changes that will bring these objectives to fruition.

THE RICH FLEE AND THE POOR TAKE THE BUS

Chapter 1

THE MOST IMPORTANT LETTER

In 430 BCE, a unique malady arrived in the Athenian port of Piraeus soon after the onset of the Peloponnesian War. Strange and fatal symptoms cursed women, men, and children of normally good health. At first, the folk of Piraeus feared that the invading Spartans had poisoned their water reservoirs. Soon, however, they realized their crisis was much worse. The illness began to appear inland and spread among the people of a narrow, walled corridor that extended six kilometers from Piraeus to Athens. Here the illness found masses of war refugees huddled in crowded makeshift dwellings, while the Spartan army pillaged their homes outside the walls. The refugees never expected to find a second lethal foe waiting inside the walls. As the disease moved onward, near chaos ensued as the entire population from Piraeus to Athens was overcome with pestilence.

Thucydides, the Athenian historian and general, was infected but survived. He described the onset of symptoms as "violent heats in the head, and redness and inflammation of the eyes, the inward parts such as the throat and tongue, becoming bloody." "Sneezing and hoarseness" followed as the strange illness moved downward from the head to the torso. Pain soon settled in the chest and produced a hard cough before progressing to the stomach. Here, "discharges of bile of every kind named by physicians ensued. . . . Ineffectual retching followed, producing violent spasms." The bodies of those afflicted appeared "reddish, livid, and breaking out into small pustules and ulcers. . . . Internally it burned so that the patient could not bear to have on him clothing or linen of even the lightest description." Death arrived to many in short order. Thucydides continued, "The catastrophe was so overwhelming that men, not knowing what would happen next to them, became indifferent to every rule of religion or of law."[1] Over the next three years, at least 25 percent of the population of Athens would die—not from war, but from disease.

The conditions that created this disaster had begun three decades prior. The epidemic was not simply a result of biology. Human behavior played a dominant role, too. In 461 BCE, as tensions mounted with Sparta, Athens began constructing a series of walls to defend its population against land invasion. When completed, the eight-meter-high, six-kilometer-long stone and brick walls formed a corridor between the port of Piraeus and the city of Athens.[2] With the weapons of the time, walls of this type were virtually impenetrable. The only hope an enemy had of overcoming such a barrier was to surround the city and then starve its people of necessities, thereby forcing surrender. The strength of the Athenian navy and its control of the surrounding seas prevented this from happening. Food and supplies arrived at Piraeus and were transported safely through the protected corridor to Athens.

When Sparta invaded the countryside and attempted to surround Athens at the start of the war, the farmers and country folk of Attica fled their homes in an attempt to gain safety inside the long walls. As the war intensified, the population inside the walls exploded from 145,000 people to an estimated half a million.[3] As the refugees' numbers increased, Athens sent its ships to raid Spartan crops along the coast of the Peloponnese and to collect items for trade. They used proceeds from these raids to feed the masses of residents and refugees trapped within the long walls.

Shortly thereafter, an epidemic arose in northern Africa near Ethiopia. It soon spread into Egypt and Libya. Given that the shipping industry was vital to the survival of Athens during the war, the epidemic soon found its way onto an Athenian ship and invaded the port at Piraeus. As people began to fall ill, some residents of Piraeus believed that their water had been poisoned by Sparta, but they soon realized that they faced a more dangerous reality: they were under attack from infectious disease. It feasted on the population crowded between the long walls. Thucydides wrote that when the war refugees arrived from the countryside, "there were no houses to receive them, they had to be lodged . . . in stifling cabins, where the mortality raged without restraint. The bodies of dying men lay one upon the other, and half dead creatures reeled about the streets."[4]

Although infectious disease had existed since time immemorial, this is the first record of the massive destruction of a population by epidemic disease. To this day, historians debate which infectious disease was responsible for the catastrophe.[5] It may have been measles, smallpox, typhus, or bubonic plague. Or it may have been another pathogen that has faded from history and may be either extinct or not recognizable today.

For centuries, episodes of infectious disease have added twists and turns to history, as well as turmoil to individual lives. The year 2019 will be remembered for the arrival of another illness. Beginning late in the year, the novel coronavirus, SARS-CoV-2, began infecting unsuspecting citizens in Wuhan, China. By early 2020, the virus had circumvented the globe and enveloped society the world over with disease and fear. Although the plague of Athens and the plague of our time are separated by twenty-five centuries, there are parallels between them.

In *On the Nature of Things*, Lucretius describes the plague of Athens as follows:

> 'Twas such a manner of disease, 'twas such
> Mortal miasma in Cecropian lands
> Whilom reduced the plains to dead men's bones,
> Unpeopled the highways, drained of citizens
> The Athenian town. For coming from afar,
> Rising in the lands of Aegypt, traversing,
> Reaches of air and floating fields of foam,
> At last on all Pandion's folk it swooped;[6]

As in this description of Athens, the COVID-19 pandemic took people off the highways and emptied our great cities. It swooped upon us and arrived from afar over air and sea. It invaded our cities, towns, schools, and homes. As it did so, everything in society changed—across health care, economics, education, and even politics.

Despite this sweep of change in our lives, where everything seemed in turmoil and everything was different, there were many historical constants in how the epidemic behaved and how we behaved in response. The COVID-19 pandemic repeated patterns that historians had noted for centuries. In the twenty-first century, however, these experiences seemed new. Not since the 1918 influenza pandemic had we seen anything similar sweep the globe.

As COVID-19 arrived, statements dotted newspapers, claiming that this new pandemic would threaten everyone. Public figures, from New York State Governor Andrew Cuomo to pop star Madonna, referred to this new plague as the *great equalizer*, where everyone was equally at risk.

We learned quickly in the spring of 2020, however, that this pandemic was no great equalizer.

In the first wave of the pandemic in the United States, people of color died at rates two to three times greater than their white counterparts. Impoverished urban neighborhoods faced higher rates of sickness and death than more affluent neighborhoods that sat only a few blocks away. Young people and women more frequently lost their jobs as a result of the pandemic than did middle-aged workers and men. Those with high levels of education often transitioned to the safety of remote work in their homes. Service-sector workers, however, if they were lucky enough to remain employed, faced a higher risk of infection in their crowded, in-person places of work. Everywhere one looked, the effects of the pandemic were unequal. Those at the margins of society paid the highest costs in terms of health and in terms of finances. This wasn't random or a case of "bad luck." It was predictable. It was history repeated.

Even the few who knew the history had hoped that this time would be different. We had more wealth and technology to fight a pandemic than ever before. Science, with its twenty-first-century understanding of viruses along with greater understanding of public health and epidemiology, might allow us to be spared. In addition, a more developed economic system and a greater social safety net sat poised to protect the economically disadvantaged. Yet these Panglossian optimists were fooled. Epidemic inequality prevailed everywhere we looked. It has been this way for centuries.

In the nineteenth century, Naples was the largest city in Italy, with a population just under 500,000 people. This population was far from evenly spread across the city. The upper city sat within the hills surrounding the port. Its residents looked down, literally and figuratively, upon those living in the lower city along the northern shore of the Gulf of Naples. The upper city was sparsely populated and affluent, while the lower city was dense and impoverished. In the regions of the lower city with the greatest concentration of people, approximately 4,500 buildings housed 300,000 residents.[7] In these small structures, as many as seven people typically occupied only five square meters, a space that was barely big enough to allow each person to lie down.[8] In addition to using these minimal dwellings for sleeping and eating, people often shared them with poultry. Running water and connections to a sewer system were nonexistent. This meant that bathing for cleanliness was not an option, and clothes were washed in large communal troughs placed in narrow streets and dark alleys. Garbage and human waste, which were dumped through windows and trickled down damp narrow alleys, pooled in the crevices of the uneven streets. One can imagine the stench. Light rarely reached inside these dwellings. It must have been like living in a cave, almost unable to see your surroundings.

In addition to having these horrid living conditions, the lower city was an economic disaster. With so many people packed on top of each other and limited job opportunities, wages were severely depressed. According to epidemiological historian Frank Snowden, during a normal ten- to twelve-hour workday, an unskilled male earned enough to buy four kilograms (about nine pounds) of pasta, and four days of labor were needed to purchase a pair of shoes. These items were luxuries, however, which large swaths of the population could not afford given that up to 40 percent of the city was permanently unemployed.[9]

When cholera arrived in Naples early in the nineteenth century, these dense and impoverished conditions within the lower city led to dramatic levels of epidemic infestation. During the 1884 epidemic, about 5,600 deaths were recorded among a population of about 460,000 people, which means that slightly more than 1 percent of the population died. These deaths were not evenly distributed across Naples. Almost 4,500 people died in the most crowded and poor lower-city boroughs: Mercato, Pendino, Porto, and Vicaria. While these were some of the most populous boroughs of Naples, they were home to about 190,000 of the 460,000 total population.[10] That is, 80 percent of the deaths occurred in an area that contained only 40 percent of the population. These horrid conditions led member of parliament Renzo De Zerbi to label this area the "Death Zone."[11] All of the nineteenth-century cholera epidemics in Naples followed this same pattern of concentration in the four most impoverished and densely populated boroughs. Economic inequality led to epidemic inequality.

Today it is easier to understand why an epidemic would spread so easily given the conditions of the lower city. Everything that leads to person-to-person contagion existed in lower Naples in this time of residential congestion and minimal sanitation. However, the population at the time did not understand how infectious diseases were spread. The germ theory of disease was only in its infancy in the late nineteenth century. While an early understanding of contagion existed, perhaps since the time of the Black Death, it wasn't until the early twentieth century that Ronald Ross developed the roots of modern mathematical epidemiology.

In 1902, Ross won a Nobel Prize for research identifying the mechanism of malaria transmission. He carefully demonstrated through a series of experiments that mosquitoes acted as a vector that transmitted malaria from human to human. He also demonstrated that reducing the population of mosquitoes and destroying stagnant bodies of water, which were their breeding grounds, could limit malaria in a local area.

Despite this success, Ross remained troubled. He recognized that one could not eliminate all mosquitoes. Did this mean that malaria could not be fully eliminated in a local area?

Based on field experience, he hypothesized that this was not true. For a better understanding, he turned away from experimentation and toward mathematics. He began by recognizing that in order for a malaria epidemic to occur, there had to be a sufficient population of mosquitoes coupled with a sufficient population of people who were not immune to being infected. He called these non-immune people *susceptible*. Further, the mosquitoes had to survive long enough for the parasite that causes malaria to reproduce within the mosquito. If there were too few susceptible people, or if there were too few mosquitoes, or if the life span of mosquitoes was too short, his mathematics showed that a local epidemic would disappear.[12]

William Kermack and Anderson McKendrick developed Ross's theories further with more exact mathematical analysis. Much of their work can be summarized in a simple manner and represented by the most important letter in epidemiology, R, which stands for the *reproduction number*. It is defined as the average number of new infections created by each infected person during the course of infection. For instance, if each infected person passes the infection to three others, on average, then the reproduction number is three.

The reproduction number of infectious disease can be thought of in the same way that an ecologist considers the growth of a species, say, rabbits, in a particular habitat, like a forest. If each rabbit in a forest has more than one offspring over the course of its life on average, then the rabbit population grows larger in each generation. If each rabbit has fewer than one offspring, on average, then the rabbit population dwindles and eventually disappears. Kermack and McKendrick showed that epidemics work the same way.

Imagine that you become infected with influenza. Before you realize that you are sick, you infect two coworkers. One of these coworkers infects a spouse and a child in their home. The other infects two people that they meet at a pub after work. In this example, the reproduction number is two. Your initial infection has grown from one infection (you), to two (your coworkers) and then to four (the spouse, child, and two friends at the pub) in each successive step of this mini-epidemic.

Whether an epidemic grows or shrinks depends on whether the reproduction number is larger or smaller than one. If each infected person creates more than one new infection, on average, then an epidemic grows. This happened with your influenza infection. If the reproduction number is less than one, then an epidemic shrinks and dies out. Suppose that eight people are infected and the reproduction number is only one-half. Eight infections become four. Four becomes two. Two becomes one, and the epidemic disappears.

Mathematical epidemiologist Adam Kucharski has a simple way of describing the key elements that compose the reproduction number with the acronym DOTS.[13] D measures the duration of the infection: the longer someone is ill, the longer the period of time that they can infect new people. O measures the opportunities for infection to spread: the more interactions with other people that someone has, the larger the number of people that they can infect. Each day an infected person has the opportunity to infect members of their household, coworkers, friends, and random people sitting at tables near them during lunch in a restaurant or sitting near them on a city bus. These are all opportunities for an infection to spread. T measures the probability of transmission: it tells the likelihood that a non-immune person is infected each time they interact with an infectious person. When someone sneezes near a coworker, sometimes the coworker becomes infected and sometimes the coworker does not become infected. S measures the fraction of the population that is susceptible (not immune) to infection: it tells the fraction of people in the population who are available to infect. If more children in a school are effectively vaccinated against measles, fewer children are able to become infected if an outbreak occurs. The size of each of these four factors helps to determine whether an infected person spreads a given infection to two people, ten people, or no one.

If we assume that people interact in a random manner, like people mixing together on a city bus or train, then the reproduction number can be calculated by multiplying these four factors. Whenever this product is larger than one, the epidemic grows; whenever it is less than one, the epidemic shrinks. Whenever one of these factors grows larger for a given infectious disease, so too does the associated epidemic.

Of course, real-world epidemics are more complex. Infectious disease involves more nuanced features of spread, such as asymptomatic transmission and latent states of disease. In addition, the interactions of people are not random. You interact with your family, neighbors, and coworkers far more frequently than others in the population. Some people, like bus drivers, interact with many people at work; a late-night janitor interacts with only a few. These complications make the reproduction number more difficult to calculate in a real-world epidemic. However, despite these complications and others like them, the reproduction number provides a guide to understanding how infectious disease spreads from person to person, how fast it does so, and how large we can expect an epidemic to be.

We saw the elements of the reproduction number present in the Naples cholera epidemics. People compressed together in a small living space created more opportunities for infections to spread. Unsanitary disposal of human waste made each of those opportunities more likely to result in transmission. The dense and unsanitary conditions of the lower city of Naples created a larger reproduction number than did the conditions in the sparsely populated and more sanitary upper city.

We saw the elements of the reproduction number in the plague of Athens, too. The area where the 355,000 refugees congregated between the port and the city had the largest density known in the world at the time. This density provided numerous opportunities for the infectious disease to spread.

This great density of Athens in the fifth century BCE was an outlier: it was ahead of its time. As society developed in the coming centuries, the new modern world evolved in two complementary directions that each favored the spread of infectious disease. As means of travel became more efficient, people moved about the world to farther distances and at a more rapid pace. In many instances, infectious diseases were traded along with goods. The Black Death arrived at the ports of Italy from Asia along the routes of trade on land and sea, as well as through military skirmishes; imperial traders and soldiers brought smallpox to the Americas and were repelled from some conquests in the Caribbean by yellow fever; and the East India Company brought cholera to England and Ireland, and from there it spread to continental Europe and the Americas. In previous episodes of history, people did not move this far, this fast. Historian Alfred W. Crosby called this intermixing of commerce and disease the *Columbian Exchange*.[14] Similarly, historian Emmanuel Le Roy Ladurie noted that this period set about the common markets of microbes and contagion.[15] The birth of international trade brought with it a larger reproduction number as new opportunities for epidemics emerged on new soils.

Yet even with the exchange of germs between the old and new worlds, these common markets would have had less influence on world history had a second effect not occurred: the great migration of the world's population to cities and the explosion of modern urban density. The congestion within the long walls of Athens and its near destruction of Athens's population by infectious disease provided a harbinger of dark days to come.

As the industrial revolution in England began, the country was a rural agrarian society. As of 1776, only a quarter of the population in England lived in urban environments. With the onset of city-based manufacturing and industrial growth, people began moving to cities to find work and wealth. By 1871, nearly two-thirds of the population in England lived in an urban environment.[16]

The United States began its history as a rural environment, too. As of 1800, there were only thirty-three cities in the United States with a population of more than 2,500 people. While today this benchmark population would be considered a small town, in the early nineteenth century, 2,500 people was urban. These thirty-three cities comprised only about 6 percent of the US population.[17] As time marched forward, international immigration and internal migration led more people to settle in cities. By the turn of the millennium, 80 percent of the US population lived in an *urban environment*—which, after 1960, was defined as "containing more than 1,000 people per square mile."[18]

While density was increasing within cities, it wasn't evenly spread across them. Late nineteenth-century Manhattan housed about 220 people per acre; however, the most-dense tenement neighborhoods in New York City had over 960 people per acre, and the most-dense block in this most-dense neighborhood had over 1,200 people per acre.[19] By comparison, a typical suburban residence in the United States today may contain a home with four people living on a quarter-acre lot. This would create a density of only sixteen people per acre. The most dense area of New York City in 1900 had 1,200 people living on one acre!

While the most-dense areas of nineteenth-century Manhattan tenements were extreme, most cities had neighborhoods that were much more dense than their city average. In this time period, Glasgow, London, Mumbai (formerly Bombay), and Paris all had a city-wide average density of between 60 and 125 people per acre. Yet each of these cities had at least one neighborhood with a density of over 350 people per acre. Mumbai had a neighborhood with 760 people per acre.[20] Many of these most-dense areas became notable for infectious disease outbreaks in the nineteenth century.

Density wasn't evenly spread across cities in the past, and it isn't evenly spread across cities today either. Many people have walked along the sidewalks of a crowded city street, passing shoulder to shoulder with others as heat radiates upward from the sidewalks and streets. On a hot summer day, this density can feel suffocating. We look up to see apartment and office buildings blocking the horizon from view. The air we breathe feels heavy. The masses of people weigh upon us in these congested quarters. On the outskirts of this same city sit far less congested residential streets. Few people populate the sidewalks there. Those that do are walking their dogs or taking a child for a stroll. On a morning walk, we can feel a brisk breeze pass over our cheeks. The air feels light. In these neighborhoods, the living spaces are larger and contain a family of a few people at most.

The people residing in these two different environments, in the same city just a short distance apart, live far different existences in terms of infectious disease risk. Density creates more opportunities for infections to spread and a larger reproduction number. This is true today and in centuries long past.

The epidemic that Athens suffered resulted as much from its congestion and density inside the long walls as it did from a novel infectious disease; they each played their role. Each was necessary to kill one-quarter of the population. Naples's densest and poorest neighborhoods suffered the most from cholera; the more spacious upper city was spared the terror that existed in the lower city during these epidemics due to differences in social and economic factors that created a larger reproduction number in the lower city. This different experience wasn't unique to Athens and Naples.

In 1894, bubonic plague broke out in the southeast Chinese mainland. Within only five months, eighty thousand people had died. Not surprisingly, the epidemic spilled over into the neighboring British colony of Hong Kong. Once there, the plague spread widely, and a full-blown epidemic took off that lasted intermittently for three decades. Each episode of the epidemic was most pronounced in the dense urban slums, where opportunities for infection were the greatest. In 1894, Hong Kong was highly segregated and bore a striking resemblance to Naples: The white Europeans lived in the hills, 800 feet above sea level, in almost total isolation from the rest of the island. Below them, the laborers lived in densely packed tenement-style housing. The district of Tai Ping Shan held over 930 residents per acre, while the more affluent European neighborhoods held about forty.[21] The slums contained a density that was twenty-three times greater than the more affluent areas of the city. The density of Tai Ping Shan provided fertile soil and many opportunities for the plague to spread.

After the 1894 epidemic, the plague receded; but it returned in 1896 and every year thereafter until 1929. In total, twenty thousand people perished. In absolute numbers, this wave of bubonic plague paled in comparison to medieval Europe, yet this epidemic in Hong Kong resulted in 10 percent of the inhabitants dying over a period of thirty-five years. Like the cholera epidemics in Naples, most of the deaths in Hong Kong were located in the densely packed, impoverished areas of the city such as Tai Ping Shan.[22] The elite of Hong Kong held a special form of immunity from infection: space. They were insulated by space from dense areas cursed by the plague.

This pandemic plague wasn't contained in Hong Kong. It continued spreading across the world and reached as far as North America. Initially it traveled along steam ship routes as rats carried it from Hong Kong to other ports. Most damaging was the arrival in Mumbai (Bombay). This third wave of pandemic plague killed over ten million people in India during the first three decades of the twentieth century.[23]

In the midst of this outbreak, India, like the rest of the world, was struck by the 1918 influenza pandemic. In 1918, influenza mortality in India was the largest in the world. Between twelve million and twenty million people died.[24]

The rate of mortality in Mumbai was far from equal across classes and neighborhoods. Europeans living in more luxurious sections of Mumbai had mortality rates of 8 deaths per 1,000 people. This was similar to the rate of mortality during the influenza pandemic in the United States of 6 deaths per 1,000. However, the lowest caste members of the Mumbai population lived in crowded urban slums. Here the rate of death was over 60 per 1,000 people.[25] By comparison, the COVID-19 pandemic had rates of mortality between 2 and 3 per 1,000 for the United States and most of Europe as of year-end 2021. The rate of death for lower-caste members of Mumbai in the 1918 pandemic was twenty to thirty times greater than the typical COVID-19 mortality rate in the United States and Europe. It has been argued that the 1918 influenza pandemic was class neutral. Clearly, it wasn't in Mumbai.[26]

Historian Svenn-Erik Mamelund argues against class neutrality of 1918 influenza mortality as well. The poorest areas in the Norwegian capital of Oslo (then known as Kristiania) had excess mortality rates that were 50 percent higher than the wealthiest areas. The congestion of the poorer neighborhoods and the fact that its residents lived in smaller dwellings led to more deaths.[27]

Across all of these epidemics in Athens, Naples, Hong Kong, Mumbai, and Oslo, the culprit that brought ruin upon the most impoverished was density. The opportunities for infection that density created brought a larger reproduction number and more risk to the most congested neighborhoods in these cities. In each case, the social and economic circumstances of the poorest residents left them to face a more severe epidemic than the wealthy.

When vaccines and medicines, such as Paxlovid, became available to prevent and treat COVID-19, views on the pandemic changed. Across the world, arguments surfaced suggesting that individuals should judge their personal risk from the pandemic and make individual choices based on that personal risk. According to this view, governments should step aside to allow people to independently choose which specific measures of safety to invoke. Because some faced less risk, it was argued that these people should not be constrained by mitigation strategies such as social distancing or mask-wearing. Eventually, this libertarian perspective came to dominate much of government response and the rhetoric of media coverage on the pandemic. This focus on individual risk missed a key part of understanding pandemics today and in the past.

When the word *risk* is employed in the context of epidemics, we need to be careful to parse out its meaning. There are two different types of risk within epidemics. I term the first type *health risk*. It measures the risk associated with what happens to someone once that person is infected: that is to say, how likely one is to get seriously ill, be hospitalized, suffer a chronic condition such as long COVID, or die. Often, health risk differs by age, comorbidities, previous exposure, or vaccination status. When people argued that individuals should be left to judge their own risk, they often meant that they should only consider what I term health risk. But this is not the only risk in epidemics.

Exposure risk is a second type of risk. It measures the likelihood that someone is infected. This differs according to an individual's number of daily personal interactions, living conditions, and job, along with that individual's behavior. It also differs according to the interactions and behavior of people around that individual. If the people near you act recklessly and infections increase in your neighborhood, then your exposure risk increases because there are more infected people around you. The circumstances and behavior of others around you determine your safety. You don't choose your exposure alone; exposure risk is a shared risk of communities and society.

Together, these two risks determine pandemic outcomes. Exposure risk determines one's likelihood of infection; health risk determines what happens after infection. Physicians often focus on individuals and health risk; public health experts and epidemiologists often focus on populations and exposure risk. Of course, each discipline considers each type of risk, but the focus is different.

The impoverished citizens of nineteenth- and early twentieth-century slums had elevated levels of both types of risk. Residential density created extra exposure risk, and lack of nutrition created extra health risk. In other situations, individuals hold one type of risk but not the other. Someone may have high health risk because of a comorbidity. That individual may be extra careful to avoid interacting with others. In limiting interactions, the individual limits their exposure risk. Importantly, the individual cannot eliminate exposure risk entirely because exposure risk depends in part on the actions of others around them.

The more important difference occurs when risks are unbalanced in the other direction. When someone has low health risk, they may not concern themselves with exposure risk if left to their own devices. A healthy twenty-year-old college student with low health risk may decide to ignore worries about being infected with influenza. They may forgo their annual influenza vaccine. They may act less cautiously than others who have a greater health risk. They may ride a city bus or go to classes while occasionally coughing. When they do so, they create exposure risk for others around them. This exposure risk is shared with the community. Someone on the bus may become infected. Before this second person is symptomatic or feeling unwell, that person may pass influenza to an elderly relative in their home or to a neighbor in their apartment building. This third person may become seriously ill. The college student with low health risk may face little harm with only a sniffle and some coughing or sneezing, but others may suffer far worse outcomes from the exposure risk that the college student created by not being careful. People like that individual who ignores exposure risk create danger for others.

In February 1519, Hernán Cortés set sail from Cuba with five hundred men headed to the Mexican mainland. The Aztec Empire and its six million citizens controlled his destination. The empire was centered on the capital city of Tenochtitlan. It was one of the largest cities in the world in 1519, a thriving metropolis with a population between 150,000 and 200,000 people. Paris was the only European city larger than Tenochtitlan at the time.

Though significantly outnumbered, the army of Cortés conquered Montezuma and the entire Aztec Empire in just over two and a half years. Cortés was a skilled and demanding general. He famously sunk his ships to avoid potential mutiny and the return of his soldiers to Cuba.[28] He created alliances with other Indigenous groups who were enemies of the Aztec. When Diego Velázquez de Cuéllar, the Cuban governor, sent troops to arrest him for treason, Cortés convinced these troops to fight alongside him against the Aztec.[29] However, no amount of skill as a military leader would have brought down the Aztec Empire given how vastly he was outnumbered by the Aztec people.

Instead, the Aztec fell to a hidden ally of Cortés: smallpox. Believed to have been brought to Europe during the eleventh-century crusades, smallpox afflicted the European continent in periodic epidemics into the twentieth century. Even though smallpox remained deadly to some Europeans, many had developed at least limited immunity due to experience with past epidemics. This mitigated the Europeans' health risk from smallpox. However, the Aztec, who lacked this history and immunity, faced severe health risk when the Europeans exposed them. The Aztec civilization was destroyed when a smallpox epidemic broke out in October of 1520. It is estimated that the population of Tenochtitlan was reduced by over 40 percent in one year, primarily due to the disease.[30] Many of those that remained alive were sick and hungry. Unable to muster a significant defense with the remaining population, the Aztec fell to Cortés and surrendered in August 1521. A population that once totaled six million people was now a part of the Spanish Empire.[31]

The spread of smallpox did not stop with the conquest of the Aztec. Smallpox spread throughout Mexico and south through Central America before continuing along the western coast of South America. There it arrived among the people of the second great empire of the Americas: the Inca. Like the Aztec Empire, the Incan Empire numbered several million people. It stretched along the Pacific Ocean from present day Ecuador in the north to Santiago, Chile, in the south. It too had a large city, Cuzco, with a population of about 150,000. When smallpox arrived, it would take two hundred thousand lives from the empire in short order. These included Incan emperor Huayna Capac, along with his eldest son and heir. Civil war and smallpox then worked together to fragment the empire. By the time conquistador Francisco Pizarro arrived, the empire was in disorder. He and his few hundred men gained control of the Incan Empire for Spain in 1533. In total, about 60 percent of the population would die from smallpox.[32]

Smallpox also ravaged Indigenous populations in Brazil, Chile, Colombia, and Venezuela. It spread northward from Mexico into other parts of North America. Here it spread in a slower fashion due to the more isolated hunter-gatherer organization of the population, who did not reside in large cities, unlike many living in the Aztec and Incan empires. Still, over a period of two centuries, two-thirds of the Catawba, Cherokee, Iroquois, Omaha, and Sioux were killed by smallpox and other newly arrived infectious diseases.[33]

During this time, imperialists were aided by superior weapons of war. However, the primary culprit for this destruction was infectious disease, not weapons. Although British officer Sir Jeffrey Amherst infamously delivered blankets infected with smallpox to Native Americans, and others may have performed similar atrocities, it wasn't biological warfare that destroyed the native population. The Aztec and Incan empires, along with the vast majority of the American Indigenous population, were already gone before Amherst's time. The primary culprit was what historian Alfred W. Crosby called a "virgin soil epidemic."[34] A series of dangerous pathogens including smallpox, measles, typhus, influenza, and others were introduced into a population that had no immunity. Almost everyone in the Indigenous population had large amounts of exposure and health risk when confronting these novel pathogens. That was all that was needed to destroy these civilizations once the virgin soil epidemic took root.

Yes, some Europeans were affected. Some became sick and died. However, they were afflicted less frequently than the Indigenous population. Although the Europeans did suffer from new diseases in the Americas such as yellow fever, they could move about more freely with minimal concern for health risk. This movement increased exposure risk for the Indigenous people. Once the people were exposed, health risk took over and destroyed their society. Nothing else was needed.

The destruction caused by Old-World germs in the New World brought about the end of two great empires and many smaller tribes and societies. They were destroyed by smallpox, with help from measles, typhus, and influenza. These pathogens upended and destroyed Indigenous civilizations throughout the North and South American continents. When Columbus arrived in 1492, the population of North and South America was between fifty million and one hundred million people; but 150 years later, this population numbered between five million and ten million. The Indigenous population of the Americas was reduced by somewhere between forty million and ninety million people in only 150 years. Historian J. N. Hays calls this destruction of life and society the "greatest demographic disaster in history."[35]

Many people puzzle over how quickly these epidemics grew. How can one infection start an epidemic in Mexico that could wipe out civilizations across two continents? The answer is *exponential growth*.

If the reproduction number for influenza is two, then your influenza infection spreads to two coworkers. Those coworkers together infect a spouse, a child, and two friends, creating four new infections. Each of these four pass it on to two more, resulting in eight infections. One becomes two, two becomes four, four becomes eight, and so on. As these infections continue to multiply, we reach over one thousand infections after ten multiplications. This does not seem too bad. However, by twenty multiplications, we reach over one million infections. In twenty-five multiplications, we have over thirty-three million infections. If each of these infections has a duration of a week, then it takes only twenty-five weeks to infect thirty-three million people. Exponential growth climbs quietly early on. The first ten periods produce only one thousand infections; the next ten produce one million. The next five yield over thirty million! In the early periods, infections multiply but they are less noticed until they explode to thousands or millions and demand attention. At this point, the epidemic is beyond control in the short term. It doesn't always take an unusual event to see infections explode; only exposure risk and time are needed.

Still, if the infections do not create significant health risk, then no one will care. If smallpox was similar to a cold and an infection just created a sniffle and headache, world history would have been different. The Aztec likely would have repelled Cortés. The Inca would still be with us. But smallpox wasn't innocuous; it was lethal. Once smallpox entered the Americas, the Indigenous people had no chance. Exponential growth of infections took over, and society and world history changed.

The reproduction number is associated with exposure risk—not health risk. If we concentrate our response to an epidemic on individual health risk, we give up hope of controlling the reproduction number. But if we concentrate on controlling exposure risk, we limit the reproduction number and fewer people face health risk. Even those with the most severe health risk can sometimes be better protected by controlling exposure risk.

Luckily for the twenty-first-century world, we knew how to slow the exponential growth of novel viruses when COVID-19 arrived. Like smallpox and other deadly diseases, COVID-19 was not just a cold. It contained a large amount of health risk. We prevented many from suffering from their health risk because we knew how to lower the reproduction number and how to control exposure risk. We isolated after infection to lower the duration of time that an infected person interacted with others. We used social distancing to reduce opportunities for infection. We wore face coverings to limit transmission. We invented new vaccines to introduce amounts of immunity and lower the fraction of susceptible people in the population. We used each of these mitigation measures, and more, to attack each element of DOTS (duration, opportunity, transmission, and susceptibility) in order to make the reproduction number smaller. In early March 2020, the United States faced a reproduction number of between three and four from SARS-CoV-2. Our early social distancing, mass gathering limits, and masking, along with other non-pharmaceutical interventions, dropped the reproduction number to around one by the end of March 2020.[36] Although the damage of this novel virus was great, it would have been much greater without intervention. If we had continued to live our lives as normal, we may have faced the fate of Athens or Tenochtitlan.

During the Columbian Exchange, the knowledge of how to limit epidemics wasn't available. In the sixteenth century, novel pathogens in the New World spread unchecked. Back then, no one understood the science of epidemiology that Ross, Kermack, and McKendrick introduced to the world in the twentieth century. Disease was spreading, and no one knew how to stop it or even how it was being spread. A novel virus ran unchecked across two continents, and millions upon millions of people died. Societies collapsed. We can only imagine that many of these societies followed the patterns of behavior that occurred in Athens and, as Thucydides wrote, became indifferent to rules of religion and law. On the other side of this divide between the civil society and chaos sat the Europeans, ready to pick up the spoils of conquest.

The COVID-19 pandemic brought similar uneven risks. The twenty-year-old student who did not care about influenza did not care about coronavirus either. Without intervening health conditions, that student had exposure risk but perhaps had limited health risk. A seventy-year-old diabetes sufferer living in the same neighborhood as the twenty-year-old had both types of risk. Both of these individuals faced exposure risk; they both could be infected. In fact, the college student likely faced more exposure risk because they had more contacts and more opportunities for infection each day than the seventy-year-old. Further, the student may have done less to limit those opportunities when the pandemic arrived. However, the student may have considered themself at low or no risk because they had minimal health risk. For the student, an infection was less likely to lead to a serious health consequence compared to the seventy-year-old. This lower health risk may have led the twenty-year-old to behave more recklessly. The student may have thought "I'm going to live my life freely because I face no risk." This view of the pandemic only contains an assessment of health risk; it neglects exposure risk. The distinction is important because each individual will share some of their exposure risk with others in the population. The college student interacts with people on a bus, in the apartment building, and on a college campus. If the student is infected, they may infect others, sometimes even before realizing they are sick. These others will pass on their infections. One becomes two, two becomes four, and so on. The student's infection may even reach someone with severe health risk, like the seventy-year-old diabetes sufferer.

The college student's exposure risk flows downstream like when a firm dumps toxic chemicals into a river, essentially sharing it with others. The pollution kills fish, destroys beaches, and contaminates drinking water. Downstream neighbors are forced to pay the cost to clean up the firm's mess. Similarly, when someone who lacks (or who perceives themselves as lacking) health risk willfully takes on exposure risk by not social distancing or wearing a mask, that person passes on part of their exposure risk to others in society. Even if an infection seems like "just a cold" for the student, they will inevitably transmit the infection to others, including vulnerable people. These new infections will be passed on too, and so it goes, on and on. Eventually the infection will reach someone with greater health risk. It is this person who will pay the cost, perhaps with their life. In this way, cavalier behaviors during a pandemic create terrible costs for others in society. Those in the community with health risks pay with their health and their lives for the cavalier person's shared exposure risk.

Economists call a situation like this an *externality*. Externalities occur when the action of one person impacts someone else who is not involved in the original action. In the case of infectious disease, a risky behavior by one person increases the exposure risk for others in society. This exposure risk is paid for by people who hold the most health risk.

Externalities create a misalignment of incentives. The college student who enjoys their life during a pandemic likely doesn't fully consider the costs of the exposure risk that they create for others. Their careless actions place too much risk on others, even those who do the most to avoid it. When externalities like this are present, society pays too high a cost. However, during a pandemic, the costs are not dead fish, dirty beaches, and unclean drinking water; here, the costs are sometimes disability and death.

These costs of exposure were not shared equally in Naples, Hong Kong, and Mumbai, nor were they shared equally during COVID-19. In each of these epidemics, the costs were borne in larger share by the least privileged of society.

At the end of April 2022, the official United States COVID-19 age-adjusted mortality rate calculated by the Centers for Disease Control and Prevention (CDC) for Black Americans was 1.7 times higher than for white Americans. It was 1.8 times higher and 2.1 times higher for the Latinx and Indigenous populations.[37] Rates of hospitalization displayed even greater disparities of 2.4 times, 2.3 times, and 3.1 times the white population.[38] In the United Kingdom, members of Black African, Black Caribbean, Bangladeshi, and Pakistani groups died at rates two to three times that of white Britons.[39] People with lower incomes and lower levels of education died at higher rates as well.[40] These outcomes were not due to specific choices that individuals within these groups made. Instead, the mortality gap resulted from the totality of choices made across all of society.

Disparities in access to health care and greater rates of comorbidities created a portion of these differences. Additional portions resulted from more complex reasons that involved exposure risk. These reasons depended upon the tangled web of personal interactions that linked people across towns, cities, countries, and continents. Exposure risk comes from our behaviors and our interactions. We are linked to people in our families, churches, schools, and places of work. We are linked to even more people through anonymous interactions in restaurants, on bus routes, and at grocery stores. Everyone in each of these locations is linked to additional people across our society, many of whom we will never meet or know. These interactions are the architecture across which exposure risk is created and shared. Exposure risk depends upon how and where we travel, and where and when we work, shop, and socialize. It also depends upon the density of our living situation both in our communities and inside our individual homes.

Sometimes our interactions come about because of choices we make, such as whether to eat in a restaurant or not. When choices determine our interactions, we mix and match in complicated ways. Sometimes individuals with extra exposure risk mix with others who also hold extra exposure risk. This creates even more exposure risk for everyone in society, even those who do the most to avoid it.

Other interactions depend upon constraints, such as whether our jobs have flexibility in terms of location and whether our wealth allows us to live in certain neighborhoods or not. Many of these constraints differ based on income and wealth levels, as well as ethnicity and race. These differences in income and wealth contain generations of unequal access to education and property.

In the United States, some of these differences were institutionalized. Jim Crow laws in the post–Civil War era of the country legalized and formalized the segregation of the Black population. The outcome of *Plessy v. Ferguson* legitimized separate but certainly not equal education. New Deal red-lining zones institutionalized urban Black ghettos, prevented Black families from getting loans to buy a home, and enabled white families to secure government-insured loans at low interest rates. In some instances, other New Deal policies created government-built housing that imposed segregation where it did not exist before.[41] All of these laws and policies enabled white families to access better education for their children and to access home loans, which they used to attain wealth and prosperity that they could share with their children and grandchildren to enable them to move up in the social hierarchy. These differences in wealth exist to this day. We often use differences in income as a measure of inequality; however, income differences are much smaller than wealth differences. In the first decades of the twenty-first century, the median wealth of white households in the United States was nearly thirteen times greater than the median wealth of Black households ($144,000 to $11,000).[42] Much of this wealth for white families was created through opportunities of home ownership decades ago when these same opportunities were not available for Black families. This feeds into other opportunities of education, employment, and socioeconomic mobility. This unequal history of race and prosperity, and of outright racism, continued to live in the shadows of the outcomes of the COVID-19 pandemic. This resultant circumstance was the prequel that led to more severe pandemic devastation for minority groups in the United States.

Collectively, economic inequality, misaligned incentives, and unequal constraints tell epidemic history throughout the ages. Indigenous people in colonial times were forced to confront exposure and health risks brought to them by others seeking wealth at their expense. Those in the lower neighborhoods in Naples and Hong Kong were constrained by economic forces to face larger burdens of cholera and bubonic plague. Those in the slums of Mumbai were constrained by economics and a rigid caste system that discriminated against them and defined a social hierarchy that limited their economic and social mobility. This led to their high rates of influenza mortality. Those who were imperiled the most in the twenty-first-century COVID-19 pandemic in the United States confronted greater exposure and health risks that were in part created by centuries of racist policies, discrimination, and unequal treatment. No one person chooses for themself in an epidemic; choices are a product of history and community. History determines constraints, and community determines risk. Together these create unequal outcomes in epidemics.

If we continue to ignore this reality, and do nothing to change it, then we will suffer similar catastrophic losses in the next pandemic, and the next, and the next . . .

Chapter 2

DIFFERENCES OF DENSITY

On March 24, 1853, a young Irishman named James Mc-Guigan boarded the British ship *Northampton* to set sail from Liverpool to New Orleans. Coming on the heels of the Great Famine, many Irish were still leaving their homeland in droves. Upon arriving in the New World, passengers like McGuigan had minimal resources to start their new life. Most were nearly destitute. Historian Patrick Brennan described the Irish arriving in America during this time as "famine refugees [who] were urban pioneers; they did not have the skills or capital to move through ports to the interior regions of North America."[1] Lacking the fare to go farther, they could settle only as far as they could walk. For many of the Irish arriving in New Orleans this meant residing in a narrow corridor along the northern shore of the Mississippi River between Napoleon and Jackson Avenues. This area near the docks where they arrived came to be known as the *Irish Channel*.

The Irish Channel was typical of urban immigrant slums of the nineteenth century—dense, dirty, and destitute. Historian Robert Reinders described the neighborhood as "filthy, cut by deep ruts, lined on each side with a narrow strip of water and bordered with low one-storey, frame-built dwellings whose roofs were old, covered with moss, jutting over footpaths—and doors and windows of solid timber, never open, that impart to the whole, a gloomy appearance."[2]

Many of the Irish who initially settled the Channel dug the New Basin Canal, which connected Lake Pontchartrain to the upper section of the city through a swamp. When completed it rivaled the Carondelet Canal located in the lower Creole section of the city. In the early 1830s thousands of Irish "ditchers" dug this 6-mile-long, 300-foot-wide canal with blistered hands, arched backs, and sweat on their brows.[3] In the years closer to McGuigan's time, labor of similar drudgery was handed to the new Irish immigrants. McGuigan expected this fate upon his arrival. Food and shelter after a hard day's labor beat the conditions back home.

For the most part, McGuigan's voyage aboard the *Northampton* was unremarkable. He was one of 314 passengers onboard. Those of his ilk were stuffed below deck in the cavernous underbelly of the ship. Favorable weather brought the ship to port in only forty-five days. A handful of deaths were recorded during the voyage, but this was common for these nineteenth-century immigrant ships filled to the brim with ill-nourished passengers escaping poverty in their homelands. In fact, the *Northampton*'s Captain Reed considered there to be less sickness during this trip than was typical during similar voyages. On May 9, the *Northampton* was moored at the foot of Josephine Street in New Orleans adjacent to the Irish Channel.[4]

Upon arrival McGuigan accepted an offer of temporary employment from the ship's stevedore and was contracted to help unload the ship. This was a lucky break for a stranger arriving in a new land. One witness claimed that McGuigan slept on deck and never left the docks during his early days in his new homeland. Another claimed that he lived on Orange Street, only a few blocks from the mooring and on the periphery of the Channel. Perhaps McGuigan was seen here after the vessel had been discharged and his work unloading the ship was complete.

Being an anonymous immigrant with no connection to the area, it was not surprising that McGuigan's whereabouts were not precisely noted. His anonymity disappeared less than two weeks later. Around May 22, he began to feel unwell. With his symptoms progressively getting worse, he arrived at Charity Hospital on May 26. According to Henry Vanderlinden, a clerk at Charity Hospital, McGuigan died at age twenty-six, "two days after his admission [to the hospital] with black vomit," a common symptom of yellow fever.[5] Medical authorities would soon denote him as the first official victim of the 1853 yellow fever epidemic that killed 8,000 of the 120,000 New Orleans residents.

Exactly how the epidemic started and how McGuigan came to be infected was never settled. The sanitary commission of New Orleans interviewed a multitude of witnesses after the epidemic had ended. At least two other ships traveled to New Orleans around this time after infestation with yellow fever on a previous voyage. Most suspicious, the *Camboden Castle* had arrived from Jamaica, a known yellow fever hot spot, and was towed up the river alongside another ship, the *Augusta*. The *Augusta* moored closest to the *Northampton* and had sailors stricken with illness simultaneously to McGuigan. However, none were recorded as yellow fever victims despite eerily similar symptoms.

Others in the city became ill at the same time as McGuigan. However, these residents had no known connection to the area of the docks. Authorities felt they were too far from the location of the *Northampton* to be linked to McGuigan. Of course, at this point in time, no one understood that yellow fever was transmitted through bites of mosquitoes from one person to another. Without clear alternatives for a source, the focus of investigation returned to the *Northampton*.

Despite the testimony of the ship's captain, who asserted that the passengers and crew had experienced good health on the voyage, others told a different story. The stevedore testified that the work of unloading the ship "was arrested by discovering what they supposed to be black vomit in the hospital of the ship," which was a partitioned space in front of the passengers' bunks. Concurrent with Mr. McGuigan's passing, several of the discharge crew took ill. One of this crew fell to the care of Dr. W. B. Lindsay, who testified to the commission, "It was said that nine persons died with black vomit on board of her, when near here, one died after the ship had arrived in the [Mississippi] river." It seemed as though Captain Reed had been misleading in his claims. In any case, whether the *Northampton*, the *Augusta*, or the *Camboden Castle* had brought yellow fever ashore, it became clear that the epidemic had arrived by sea.

Once the disease arrived, the Irish Channel provided fertile ground for yellow fever to spread. The dampness in the docklands and the neighborhood provided ideal breeding grounds for the mosquitoes. The density of the residents' quarters, which were tightly packed in narrow streets adjacent to the docklands, made it easy for mosquitoes to pass between the residential areas and ships where dockworkers, seamen, and laborers lived, worked, and intermixed. Once yellow fever took root, the epidemic grew very widely and very quickly in these near ideal conditions.

New Orleans was a center of commerce for the New World during this time. Ships continually arrived from and departed to ports throughout Africa, the Caribbean, and Europe. Trade flourished from access to goods brought down the Mississippi River from the North American heartland. The population of New Orleans rose to nearly 120,000 people as of 1850. It was now the fifth-largest city in the

United States. Just forty years earlier, it had contained only 17,000 people.

As the population grew and more ships arrived every year, the city was more frequently visited by yellow fever and other diseases brought ashore by seafarers. In the thirty-five years between 1825 and 1860, there would be twelve yellow fever epidemics, each with at least 1,000 deaths.[6] Yet 1853 was an outlier compared to the most recent years. A major outbreak had not occurred since 1847 when 2,000 people had died.

Even as McGuigan and other early cases appeared in the summer of 1853, city officials and medical professionals were reluctant to admit that a yellow fever epidemic had arrived. Dr. Erasmus Darwin Fenner described the diagnostic objections of some of his fellow physicians in his 1854 recounting of the epidemic. He detailed comments of other physicians who described victims as "too yellow" or not the "right hue," or who claimed that the characteristic black vomit was "not dark enough" or that it was "too black." Others simply thought it was too early in the season to be yellow fever, which traditionally arrived later in the summer.[7]

Businesspeople and newspapers were equally unwilling to give the epidemic credence. During colonial times, cities suspected of pestilence faced quarantines and blockades. Trade stopped. Money was lost. Commercial activity ground to a halt whenever and wherever disease was identified. Finance also provided a reason for the ship captain's dishonesty when misrepresenting the good health of the *Northampton*'s voyage. Captaining an infected ship may cause delays in finding his next passage.

In the early weeks of the epidemic local newspapers tried to stifle news of the danger and published corrections and clarifications when rumors of the outbreak began to swirl in the population at large. Other newspapers in the United

States reported openly of the epidemic before those in New Orleans. Historian Patrick Brennan quotes the *Philadelphia Ledger*: "Northern newspapers and those printed in New Orleans appear to have a different appreciation for the gravity of the epidemic at hand. [In New Orleans] there is scarcely anything to indicate the presence of an epidemic."[8] The suffocation of the story lasted into the summer.[9]

Eventually, after more than 300 people had died, the news could no longer be held in check. The epidemic took off, marching from 200 deaths per week to a high of 1,400 deaths in one week at the end of August. This latest round of yellow fever overtook the city. The conditions were so dire that the city council adjourned in July in order to keep themselves safe; they did not return to meet until October when the danger had fully passed.[10]

As with other epidemics, much of the damage was centered on the least fortunate citizens, particularly those in the Irish Channel. Despite its name this enclave included immigrants of many ethnicities in large numbers, particularly German, Italian, and French. It also included a significant free Black population. One can see the diversity of the neighborhood in the existence of the "Three Churches" of the Irish Channel. In the mid-1850s the Redemptorists made the decision to build three separate Catholic churches in proximity of each other in the eastern end of the Channel. St. Mary's Assumption served the German population and St. Alphonsus served the Irish. They were built less than 100 meters from each other. The third church, the Notre Dame de Bon Secours (the "Old French Church"), built for the French, sat only two blocks away. All three churches were completed within a decade and stood less than a five-minute walk from each other.

The residences of their parishioners were small and crowded together. Slim shotgun houses were the norm. Each one-story home sat about 12 feet wide with rooms stacked in a corridor like a train car, passing from one to the next without a hallway. The entry led to a living space followed by a bedroom or two; last came a kitchen at the rear. Sometimes two houses were combined into a double shotgun, with a shared wall separating the two homes. This allowed developers to skimp on construction costs and pack more homes into the tight building lots. It was within this congestion of minimal dwellings that the yellow fever epidemic spread most violently.

During the epidemic, one out of fifteen residents of New Orleans died. However, more than 5,000 of the 8,000 killed were born in either Ireland or Germany. The Irish and German rate of mortality was about one in five.[11] Death rates for these groups were over twenty times higher than for those considered natives of New Orleans. The two populations that fared the best were white residents born in New Orleans and the Black enslaved population, many of whom had been in New Orleans for a number of years. Many from these two groups had survived previous yellow fever epidemics and gained at least limited immunity. From this they had lower exposure and health risk.

Three factors helped to create these disproportionate rates of mortality between the newly arrived immigrants and those who had lived through previous epidemics. First, poverty led to small dwellings, increased density, and poor nutrition. These effects made the Channel little different than the death zone of Naples and the slums of Tai Ping Shan in Hong Kong during the same time period. Second, many New Orleans natives had some immunity from the frequent yellow fever epidemics that cursed the city in years prior. Most Irish and German immigrants had never encountered yellow fever in their homelands and were more susceptible to its perils. As the locals would say, they had not yet *acclimated*. Historian Jonathan Pritchett attributes most of the disproportionate rates of death to these two factors, basing his conclusion on a study of internment records from Lafayette Cemetery where one out of five epidemic victims were buried.[12] What made the Irish and other recent immigrants different was their abject poverty and recent arrival to New Orleans. They were frequently singled out as both the victim and the cause of what came to be known locally as the *stranger's disease*. Of course, the new immigrants had done nothing wrong. They didn't choose to live in these quarters because of preference. It was all they could afford. Further, most had not brought yellow fever with them from their homelands. In most every circumstance, they were infected after arrival, although some became sick during their voyage. They were true victims.

There was a third factor that also made the immigrants of the Channel different. They were tasked with the foulest labor in the city. They dug ditches and canals in swamps infested with mosquitoes. The labor was so dangerous that even owners rejected it for enslaved people, who were considered an investment by their owners, one that needed to be protected. The Irish, German, and other immigrants like them were cheap labor; they were considered expendable in the eyes of many.[13] Ultimately, few in the wider society of New Orleans cared about lives lost in the Channel. Immigrant labor provided insulation to keep the rest of the city safe from the infections that doomed the lower classes.

While they happened centuries apart, the arrival of yellow fever in New Orleans had similarities to COVID-19 in New York. In late 2019 and early 2020 all eyes turned toward Wuhan, China. In late January 2020, the World Health Organization and the United States Secretary of Health and Human Services each declared public health emergencies due to the rise of what would come to be called COVID-19. The world sat hopeful that the health emergency in China would be contained. On February 2, as a response to the crisis, President Donald J. Trump implemented a limited travel ban on persons arriving from China. Despite these limits, a smattering of infections began to pop up across the United States during the month of February. Yet there still seemed to be hope that a widespread outbreak could be avoided outside of Asia. People wished, perhaps naively, that SARS-CoV-2 would fizzle out as SARS-CoV-1 had in 2003.

Nerves began to fray in the United States and Europe as the calendar moved forward. A Chinese tourist died in France on February 15. This was the first known COVID death outside of China.[14] In the United States, the first COVID-19 death was announced in Washington State on the last day of February.[15] From here, things accelerated at a pace that only the most pessimistic anticipated.

In the United States, the New York City metro area became the epicenter for the pandemic despite earlier infections on the West Coast. While he was not the first case in the New York City metro area, New York attorney Lawrence Garbuz received a great deal of media attention. He was hospitalized on February 27, 2020, and treated for pneumonia after a chest x-ray revealed lungs "full of cobwebs."[16] As his condition deteriorated, he was intubated and placed on a ventilator. With his condition still not improving, he was transferred to a larger hospital in Manhattan. On March 2, he was finally tested and diagnosed with COVID-19.[17] He had been in a hospital for four days before anyone knew the true cause of his illness.[18]

This delay in testing, even after hospitalization, hinted at the lack of preparation in the American health care system. Despite concern in the population, President Trump attempted to calm the country. On March 10 he stated, "We're prepared, and we're doing a great job with it. And it will go away. Just stay calm and it will go away."[19] Like newspapers in nineteenth-century New Orleans, he was trying to stifle the story. The situation was not under control. Officials couldn't identify the person who infected Garbuz, and other cases like his, those without a known exposure, began to appear. Undetected community spread had arrived in New York.

Just one day after President Trump's statement, the World Health Organization declared a global pandemic and Dr. Anthony Fauci and Dr. Robert Redfield, not yet household names, testified to the United States Congress. In response to the question from Representative Carolyn Maloney—"Is the worst yet to come?"—Dr. Fauci replied, "Yes, it is."[20] Two days later most schools in the New York City metro area closed. Many thought these changes would be short-lived. Parents expected their children to be back in school in a few weeks at most, but they were wrong. It seemed as though a new world had arrived.

Despite the increased anxiety, as of March 15, 2020, there were fewer than 4,000 known cases of COVID-19 across the entire United States. At the time, these numbers seemed huge. Yet few in the general population expected what was to come. Most did not understand how undetected community spread, lack of testing and identification, and exponential growth would cause the pandemic to spiral far beyond control.

Stay-at-home recommendations, limits on mass gatherings, and closing of non-essential businesses, restaurants, and schools were soon implemented far and wide across the country as case numbers increased in an exponential explosion.

Cases would quickly grow to a point where we would not have a single day with fewer than 4,000 *new* infections for the remainder of 2020 and all of 2021. Once the epidemic took off in full, some days would tally over 100,000 new infections. Even further, the United States would record over 4,000 *death*—not cases—in single days during the winter in early 2021.

On March 30, there were slightly more than 170,000 cases across the entire United States. One-half of these were in the New York City metro area. Other large metro areas such as Detroit and New Orleans were seeing large outbreaks by mid-April.[21]

Why these cities? Was there something unique about them? New York City's exorbitant density quickly became an easy scapegoat to answer these questions. It was singled out as unique, as the following quote from the *New York Times* makes clear:

> New York has tried to slow the spread of the coronavirus by closing its schools, shutting down its nonessential businesses and urging its residents to stay home almost around the clock. But it faces a distinct obstacle in trying to stem new cases: its cheek-by-jowl density.[22]

The author was not alone in this opinion. Many people saw density as New York's main problem. This notion also provided false hope that less dense and more rural areas of the country could still be spared the trauma that everyone saw in New York. Even Governor Cuomo piled on with concern about the density of New York City. He tweeted on March 22 at 11:36 a.m., "This is not life as usual. There is a density level in NYC that is destructive. It has to stop and it has to stop now. NYC must develop an immediate plan to reduce density. #StayAtHome."

On first consideration this argument made sense. Density creates more opportunities for an infectious disease to spread. It increases exposure risk. New York City had the same problem as Hong Kong, Mumbai, Naples, and New

Orleans more than a century earlier. Yet there were subtleties within this density that had yet to be appreciated and that also tied past epidemics to the present.

Governor Cuomo and others who concentrated on density as a cause of spread missed two important issues. One issue concerned the patterns of arrival of infectious disease. The other concerned different types of density and how standard descriptions of density missed a key point about the spread of infectious disease. These two issues would define the path of the New York City epidemic and repeat the history of yellow fever in New Orleans.

New Orleans had masses arriving by ship in the nineteenth century; New York had masses arriving by plane in the twenty-first. Atlanta's Hartsfield-Jackson International Airport had the most domestic and total passenger volume of any airport in the United States. However, the New York City metro area had by far the most *international* air travel of any location in the United States. In 2018, New York's John F. Kennedy International Airport and Newark's Liberty International Airport ranked first and fourth in the United States in terms of the number of international air passengers.[23] Together they transported more than twenty-three million international passengers to or from the New York City metro area.[24] Second on the list, Los Angeles International had only 12.5 million—slightly more than one-half of the total for New York City.

In late March 2020, urban economist Jason Barr and I compared the effect of density to other factors, including air travel, on the incidence of COVID-19 cases across United States counties. Not surprisingly, density was a factor contributing to the number of cases within a county. Counties that were 10 percent more dense had about 6 percent more cases in late March. However, the presence of a very large airport had an even bigger impact on the number of new cases. If a county had an airport that served at least one million passengers, that county had, on average, twice as many COVID-19 cases in late March compared to a similar county without a large airport. Along with this, counties that had early cases had much larger epidemics than counties without early cases. Counties that had at least one case by March 1 had twice as many cases as counties with an outbreak starting after this date. The arrival of cases early in the pandemic was the most important part of this initial spread.[25]

Part of the reason for this was the missed early cases and the start of undetected community spread. The virus had taken hold in areas with early cases partly because of scant and delayed testing. There were far more undetected cases that were infecting people like Lawrence Garbuz than officials realized. Exponential growth took over once the pandemic arrived in these areas. Places like Detroit, New Orleans, and New York City were caught unaware.

Like New Orleans was a yellow fever port, New York City was a COVID-19 port. There was a difference, however. The nineteenth-century arrivals to New Orleans were impoverished immigrants scuffling across the globe on a forty-five-day odyssey to start a new life. These were desperate people. In contrast, the arrivals to New York were business travelers and jetsetters on vacation to and from Europe. Many of these people had high incomes. The social status of these nineteenth- and twenty-first-century travelers was different, but their effect was the same.

Epidemics like those of New Orleans and New York are like lightning strikes in a forest.[26] A bolt lands and a tree is set aflame. The fire passes from tree to tree until it runs out of wood and the reproduction number drops below one. Not all lightning strikes start a fire. However, a forest with more lightning strikes is more likely to be set ablaze. In much the same way, a city with more arrivals by sea or air is more likely to contain the early spark that starts an epidemic. It doesn't matter if the arrivals are nineteenth-century immigrants or twenty-first-century business travelers or tourists. New York City was a likely place for the first pandemic fire with its many travelers. It didn't have to be New York City, but it was most likely to be the first city set on fire in the United States.

Because these cities and ports are heavily populated, density appears to be the primary cause of their intense affliction. Instead, it is because cities get the earliest cases, which dwarf the infection rates in smaller places. This makes it appear that *only* dense big cities face danger. However, their prominence is temporary. The epidemic will eventually visit smaller cities and rural lands as well. These rural locations are at more risk than they realize when they see only large cities like New York burning.[27] They too will be visited by the fire as it spreads away from the port.[28]

There is a regular pattern of cities and ports being struck first by epidemics, followed by movement to more rural areas second. By the end of 2020 the United States epidemic, in terms of cases per capita, was not centered in cities at all. As of January 5, 2021, the top five states in terms of cumulative cases per capita were North and South Dakota, Iowa, Tennessee, and Utah. At the same date, North Dakota, South Dakota, and Mississippi ranked among the top ten in deaths per capita. Similarly, the port of Piraeus was struck before Athens. The fourteenth-century Black Death spread to the European interior after entering through ports such as Genoa, Venice, and Sicily.[29] The earliest yellow fever outbreaks in Europe started in Spanish ports from ships arriving from the New World.[30]

Yellow fever epidemics were a persistent source of danger in North America, including the United States. All of these epidemics began in ports. Charleston was struck in 1699, and 15 percent of the population died. Numerous eighteenth- and nineteenth-century epidemics would follow in Charleston and nearby Savannah.[31] Yellow fever also struck northern ports—Philadelphia in 1783 and 1798, New York City in 1795 and 1798, Boston in 1798, and Baltimore in 1800. However, no port was visited more frequently by yellow fever than New Orleans, with a dozen major epidemics in the 1800s.

As an attempt to stop these recurrent epidemic arrivals in ports, President Rutherford B. Hayes signed the National Quarantine Act into law on April 29, 1878. It gave the Marine Hospital Service the authority to govern the retention of ships having cases onboard or arriving from ports where infectious diseases were present. It was passed largely to stop infectious disease from coming to the United States' shore through infected sailors and ship passengers.[32] This was a particular issue at the time in the North American south, as thousands of refugees had fled Cuba following a war for independence with Spain. In particular, hundreds of refugees were arriving in New Orleans during this time.

However, passing the National Quarantine Act would not be sufficient. There were delays in implementation and enforcement. New Orleans had weakened its own quarantine standards two years earlier. Instead of a mandatory ten-day quarantine, the New Orleans Chamber of Commerce pressured the Louisiana Legislature to allow ships to pass at the discretion of an inspector. Local businesses threatened lawsuits when perishable goods like fruit began to spoil on ships. In May the ship *Emily B. Souder* arrived in New Orleans after departing Havana, where yellow fever currently roiled the population. Upon inspection of the *Souder*, one sailor was removed and sent to the quarantine hospital. Another sailor, John Clark, appeared ill. His shipmates argued that he was simply unwell from drinking the night before. He was let to pass with the ship after a short inspection. Clark would die shortly after with symptoms matching yellow fever. However, his death was recorded as malarial fever by the board of health. Shortly after, two subsequent passengers on the *Souder* would die of fever as well.[33] The records made no mention of yellow fever at the time. It appeared that New Orleans was trying to stifle news of another epidemic, just as they had in the past.

Early in the summer the ship *Charles B. Woods* arrived in New Orleans after passing through the quarantine station south of the city. Within six weeks, all members of the families of the captain and engineer had fallen ill. All survived. However, a four-year-old girl living near them would not. She was the first official fatality of yellow fever that summer. The epidemic lightning bolt had arrived once again on either the *Souder* or the *Charles B. Woods*, and it eventually spread throughout New Orleans, this time claiming 4,000 lives throughout the city.[34]

The epidemic didn't stop in the vicinity of New Orleans like it did two decades earlier. Instead, it crept four hundred miles northward up the Mississippi River to Memphis. Until this point in time, Memphis hadn't been stricken with yellow fever to the extent of New Orleans. Seventy-five people died there in 1855 and another two hundred fifty in 1867. It wasn't until 1873, when 2,000 people died, that a large epidemic occurred.[35] During this time period Memphis grew from 22,000 residents in 1860 to 48,000 in 1878. With the population growth and increased density came a decrease in the sanitary conditions of the city. In the Gayoso Bayou in the northern part of the city, the "once clear running water" had become "a series of stagnant pools, clogged with debris."

This area made a fertile environment for the mosquitoes that spread yellow fever and contributed to the rising size of the epidemics in Memphis.[36]

When Memphis learned of the most recent outbreak in New Orleans, the city established quarantine stations for people and goods arriving from the southern Mississippi River.[37] But as in New Orleans, quarantine did not stave off the coming epidemic.

Two crew members on a Mississippi towboat were infected. In order to prevent their infection from spreading to the rest of the crew, the infected men were set ashore in Vicksburg, Mississippi.[38] Cases soon broke out 150 miles inland in Grenada, Mississippi. Yellow fever was only one hundred miles from Memphis.[39] The city enacted a full shipping blockade.

Kate Bionda and her husband owned a small snack shop on Front Row near the steamboat landing and adjacent to the slum section of Memphis that was referred to as "Pinch" or "Pinchguts." This area was so named due to the emaciated condition of many of the Irish immigrants who lived in the area. The Biondas lived above the snack shop with their two children. On August 9, Mrs. Bionda became ill. By August 13, she was dead at age thirty-four.[40] After a physician's examination of her body, the city announced that she was the first official yellow fever death in Memphis in 1878.[41] Later it was discovered that there were at least ten previous cases of yellow fever and four deaths prior to Mrs. Bionda. One of these was a steamboat worker who had evaded quarantine upon his arrival.[42] Perhaps his arrival to the steamboat landing brought the disease to Mrs. Bionda and the rest of Memphis.

Panic ensued across Memphis when city officials announced Mrs. Bionda's death. While Memphis had not suffered as strongly as New Orleans in past epidemics, its residents knew how quickly and savagely yellow fever could spread. They began to flee the city by whatever means possible. Historian Thomas Baker quotes a nun who witnessed the exodus: "On any road leading out of Memphis could be seen a procession of wagons, piled high with beds, trunks, and small furniture. . . . Beside these walked groups of men, some riotous with the wild excitement, others moody and silent from anxiety and dread."[43] In total it is estimated that only 20,000 inhabitants of the original 48,000 remained in Memphis that summer. There was a vast discrepancy in those who remained and those who left: 14,000 of the 15,000 Black residents of Memphis stayed in the city—only 1,000 were able to flee. Barely two decades after the Civil War, one can imagine that for many Black residents, continuing to live in Memphis was less a choice and more a constraint imposed by racial segregation, limited finances, and the lack of opportunity to flee.

The city was barren during the epidemic. As Baker writes, "The city appeared to be desolate and deserted, almost literally a tomb. Few ventured into the streets; doctors, nurses, and volunteer workers on their rounds met only each other."[44] Businesses were shuttered. Food and other supplies were scarce. In describing the scene in Memphis, historian Molly Caldwell Crosby wrote, "Main Street now held piles of coffins, stacked one atop the other, so that walking the thoroughfare felt like entering a tomb."[45] Memphis re-enacted the description of Athens, nearly deserted except for bodies piled on bodies in the streets. In total 5,000 of the remaining Memphis residents would die over the coming weeks and 17,000, almost the entire population left in the city, were infected. The epidemic was most severe in the impoverished Pinch section of the city.[46] Just as in the yellow fever epidemics of New Orleans, poor immigrants who were newly arrived to Memphis once again faced the brunt of the epidemic attack.

Infectious disease still enters through ports today. It ferments and grows there before eventually spreading outward to other, less suspecting, less aware, and less prepared areas. This happened in 2020, first in New York City, and then the rest of the country. In the past, when travel was less frequent, travel bans, blockades, and quarantines could play a role in slowing epidemic arrival. But because only one infection or two was needed to spark an epidemic, these methods were unlikely to offer full protection. They are even less effective today with mass global travel that occurs at hyper-speed.

In 2020, when many people pointed to New York City's density as the primary cause of the pandemic's severity, they overlooked the importance of New York City's role as a port. They also lacked understanding of the nuance of density. Density is not distributed evenly across a city. Additionally, not all density is the same. Cholera, plague, and influenza were concentrated in the most dense and poor sections of Naples, Hong Kong, and Mumbai. Yellow fever was concentrated in the Irish Channel of New Orleans and the Pinch district of Memphis. These areas were dense in general, but they also had a special kind of density that made their epidemics more severe, which results from poverty.

People frequently think of dense inner-city ghettos when the word poverty comes to mind. However, the most poverty-stricken areas of the United States are in some of its most rural areas. The most impoverished counties within the United States are located in Alabama, Arkansas, Louisiana, Mississippi, and South Dakota. The most poverty-stricken location is Todd County, South Dakota, with a population of just over 10,000 people. More than half of its residents live below the poverty line.

This, of course, is not to say that cities don't have poverty. The interaction between density and poverty in New York City illustrates how some types of density are more damaging than others when epidemics strike.

Density and poverty vary across neighborhoods within New York City.[47] Some areas have over 100,000 people per square mile. The areas this dense are all located in Manhattan. Most of these dense areas are very wealthy, with poverty rates of less than 5 percent. However, Central Harlem in northern Manhattan contains more than 100,000 people per square mile and has a poverty rate above 25 percent. Morris Heights, Highbridge, and Claremont in the Bronx, along with Jackson Heights in Queens and Flatbush in Brooklyn, are all similar to Central Harlem in their concentration of people and poverty. Each of these areas contains density of over 80,000 people per square mile and poverty rates between 16 and 37 percent. There is diversity in the relationship between poverty and density. Some dense neighborhoods are impoverished, and some are affluent.

The dense high-income neighborhoods in New York City are proximate to Central Park, hubs of transportation, and financial and commercial centers. In Manhattan, a glance across the skyline easily identifies these dense locations. They are populated with tall skyscrapers holding a mix of residential and commercial building space. Some of these skyscrapers house thousands of people. Most of these neighborhoods also contain high-level amenities and attractions. Parks, restaurants, and high-end shops and groceries live alongside these massive residential buildings. An appended description for a newly built condominium building in one of these neighborhoods reads, "The graceful tower offers views spanning from the East River to Central Park, and every residence is wrapped in deep, continuous private terraces that extend living and entertainment space into the skyline. . . . [This building] places residents where Manhattan's most prestigious residential neighborhood and its premier business district come together."[48] This description, and thousands of other real estate listings like it, sounds utopian to many. Although people are piled high on top of each other in these luxurious buildings, and the neighborhoods that contain them are dense, the apartments can be lush with space inside the living quarters, in nearby parks, and in streets with wide sidewalks. Author Jay Pitter refers to this type of density, dreamed of by many urbanists, as *dominant density*.[49] It is built for and populated by the privileged.

This is not the case for other dense urban neighborhoods, which more closely match the stereotype of densely packed inner-city life interlaced with poverty. Pitter refers to these dense conditions as *forgotten density*. They encompass places where privilege is rare—shanty towns, factory dormitories, public housing, and shelters. This density is crowded in a way that dominant density is not. Spacious stores, wide sidewalks, palatial condominium lobbies, private terraces, and parks do not exist here to the same degree they do in dominant density neighborhoods. Here, we see poverty. We also see overcrowded housing and minimal infrastructure.

When we combine the reproduction number with density, we expect that more people in the same geographic location will lead to more opportunities for a virus to spread. Traditionally, density is measured in terms of people per acre, square mile, or kilometer. However, a virus doesn't spread across acres, miles, and kilometers. It spreads across feet and meters. The distinction between types of density reveals more clearly how density and disease are related. The number of people that live within a small apartment matters much more for the spread of infectious disease than the number of people that live within a square mile of land. This is why diseases spread most severely in the impoverished sections of cities like Naples, Hong Kong, Mumbai, New Orleans, and Memphis. The relationship between disease spread and density concerns how people interact within *small* spaces.

Interactions within dense affluent neighborhoods are different than interactions in dense impoverished neighborhoods. Of the densest neighborhoods in New York City, those that are in affluent neighborhoods of Manhattan, such as the Upper West Side, all have far fewer people per household on average than the dense neighborhoods with higher rates of poverty in the outer boroughs such as Morris Heights in the Bronx, Flatbush in Brooklyn, or Jackson Heights in Queens. These dense impoverished neighborhoods also have much higher rates of overcrowding (defined as more than one person per room within the dwelling).[50] The people in these impoverished dense areas have more person-to-person contact than people from affluent dense areas.

Yet this too understates the situation. Not only are there more people per home and more people per room in overcrowded areas, but, not surprisingly, the overall living space is also smaller. More people cram into fewer rooms with less space in each room. If we compare high-income neighborhoods to low-income neighborhoods the distinction is striking. New York City neighborhoods in the top quarter of income have residential living spaces that are 29 percent larger than neighborhoods in the bottom quarter of income.[51] Low-income neighborhoods contain households with more people per residence, and the residences are significantly smaller.[52] These are the type of dense conditions that allow infectious disease to spread.

I call this type of density *inward density*. It is density created by cramming people into small spaces. Inward density is most common among the urban poor and multi-generational families. In contrast, density is created in affluent urban neighborhoods by building up. The buildings in the neighborhoods ranking in the top decile of income within New York City contain 80 percent more floors than those of the buildings in the neighborhoods in the bottom decile.[53] The buildings are almost twice as tall in affluent neighborhoods than impoverished neighborhoods. Density in affluent areas is created vertically. I call this type of density *upward density*.

The story of density and infectious disease is not about the number of people per unit of land area, but rather it is about how people mix within the area. Upwardly dense neighborhoods that have larger living spaces, more rooms, and easy access to parks nearby were harmed far less early in the COVID-19 pandemic. These neighborhoods, although dense by traditional measures like people per square mile, have space for a loved one to remain isolated when ill, and this reduces the likelihood that other household members are infected. They also have space outside for parks and walks in fresh air. When confronting a pandemic, they have more space inside and outside to remain safe and to isolate from exposure.

The density of impoverished neighborhoods does not provide this safety because of its crowded and congested inward density. Greater numbers of people are packed into smaller apartments with shared bedrooms and bathrooms. Distance and isolation are not possible when someone is ill. Infections spread easily from person to person within a small apartment when rooms must be shared. Inward density is common in many urban neighborhoods today and in the past. The lower city of Naples, the Tai Ping Shan district of

Hong Kong, and the slums of Mumbai all were inwardly dense. So too was the Irish Channel of New Orleans, with row upon row of small shotgun houses, and the Pinch district of Memphis. Inwardly dense neighborhoods allow epidemics to spread quickly and easily.

To provide yet another protection against exposure for affluent areas of Manhattan non-essential businesses closed when the city shut down and those able to work from home did so. Commuters, tourists, and shoppers from surrounding areas did not enter Manhattan. This provided even more space in Manhattan's upwardly dense neighborhoods. It is estimated that the population of Manhattan grows from about 1.6 million people to four million people during a typical workday. Even on weekends the total number of people within the city is about 80 percent larger than the number of residents.[54] The stores, sidewalks, parks, businesses, and everything else in Manhattan's hubs of commerce and tourism are organized to accommodate far more people than actually live there. Once much of Manhattan closed in the spring of 2020, these non-residents did not enter the city. All the space that commuters, tourists, and shoppers normally take up during the day was vacant and became available for socially distant residents. Overnight there was extra space in the wealthy upwardly dense neighborhoods within Manhattan that surrounded the commercial centers.

At the same time, little changed within the less wealthy neighborhoods that contained inward density. People remained overcrowded in their small apartments where they shared rooms with multigenerational family members. They shopped in stores with narrow aisles that contained pre-pandemic resident populations. They continued to commute to minimum wage and essential-worker jobs that could not be performed on Zoom. Most did so on still-crowded public transportation. They didn't gain safety when the rest of the city shut down. They continued to move about the city for work, and they came home to their crowded neighborhoods to shop and live amongst others who had also traveled to work on crowded city busses and subway cars. All of these experiences created heightened exposure risk for these individuals. Residents of inwardly dense neighborhoods faced greater exposure risk in their homes, in the shops around their homes, in their workplace, and in the commute to their workplace. Others around them faced this greater exposure risk too. Externalities built upon externalities and the exposure risk grew in these neighborhoods even more.

Once New York City was struck by the pandemic lightning bolt, the exposure risk in these inwardly dense neighborhoods ignited the largest pandemic fires. Each infection had a greater chance to spread to others in the congested and crowded conditions within these neighborhoods. This created a larger reproduction number in inwardly dense neighborhoods than in upwardly dense neighborhoods. As these fires grew in the inwardly dense areas, not enough was done to stop them. These areas with the most exposure risk and the largest pandemic fires were shorted on mitigation and monitoring measures such as tests for the virus that causes COVID-19.

The United States initially had a severe testing shortage across the country. One couldn't just pop into a local urgent care center or pharmacy and receive a quick and easy test. At-home tests did not exist yet. In New York City, even patients presenting with symptoms consistent with COVID-19 were not tested because tests were so scarce. As one physician told the *New York Times*, "From a medical standpoint, the testing in the . . . moderate patient is not going to make much of a difference in our medical management."[55] If the treatment and recommendations for isolation and care did not depend upon a specific COVID-19 diagnosis, a patient was not tested.

Dr. Anjali Viswanathan discussed her frustrations with *ABC News*. She commented on her patient who worked at a New York City area airport and had traveled to Italy for ten days in early March when the pandemic exploded there. The patient developed the common symptoms of COVID-19 including shortness of breath and a fever. Dr. Viswanathan was unable to acquire a test for her patient because she was only twenty-eight years old and not considered high risk.[56] This, of course, meant health risk and not exposure risk. Dr. Viswanathan stated that other physicians had similar experiences and correctly pointed out, "It's even more important to know which patients carry the virus who don't fit the typical profile. That's the only way to protect the community at large."[57] The testing policy ignored exposure risk.

When faced with a shortage of tests, the protocols may have made sense from a perspective of managing treatment and health risk for physicians, but they didn't make sense from the perspective of managing exposure risk and improving public health. We needed to do more than simply identifying cases for treatment. The epidemiological rationale for controlling the pandemic depended upon lowering the reproduction number. We needed to be able to limit the additional infections that resulted from each new infection. If we had been able to test widely, we would have found more infections more quickly. Once found we could have isolated those infected before they generated additional infections. With sufficient testing we could have lowered the reproduction number more quickly and stifled the epidemic fire. Economist Joshua Gans argued this point early in the pandemic. The key to controlling exposure was information gained from testing.[58] The testing shortage created even more damage because we failed to realize how frequently asymptomatic individuals unknowingly transmitted the virus.

It took four days after hospitalization before doctors knew that attorney Lawrence Garbuz was infected. Before this information was known he likely infected numerous people within his hometown and in the hospital. This wasn't his fault. Others like him were not being tested either. One of these untested people infected him. If his case hadn't become so serious, he would have continued infecting others through no fault of his own. Others were doing the same when tests were only being used for those with the greatest health risk. In addition, there were large numbers of asymptomatic infections walking about the street, infecting others without knowing it. As these infections built up, New York City's pandemic fire grew out of control before the smoke alarm went off. By the time we saw the fire it was too large to quickly extinguish.

Other countries did a much better job with testing than the United States. As of March 12, 2020, European countries such as Italy, the Netherlands, and the United Kingdom, along with Israel, were testing at rates over fifteen times greater than the United States. South Korea was testing at rates over 150 times that of the United States. By not being prepared to implement widespread testing, the United States botched the early period of the pandemic, particularly in New York City where the virus was concentrated. This lack of preparation harmed vulnerable citizens the most and cost them their lives.

With cases rising, the testing shortfall caused the most acute damage in New York City's inwardly dense neighborhoods.[59] Data over the first month of the pandemic, provided by the New York City Department of Health and Mental Hygiene, shows that the limited tests that were performed were not evenly spread across the city. Neighborhoods with the least poverty had the most tests. Their rates of testing were 34 percent higher than neighborhoods with the most poverty.[60] If infections were more prominent in these low-poverty neighborhoods and tests were performed in proportion to rates of infection, this wouldn't have been a problem. However, the opposite was true—rates of infection were higher in the high-poverty neighborhoods that weren't being tested. More infections but fewer tests meant that more people were unaware of their infected status and were spreading infections across these high-poverty neighborhoods. Pre-symptomatic exposures and asymptomatic exposures made this problem worse. This becomes clear when one examines the rate of test *positivity*.

Positivity is the fraction of tests that return a positive result. However, this statistic is a function of the rates of testing. An area that has fewer tests must ration them more strictly than an area with many tests. The area with fewer tests can only test the most important cases that are most likely to be COVID-19. Thus, an area that has a large number of infections but few tests will return a higher level of positivity than an area with an equal number of infections but many tests that they can use in more uncertain situations.

If testing was performed at equal rates for each neighborhood in the city, positivity would be very informative because it would identify the most infected neighborhoods. This wasn't the case in New York City. High-poverty, inwardly dense neighborhoods had more cases but lower rates of testing. This meant that more infections in these neighborhoods were left undetected. These undetected infections created even more exposure risk for others in these neighborhoods that already contained more exposure risk because they were inwardly dense. These unidentified cases are the most important part of positivity from a public health perspective.

If we ration tests to the most serious cases of health risk, and do not test the less serious cases, as New York City was doing, then we allow all the less serious cases to continue spreading the virus. As we increase testing rates, the positivity drops because more test subjects will come from parts of the population less likely to be infected. For COVID-19, the World Health Organization (WHO) recommended that rates of testing needed to be high enough to yield rates of positivity not greater than 3 to 5 percent.[61] Keeping positivity this low would help to ensure that few cases went unidentified in the general population and that secondary cases were not developing outside of the knowledge of public health officials. In the spring of 2020, New York City rates of positivity were above 50 percent, more than ten times higher than the recommendation of the WHO.[62] Some of the highest poverty neighborhoods had much higher rates of positivity.[63]

Jackson Heights, a cultural gem of New York City, sits in Queens just to the south of LaGuardia Airport. It is one of the most diverse, inwardly dense, and impoverished neighborhoods in New York City. In 2020, more than 60 percent of the population was Hispanic, and more than 40 percent of this Hispanic population was living in poverty. In addition to a multifaceted Hispanic population, the neighborhood also contained a large Asian population with varied ethnic backgrounds. Many residents of Jackson Heights were recent immigrants. About 60 percent of Jackson Heights residents were born outside of the country. This created the fifth-largest immigrant neighborhood in New York City.

The neighborhoods of Corona and Elmhurst, which sit adjacent to Jackson Heights, are similar in demographic profile. They too have high rates of poverty and large populations of immigrants. Together, these three neighborhoods made up the largest area of immigrants anywhere in New York City in 2020.[64] In addition, they each ranked in the top five neighborhoods in New York City in terms of overcrowded housing.[65] These neighborhoods were inwardly dense and poor. Early in the pandemic, each of these three neighborhoods had positivity rates near 70 percent.

The neighborhood with the lowest positivity at this time was the Financial District in the areas around Wall Street. This area was affluent, with a median household income twice as large as Jackson Heights, Corona, and Elmhurst. The population in this neighborhood was 70 percent white. Both Jackson Heights and the Financial District had density of more than 90,000 people per square mile living within them. However, their density was of different types. Jackson Heights was inwardly dense, while Wall Street was upwardly dense. Further, when the pandemic arrived, the Financial District became a ghost town. In addition to residences, most of the buildings in this neighborhood supplied office space to white-collar firms. The buildings in this neighborhood contained twice as much commercial space as residential space. Much of the commercial space became vacant when the pandemic hit as people converted to working from home. Retail shops and restaurants closed, and tourists disappeared. Exposure risk was now even lower than before. Their rate of positivity was less than 30 percent. This was still a huge number—much larger than was ideal. Yet their situation was far better than in Jackson Heights.

It wasn't just these two neighborhoods. Across the city, neighborhoods with the highest positivity had an average household size that was 60 percent larger than the neighborhoods with the lowest positivity. These high-positivity neighborhoods were the same neighborhoods that had less living space. Infections in these neighborhoods were entering small households that had more people in them. They had fewer rooms and people couldn't isolate once infected. If they weren't tested and didn't know that they were infected, the virus spread more easily. These were the neighborhoods where tests were urgently needed to control exposure risk. They didn't get them. They were neglected.

Conversely, the low-positivity neighborhoods were upwardly dense. They contained average building heights over three times as tall as the high-positivity neighborhoods. They had fewer people in larger residences with more rooms. People could more easily isolate themselves when ill. These were the neighborhoods where tests were performed most frequently.

The pandemic ran amuck in the neighborhoods with the most dangerous form of density. Inwardly dense neighborhoods were already economically disadvantaged. Everything was running against these populations in the pandemic. Our lack of testing in low-income, inwardly dense neighborhoods exponentially increased their hardship. One missed, untested infection became two, and two became four, and so on. Every time we missed diagnosing a case because we didn't have a test to give or because we intentionally or unintentionally rationed it away from these neighborhoods and into a more affluent neighborhood, we let the pandemic spread a bit more out of control for the people who could least afford to be infected. The testing protocols didn't control the exposure risk within these neighborhoods—instead, it grew larger by the day. Illness and death mounted in these neighborhoods that had the least power to put out the epidemic fire.

When the first data describing differences in racial and ethnic outcomes arrived in early April of 2020, the rate of death among the Black and Latinx populations was nearly twice as large as that for the white population of New York

City.[66] Other cities were experiencing the same unequal harm.[67] We should have recognized the excessive danger present in these inwardly dense neighborhoods when the pandemic began and allocated extra resources to them, such as tests and medical care. That was the humane and efficient thing to do. Give greater resources to the neighborhoods where the exposure and health risks were the greatest. Instead, we did the opposite. We tested more widely in other areas of the city that were already more safe. In doing so, people living in inwardly dense neighborhoods faced even more danger because of society's neglect.

Impoverished immigrant populations in nineteenth-century New Orleans faced similar neglect. The 1853 yellow fever epidemic in New Orleans was one of many to hit the city. New Orleans was so frequently stricken that it received the nickname of *necropolis*, city of the dead.[68] As with many viruses, if someone contracts yellow fever and recovers, then partial or full immunity is granted. This is one reason why those born in New Orleans and enslaved people who had lived for significant periods of time in the city were less likely to die during the nineteenth-century yellow fever epidemics. As a corollary, this contributed to the higher rates of death among newly immigrated groups who didn't come from tropical areas. While the population of New Orleans did not understand the mechanism by which immunity came about, it was well aware of the differences in mortality among those native to the area and those not.

The knowledge was so strong that it pervaded the culture and created a class hierarchy within the city. Historian Kathryn Meyer Olivarius is an expert in the construction of this hierarchy and its link to yellow fever. One who could demonstrate that they had been afflicted but survived was said to be "acclimated." This placed recent immigrants below natives of New Orleans in the social hierarchy of the city. It also played a role in the use of slavery and the working roles of immigrants.

In one respect, enslaved labor was used as insulation from disease. It provided the white population protection from labor that exposed them to infection. Enslaved people did the dangerous work. White immigrants tasked with similar work died at high rates. Jo Ann Carrigan quotes the *New Orleans Weekly Delta*, which argued that "White laborers violated the laws of nature 'in making negroes of themselves by doing the work in hot noon-day sun that negroes ought to do.'"[69]

Because the new immigrants were not acclimated, they were forced into dangerous labor and exposed to infectious disease. They couldn't get other jobs. As Olivarius told an interviewer at National Public Radio, "Bosses will not hire clerks and bookkeepers who are not expressly acclimated. Women will not marry men not described as acclimated. You can't live in certain neighborhoods, and people will not rent rooms unless you're acclimated. Certain social circles will exclude you."[70]

The commonly stated belief that Black people were naturally immune was a convenient lie. Olivarius's research shows that owners of enslaved people paid 25 to 50 percent more for enslaved people with proof of acclimation than for those without proof.[71] The owners were aware of the danger posed to Black and white people who were newly arrived to the area. Their wealth gave them power to dictate where people worked, and they used it to their advantage to keep themselves and others like them safe. They also used it to their financial advantage.

As immigrants began flooding New Orleans, the jobs given to enslaved people changed. Before immigrant labor became widely available, the Spanish used enslaved people to build the Carondelet Canal in the Creole section of the city at the end of the eighteenth century. However, enslaved people were an investment in the eyes of their owners. When Irish and other immigrant laborers arrived, these new immigrants were seen as expendable. They were easily and affordably replaced. "A steamship captain spelled out the simple economics . . . in 1852. 'Every time a boiler bursts . . . they would lose so many dollars' worth of slaves; whereas by getting Irishmen at a dollar-a-day they pay for the article as they get it, and if [the Irish laborer] is blown up, they get another.' "[72] With the flood of immigrants in the 1830s, the investors who built the New Basin Canal saw that immigrant labor was less expensive and provided less risk to a loss of investment. The new immigrants were at the lowest levels of the white social hierarchy because of their lack of acclimation and their poverty. They lacked opportunities for other employment and their large numbers competed wages down to minimal levels. It made no financial sense to the owner to send an enslaved person into a risky environment when cheap immigrant day labor was available. These immigrants were readily hired day by day to dig at these low wages. If they became ill or died, they wouldn't be paid. By using day labor, the canal company shifted all of the risk onto workers. The firms faced no financial risk from disease as long as there were cheap immigrant laborers lined up to take the job each day.

Thousands died digging the New Basin Canal, while working in pools of stagnant water filled with mosquitoes that transmitted yellow fever and malaria, or from cholera that had just arrived in North America. The victims were buried in mass graves, such as in Girod Street Cemetery, only two blocks from the basin.[73] Legend claims that 10,000 men died from infectious disease while digging the canal.

Although twenty-first-century New York City is far different than nineteenth-century New Orleans, there are similarities when considering their epidemics. It is going too far to say the urban poor of twenty-first-century New York City were exploited to the same extent as nineteenth-century immigrants in New Orleans, who were treated no better than disposable tools. However, the parallels exist no matter how difficult they are to admit. The affluent in New York City remained sheltered and received more tests when ill. Those from more impoverished neighborhoods continued to travel to jobs deemed essential, often on crowded public transit, and returned to crowded inwardly dense housing with little space to isolate if infected. When they became ill, they less frequently received tests and because they were not tested infections spread more widely in these neighborhoods. The result—more people died in these inwardly dense neighborhoods. They didn't die at the same rates as Irish immigrants in nineteenth-century New Orleans. Yet they died at significantly higher rates than those more affluent who lived only a neighborhood or two away.

While there were many parallels between New Orleans's yellow fever epidemics and New York City's COVID-19 epidemic, one salient difference stands out. The arrival of disease through a port came from very different groups of people. In New York City, it wasn't poor immigrants arriving on a ship who brought lightning ashore. It was affluent businesspeople and tourists traveling about the world to Europe and other exclusive destinations. Yet this distinction didn't matter for where the epidemic concentrated its destruction. No matter where it arrived or who brought disease to these cities, disease found the inwardly dense neighborhoods whose residents face the most danger during pandemics. They need to be protected and not neglected. In New Orleans, neglect came about through profiteering strategies of labor use. In New York City, it came about through misallocation of resources that could have been used to protect the most vulnerable.

In hindsight, as a society in the twenty-first century, we failed those who lived in inwardly dense neighborhoods. We didn't protect these most vulnerable populations from the exposure risk that took too many to the mass graves of the potter's field on Hart Island, the site where those too poor to pay for a funeral were buried in New York City. In the first year of the pandemic, these mass graves became the burial location for nearly 3,000 COVID-19 victims in the city.[74] While they are not the only ones impacted, it is the poor who live in inwardly dense areas that face the most destruction whenever and wherever lightning strikes.

Chapter 3

ONE (UNLUCKY) SPARK

In the summer of 1906, banker Charles Henry Warren rented a vacation home for his family in Oyster Bay, Long Island. After a glorious summer on the beach, things turned sour in late August. Warren's young daughter became seriously ill. She developed a soaring fever. Aches, pains, and digestive issues mounted. Within a few days, Mrs. Warren, a second daughter, two maids, and a gardener presented the same symptoms. In total, six of the eleven people within the residence fell ill. After study by medical experts, no source of the outbreak was found. The home's owner, Mr. Thompson, feared that if the source was not identified, he would not be able to rent the home in the future.

To solve the mystery, he hired George Soper, a sanitary engineer, to investigate further. Soper initially focused on the water supply along with the single indoor toilet, the outhouse, and the manure pit. None of these revealed a cause. He next moved to the possibility that contaminated clams purchased from a local woman who lived on the beach had sickened the family. When he learned that not all of the ill had eaten the clams, Soper discarded this hypothesis too. Eventually, his focus turned to a cook who had been newly hired in August two weeks before the outbreak. This cook was an immigrant from Cookstown, Ireland, who had arrived in the United States in 1884 at the age of 15. Initially she had found employment as a domestic servant before eventually being promoted to cook.

Soper traced her work history over the previous decades. He found that she had cooked for many wealthy families throughout New York City during this time. Soon he discovered that the same illness had appeared in seven of these families. While it seems obvious in retrospect, until Soper's investigation, no one saw a common element in these outbreaks. Soper was the first to put the pieces together; he identified Mary Mallon as the source of each of these typhoid fever outbreaks. Henceforth, Mary Mallon would live in infamy as *Typhoid Mary.*

Because of her probable connection to many cases of typhoid fever, Mary was detained by the New York Department of Health for testing. Although consistently asymptomatic throughout her life, she tested positive for *Salmonella typhi,* the bacteria that causes typhoid fever. She was the first known healthy carrier of the disease. As a result of the exposure risk that she created for others, she was forcibly isolated in a cottage on North Brother Island, which sits in the East River between Manhattan and Queens.

In 1909, Mary sued the health department for release. Her appeal failed, largely due to her constantly testing positive despite undergoing several attempts at treatment. Finally in 1910, Mary was released on the condition that she not accept employment as a cook. With limited employment opportunities for a woman at that time, cooking provided her the best opportunity for a significant and consistent income. She soon went back on her word.

In 1915, an outbreak of typhoid fever occurred at Sloane Maternity Ward in Manhattan. Over the course of three months, twenty-five people became ill and two died. Investigators eventually discovered Mary cooking in the hospital under the name Mary Brown. Typhoid Mary was returned to North Brother Island. There she lived, alone and isolated, until her death in 1938.[1]

Typhoid Mary lives in historical lore for a number of reasons. She refused to admit her role as an asymptomatic carrier.[2] She was the focus of ethical concerns for forced isolation during the two decades of her second containment. Most infamously, she was a super-spreader of a deadly infectious disease.

There are two types of super-spreaders. The first type is an infectious person who interacts with a large number of people in their daily life. This type of super-spreader comes into daily contact with many friends and family members and may have a job that requires a lot of person-to-person interaction, such as driving a bus, running a reception desk at a hotel, or acting as a clerk in a retail store. The second type of super-spreader is a large event, such as a wedding, funeral, business conference, or party that brings together a number of people. These events put each person in attendance into contact with a big group of people on a temporary basis. If a single infectious person is present at one of these events, then all the attendees face the possibility of becoming infected. Mary Mallon was the first type of super-spreader, as she moved about in her daily life in homes containing large families and multiple service workers. In total, 122 cases of infection and 5 deaths were directly tied to Mary during her life.[3] It is unknown how many additional direct infections went undetected or how many additional secondary infections she caused.

Typhoid fever has a reproduction number of a little under three.[4] Mary, having infected at least 122 people, was clearly an outlier. She was a super-spreader in the truest sense of the word, and to this day remains the most infamous super-spreader in United States, and perhaps in world, history. However, the existence of super-spreaders like Mary is not unusual. In most epidemic outbreaks, there are super-spreaders like Mary who far exceed the typical reproduction number and play a disproportionate role in the spread of an epidemic. Controlling super-spreading is one key to stopping epidemics and keeping populations safe.

About the same time that Mary was spreading typhoid fever across New York City, an Italian engineer and economist named Vilfredo Pareto discovered something that he found peculiar.[5] Like the anecdote of Newton recognizing gravity after observing an apple falling from a tree, Pareto had an epiphany while he was observing nature. He realized that the healthier and more productive plants in his garden provided an excess of peas, while others languished with minimal production. When he counted the output of each plant, he found that 20 percent of his pea plants produced 80 percent of his peas.[6] With his pea plants as inspiration, Pareto investigated other issues of uneven distribution. Most famously he discovered that the distribution of land in Italy was highly skewed; 80 percent of land in Italy was owned by only 20 percent of the population. Following Pareto, several other distributional inequities were found, most notably within distributions of income and wealth, but also in many other areas of society.[7] The pervasiveness of this ratio became known as the Pareto principle or the *80/20 rule*.

In ensuing years other examples of the 80/20 rule were discovered. The 80/20 rule applies (approximately) in epidemiology as well. A number of infectious disease outbreaks involving HIV, malaria, SARS-1, measles, and smallpox followed a similar pattern, in which large outbreaks and the majority of new infections could be traced to a small set of individuals or events.[8] This small set of individuals who generated a large percentage of new infections were the *super-spreaders*, of whom Mary Mallon is the most famous.

In the case of typhoid fever, a reproduction number of three means that each person infected with typhoid fever will, on average, infect three additional people. With a reproduction number of three, how is it possible then to have super-spreading such that one person infects as many as 122 people? Because it is an average, a reproduction number of three can be attained in several different ways. Every infectious person in the population could infect three others. Or one-half of the infected population could each infect six people and the other half could infect no one. Or 20 percent of the population each could infect twelve others, 60 percent each could infect one other person, and 20 percent each could infect no one. All of these examples result in a reproduction number of three. The last example conforms to the 80/20 rule.

Thus, while the reproduction number is useful, it veils super-spreading because it only considers the average number of new infections that are likely to occur from each existing infection. It does not consider the variance in the distribution of new infections created. It does not consider the fact that some infected people will not transmit the disease to anyone while outliers such as Mary Mallon might transmit the disease to hundreds of people. Epidemiologists call the variance in the distribution of the number of infections created *dispersion*. This concept was developed by James Lloyd-Smith, a disease ecologist, as a way to better understand infectious disease dynamics and super-spreading.[9]

Despite knowledge of people like Typhoid Mary, it wasn't until the severe acute respiratory syndrome (SARS) pandemic of 2003 that super-spreading came to be better understood. On February 21, 2003, Dr. Liu Jianlun, a sixty-four-year-old medical professor, traveled from mainland China to Hong Kong to attend the wedding of his nephew.

Upon arrival, he checked into his room on the ninth floor of the Hong Kong Metropole Hotel. He was feeling unwell but not experiencing symptoms that he felt significant enough to prevent travel or prevent attendance at the wedding. However, before the wedding took place, his symptoms worsened, and he entered a local hospital. Less than two weeks later, on March 4, 2003, he died as the first known case of SARS in Hong Kong.

While tragic, the story does not end there.[10] At least seven additional people staying on the same floor as Dr. Jianlun were infected, and it is unknown how many additional people he infected near his home or while traveling to Hong Kong. Among those linked to the Metropole, twenty-six-year-old Esther Mok was in Hong Kong on a brief shopping trip. She took SARS home with her to Singapore and infected 160 others. Johnny Chen, a forty-eight-year-old American businessman, was also staying on the ninth floor of the Metropole. He infected dozens of hospital workers after traveling to Vietnam.[11] Another guest, Kwan Sui-chu, returned from Hong Kong to her home in Toronto, where she would die of SARS on March 5. Before dying, she infected at least nine others. These nine infected 257 additional people in Toronto. In total over 70 percent of the SARS cases in Toronto would be linked to this chain of infections beginning with Kwan Sui-chu. Finally, while not a guest at the hotel, a twenty-seven-year-old man who had visited a guest at the Metropole during Dr. Jianlun's stay infected over 100 heath care workers at Prince of Wales Hospital in Hong Kong.[12] This particular outbreak of SARS had super-spreaders on top of super-spreaders.

The COVID-19 pandemic also had patterns of infection and levels of dispersion that indicated super-spreading. One study found that about 10 percent of cases created 80 percent of new infections.[13] Another group of researchers who studied the transmission of COVID-19 found that just 2 percent of infected individuals created 20 percent of new infections.[14] The results of another study almost exactly matched the 80/20 rule.[15]

These examples of the 80/20 rule—where many infections are linked to individuals like Mary Mallon, Liu Jianlun, or the other guests of the Metropole—are different from the second type of super-spreader: a large number of cases linked to one event. Throughout 2020 and 2021, COVID-19 super-spreading events were documented at churches, ski resorts, restaurants, nursing homes, prisons, and even Zumba classes.[16] Many times super-spreading occurred at events that seemed innocent enough at the outset, like weddings and funerals.

Andrew Jerome Mitchell passed away in Albany, Georgia, on February 24, 2020.[17] A lifelong resident of Albany, he plied his trade as a janitor and took pride in his work. He was described in his obituary as someone with "an engaging personality; a gigantic heart . . . a friend you could always depend on and [who] was always ready to lend a helping hand whenever needed."[18] More than 200 people attended his funeral.

Shortly following the funeral, one attendee began to feel unwell. He was admitted to the local hospital, Phoebe Putney Memorial, with shortness of breath. With a history of lung disease and no unusual travel history, this man's case did not seem unique. He spent a week in the hospital, where he was cared for by fifty different medical workers who took no special precautions. When his condition deteriorated, he was transferred to a larger hospital in Atlanta, three hours away. In rural areas of the United States, it is common to have vast areas with limited medical care. That a hospital in rural Georgia needed to transfer someone three hours away for more advanced medical care was not unusual for this part of the country. Upon arrival, he was tested and found to be suffering from COVID-19. That evening the staff of Phoebe Putney learned that they had been caring for a COVID-19 patient for almost two weeks without knowing it. Two days later this man died as Georgia's first COVID-19 fatality.[19]

During the days between the original funeral and the funeral attendee's passing, another funeral took place in Albany. Like Mr. Mitchell, Johnny B. Carter was born in Albany. A retired Norfolk Southern Railroad worker and active church member, "he was a straight-shooting man of integrity . . . [who was] known for his gracious and generous demeanor."[20] Mr. Carter passed away on February 28, 2020. His funeral service was held in Albany on March 7, three days prior to anyone knowing that COVID-19 had arrived in the town at Mr. Mitchell's funeral. Mr. Carter's funeral was also widely attended.[21]

Within a week, what was expected to be a six-month stockpile of medical equipment was exhausted and all ICU beds were full at Phoebe Putney. COVID-19 had invaded this small town in full force. All twenty-three of the first COVID-19 patients in Albany had attended one of the two funerals.[22] As the days and weeks moved forward, Albany remained one of the hottest of hot spots in the nation, yet it received little media attention compared to New York and other major cities. By March 30, Dougherty County, within which Albany sits, had 278 cases of COVID-19 and eighteen deaths out of a population of 90,000. This was two more than nearby Fulton County, Georgia, home to Atlanta, with a population of over one million people.

At this time, with the focus on New York City as the epicenter of the US pandemic, Albany, Georgia, was barely noticed by most. Yet it rivaled New York City on a per-capita basis as the center of the pandemic. As of March 30, 2020,

New York City had about 4,500 cases per million residents, eclipsing Dougherty County, which had about 3,000 cases per million. However, Dougherty County had almost 200 deaths per million people, while New York City had under 100 deaths per million at this time. People were dying in Dougherty County at rates twice as great as New York City despite it having 50 percent fewer cases per capita. Nevertheless, almost no attention was called to Dougherty County's desperate situation. Perhaps this lack of attention was due in part to its 74 percent Black population and its poverty.

Albany, Georgia, is sparsely populated and poor in comparison to New York City. Yet the high rate of mortality in Albany, from a lower per capita caseload, was predictable. According to the US Census Bureau, about 30 percent of Albany's residents live below the poverty line, and 20 percent lack health insurance. In contrast, only 17 percent of New York City's residents live in poverty and only 8 percent lack health insurance, a value close to the national average of 10 percent.[23] New York City was better off than Albany across every metric commonly used to predict health risk and comorbidities for severe COVID-19 outcomes.[24] Albany is financially poor and rural, and its residents died at higher rates than even residents of New York City at the height of the spring 2020 pandemic wave.

The impact on rural areas like Albany would not be unusual later in the pandemic. After disease enters through ports, it travels to rural areas. However, as chance would have it, lightning struck early in Albany. It was an unlikely strike; most other pandemic epicenters in the United States in March 2020 were urban locations that served as entry points for travel and tourism. Because Albany was poor and rural, few paid notice—a sign of times to come.

The people attending the two funerals in Albany did nothing wrong, given how early in the pandemic these events took place and given that they had no indication that COVID-19 was among them. Funerals, church services, sporting events, and other mass gatherings were still common across the country when these funerals took place in late February and early March. One unlucky spark at any one of them could have lit a fire. That spark hit an Albany funeral, and super-spreading resulted.

Ben Althouse of the Institute for Disease Modeling offers a metaphor of super-spreading that helps describe it: "You can think about throwing a match at kindling. . . . You throw one match, it may not light the kindling. You throw another match it may not light the kindling. But then one match hits in the right spot and all of a sudden the fire goes up."[25] Most times we are lucky and an individual case doesn't lead to a large outbreak, just like most lightning strikes don't cause a forest fire. Occasionally we are unlucky. Then poor and vulnerable communities like Albany are devastated by disease and death.

Human psychology interacts here as well. When people see match after match being thrown into kindling without observing any effect, they begin to discount the danger of a fire. A child who throws ten lit matches on a lawn doubts their parents' advice about the danger if the child doesn't witness a fire. Experience tells the child that nothing is wrong with that behavior. Yet in a different lawn, one unlucky match sets the yard on fire, and the house goes up in flames with it. As with the pandemic, because of the variance in the distribution of infections created, most infections don't create large numbers of new cases. But some do—and when they do, the effects can be catastrophic.

However, chance is only one part of the story. Mary Mallon was an asymptomatic carrier of a deadly infectious disease who interacted with many people over the course of the inferno that she created. Once unknowingly infected, she became a super-spreader because she interacted with the families that she cooked for every day, along with other service workers in the households where she cooked. At events like weddings and funerals, large groups of people congregate together in congested spaces. When someone enters this space with an infectious disease, it almost certainly will spread to others at the event. There is more order to super-spreading than the kindling-and-match metaphor leads one to believe. However, this order often lies more hidden than one expects.

What ties together Mary Mallon as a super-spreading individual and the Albany, Georgia, funerals as super-spreading events are the large number of interactions that they each enabled. If Mary Mallon had worked alone in her home as a seamstress, she would not have become Typhoid Mary, even with her asymptomatic infection. If the Albany, Georgia, funerals had been less well attended, COVID-19 may not have spread so widely in this small town. Some individuals, such as bus drivers, have many interactions throughout the course of a day. Others, like at-home school tutors, do not. Some events are large gatherings, like weddings and funerals, while others, like dental appointments, are not. Regularity exists in the patterns of interactions within our social lives and in the pattern of our connections to each other through friendships, jobs, and family. These patterns determine the number of matches struck, the placement of their landing in the kindling pile, and the size of the kindling pile. More than luck, super-spreading depends on the patterns of interactions in individual lives and society.

To understand super-spreading, we need to understand these patterns of social-network organization and the patterns of our connections to each other. We start with one of the greatest social networkers of all time. Bill Clinton knows a boundless number of people and a litany of facts about each. He famously recorded meetings in a black notebook that he carried with him when he was a Rhodes Scholar at Oxford and was rumored to have index cards with names, addresses, and personal information on over 10,000 personal contacts by 1980—well before his political career took off.[26]

Not everyone is as socially connected as Bill Clinton. My iPhone contact list contains only 200 people. As my children will attest, I'm not popular. Most people are somewhere between Bill Clinton and me. Sometimes Facebook is used to measure the size of someone's social network. The average Facebook user has a little under 350 "friends."[27] Yet a small number of users have numbers of friends approaching the 5,000-friend Facebook limit. The discrepancy between these few people and the average of 350 friends, as well as the difference in popularity between Bill Clinton and me, gives us a hint as to the wide variety of differences in social connections.

Facebook friends are not always friends in the traditional sense of the word. Possibly some have not been met in person. However, the way in which social-media friends are connected shares similarities to real-world contact networks. Some individuals come into contact with huge numbers of people over the course of a given day, while others interact with only a few individuals. A bus driver may interact with hundreds of people per hour. A telemarketer working from a home office may interact with no one in person. Neither of these extremes represents the typical case. The average number of contacts per day that are both of a long enough duration and close enough proximity to spread an infectious disease, such as influenza, is a little over twenty people for individuals between twenty and fifty years of age.[28] However, the average number of contacts is less important than the extremes in the spread of a contagious disease. Airline routes help to explain why.

On a long flight, most of us have at one time become bored and flipped through the airline magazine placed at our seat. The magazine probably contained a map of routes between different airports. When we looked at these maps, we noticed that *most* airports connect to only a handful of others. However, there exist a small number of airports that have an extraordinary number of flights coming and going each day. These are the airline *hubs* in major cities such as Atlanta, Beijing, Chicago, London, and Paris. When we think of airports, these locations immediately spring to mind. Yet there are hundreds of other smaller commercial airports in the United States and thousands across the world.

In the United States, the Federal Aviation Administration lists about 500 primary commercial airports. In 2019, the Atlanta airport had about fifty million passengers pass through it. The eighth-ranked airport, which had about one-half of Atlanta's total, is in Seattle, Washington. Only twenty-eight airports had over ten million passengers, and only ninety-six of the 500 had over one million. This ninety-sixth-ranked airport is Piedmont Triad International near Greensboro, North Carolina. This airport in Greensboro is already a smaller airport than the ones typical travelers pass through, but there are over 400 commercial airports smaller than it in the United States.[29]

With the vast majority of airports being this small, it may seem amazing that we can get anywhere other than a major city without spending days traveling. The key is in the organization of the hubs and the flights between airports. We don't typically fly from small airport to small airport, piggybacking across the country or continent. Typically, even if starting in a small town, we fly to a hub near our departure or destination, or somewhere in between. I grew up in a small town in northern Michigan named Cedarville. The nearest airport is 30 miles away in Sault Ste. Marie. This airport has only 25,000 passengers per year. The nearest airport to my current residence is in White Plains, New York. It too isn't a major airport, yet I can pass from my new home to my old home in only two flights: White Plains to Detroit and Detroit to Sault Ste. Marie. This is typical of most flights anywhere we want to travel. Most airports connect to at least one hub, and the hubs connect to each other. In almost all cases, the worst domestic flight situation results in three flights: small airport to hub, hub to another hub, and that hub to a final small airport.

Airlines set such routes deliberately because their hub-and-spoke format is efficient. Although no one plans it, our social networks follow a similar organizational pattern. Just like an airline routing pattern, almost all people are connected to at least one, and often more than one, social hub. A social hub can be a person like Bill Clinton, or it can be a location like a place of employment, a gym, a school, or a place of worship. Like airport hubs, social-network hubs are connected to each other, but not by planes; they connect by people. Consider this example: On a Friday, a student travels to school on a crowded bus, attends classes throughout the day, and participates in an athletic event after school.[30] The gym is packed with parents, who each arrive after interacting with dozens of people at work during the day. The student's family then attends a weekend church service in a neighboring town.

This student is a social hub, and each of the locations to which the student travels is a social hub. There are 100 students on the bus who interact with each other. Each interacts with dozens more students and teachers throughout the school day. Many breathe the same air as each parent at the athletic event. All these parents connect each of these students to everyone at their various places of work. Dozens of new people at the church connect to them all. Hubs are connected to hubs. Social-network scientists call this hub-to-hub contact pattern *assortative mixing*.[31] Assortative mixing is dangerous for infectious disease spread. As soon as one person is infected, everyone is exposed across all of these hubs. The hub-to-hub contacts sustain an epidemic through super-spreading.

Because of their large numbers of connections, hubs have more exposure risk and are likely to contact someone with an infectious disease. Once infected, these highly connected social hubs connect to other hubs and unknowingly spread infections far and wide. They are the super-spreaders. Some, but not all, of the people they infect will also be social hubs. Liu Jianlun was a super-spreader who unknowingly infected other super-spreaders—the other guests who also stayed on the ninth floor of the Metropole Hotel—who then triggered SARS outbreaks in Singapore, Canada, and Vietnam. This is the manner through which infectious disease spreads widely.

Yet many of the infections that the hubs create stop after just one infection. Imagine a wagon wheel without the rim attached to it. There is a center hub with a large number of spokes. The hub passes its infection to the spokes, but the spokes aren't connected to anything else. The chain of infections appears to stop there. Many who criticize school closures and mass-gathering limits fail to consider the secondary infections that emanate in this process. They see most infections stop at the end of a spoke. Most of these typical or "average" infections don't super-spread. We see infection after infection from which nothing substantial results.

But then, sometimes, one infection lands in just the wrong place at just the wrong time, and we get one unlucky spark. The result is super-spreading. These events, which create chaos, might not be easily linked to the source. A child is infected by a teacher at school. The child isn't yet symptomatic but infects a friend from another school at a church service. This second student volunteers at an inwardly dense shelter, and two dozen people are infected. Later in the week, the first student may feel as though they have a cold. The student tests positive for COVID-19 and isolates. The student infects no one else at the school. It seems as though the infection caused no harm to others. But it did. The student's infection led to two dozen infections at the shelter. These infections may never be connected to that student. However, the student may have started a chain of infections that will number in the hundreds or thousands.

Biogen is a biopharmaceutical company founded in 1978 in Geneva, Switzerland, by a group of prominent scientists, two of whom subsequently won Nobel Prizes. In late February 2020, the company held a leadership meeting at the Marriott Long Wharf Hotel in Boston. The meeting was attended by about 175 employees of the company, some of whom had traveled from cities across the United States and Europe. Shortly after the conference ended, initial reports circulated that a small number of people at the conference had tested positive for COVID-19. By March 6, seventy of the ninety-two COVID-19 cases in Massachusetts had been linked to the conference. Additional cases connected to attendees were subsequently reported in Indiana and North Carolina after the attendees returned home.[32]

At the time, this conference was *the* super-spreading event of the US pandemic. It had all the hallmark characteristics of a super-spreading event: It gathered together a large number of people, most of whom had high numbers of contacts during the four-day conference. And some attendees came from outside the United States, most notably Europe, where significant outbreaks in Italy and Spain were already erupting. In hindsight, we now understand that early reports of the size of the spread were greatly understated in March.

In August 2020, a group of researchers from the Broad Institute, a collaboration between MIT and Harvard University, began tracking infections from the Biogen conference. As a virus spreads and reproduces, it slowly mutates. Genetic researchers can track individual strains of the virus as one would track the genetic lineage of a family. Sometimes there are large accumulations of mutations that lead to new strains. The well-known Delta and Omicron strains of COVID-19 are famous examples. Most of the time, there are only subtle differences between strains. In the case of Biogen, researchers believe that the initial strain present at the conference came from Europe but quickly experienced a unique mutation. They were able to track this mutation throughout the United States and other countries of the world after the conference.

This tracking led to a startling discovery: By August 2020, 20,000 cases across the world were linked to the Biogen conference. Locally, researchers believe that 40 percent of all COVID-19 infections that occurred in the Boston area before July 1, 2020, were linked to the Biogen conference.[33] An update with data collected until November 1, 2020, indicated that 45,000 cases in the United States and nearly 250,000 across the world were linked to the conference.[34] This was an unlucky spark that could be traced only because of its unique mutation. There were many other superspreading events like this that will never be known. They started in schools, churches, hotels, and funeral parlors, among other places. But these locations will never be identified because the pandemic became so widespread.

Just weeks after it began spreading, the strain present at the Biogen conference entered the population of people experiencing housing insecurity in Boston.[35] In the first three months of the pandemic, 900 people experiencing housing insecurity were diagnosed with COVID-19.[36] With many in this population lacking access to health care, many infections may have been missed. In early April, a widespread testing program was instituted over two nights within Boston shelters, and 37 percent of people tested positive.[37]

Like other vulnerable populations, people experiencing housing insecurity are particularly at risk, both in terms of exposure and in terms of health. Across the United States, there are nearly 570,000 people without stable housing options. That is slightly less than one out of every 500 Americans. About five out of eight of these people sleep in shelters; others sleep on the streets or at other unsheltered locations. About 35,000 of these people are unaccompanied youth. Two out of five are Black—three times the percentage of the Black population in the country.[38] Over 6 percent are military veterans.[39] Mental health issues are common. A 2009 study by the National Coalition for the Homeless found 20 to 25 percent of people experiencing housing insecurity in the United States suffer from some form of severe mental illness.[40] This is three to four times greater than the average for the United States.

It is difficult to find a more vulnerable group than people experiencing housing insecurity. Outbreaks of infectious disease are common in this population, and access to health care is severely limited. As a response to the dual AIDS and tuberculosis crisis in Boston, the Boston Health Care for the Homeless Program (BHCHP) was created in the mid-1980s from a pilot program funded by the Robert Wood Johnson Foundation and the Pew Charitable Trust. In April 2020, this program led the call for increased testing among people experiencing housing insecurity and provided a massive influx of resources to help combat the pandemic.

The problems the BHCHP faced when attempting to protect this population from exposure were numerous. The standard protocols for fighting the pandemic were difficult to implement in shelters. How was one to organize a shelter to accommodate physical distancing, isolation, and quarantine? In an interview with CNN, Dr. Jim O'Connell, president of the BHCHP, stated, "All these things we are recommending for social distancing, you can't do that when you walk into a shelter." Crowded and overrun, the shelters were inwardly dense and, without additional resources, little could be done about it.

Yet despite the challenges, the BHCHP enacted a plan to limit exposure risk for people experiencing housing insecurity. They performed over 16,000 tests through July 2021. They screened all shelter guests daily for symptoms. They put up tents for quarantine and isolation to increase social distancing. They arranged for an allocation of 500 beds at the Boston Convention and Exhibition Center, which had been refitted as a COVID-19 field hospital. They created another fifty-two-bed COVID-19 unit at their 24/7 Barbara McInnis House. They moved older and at-risk persons living in shelters to a college dormitory to isolate them and provide more opportunities for social distancing.[41] Finally, they administered over 8,000 doses of vaccine, once available, to patients, staff, and employees of their shelter partners.

Repeatedly throughout the pandemic vulnerable populations needed direct assistance. Status quo health care and pandemic response left holes that vulnerable people fell through. The Biogen super-spreader event left people in Boston experiencing housing insecurity even more vulnerable than normal. BHCHP was a lifeline that dramatically decreased exposure to the pandemic for these people and provided care that they would not have received otherwise.

The Biogen conference was the leader of all known super-spreader events in terms of cases. Of course, there may have been even larger events that went undetected. Both the Albany, Georgia, funerals and the Biogen conference occurred very early in the US pandemic. Researchers and public health officials were able to link them to the genesis of their local outbreak. Then, through contact tracing in Georgia and through genetic analysis in Boston, the subsequent infections were able to be tracked. If either of these events had occurred in April or May when levels of infections were much higher, then the high levels of community transmission may have prevented contact tracers and genetic researchers from tracking the pool of infections to a common source. The high number of infections throughout the middle months of the first year of the pandemic made this type of tracking virtually impossible.

However, another super-spreading event came to attention in early fall of 2020. It was noticed because of the prominence of those involved. On Saturday, September 26, 2020, the White House hosted a ceremony in the Rose Garden to celebrate the announcement of Judge Amy Coney Barrett's nomination to the US Supreme Court. Photographs from the event show over 200 people seated shoulder to shoulder as President Trump introduced Judge Barrett.[42] Most of the attendees were not wearing masks.

Prior to the ceremony in the Rose Garden, a reception was held inside the White House. Photographs from this event also show attendees talking in close proximity, again without masks.[43] By mid-October, at least thirteen people present at the ceremony had tested positive for COVID-19, including President Trump and the first lady, two US senators, the president's press secretary, two assistant press secretaries, and the president of the University of Notre Dame, Judge Barrett's alma mater. Following the ceremony, numerous other people tested positive within President Trump's orbit, including campaign and policy advisors and journalists who had been in close contact with those who attended the event.[44]

An event like this is a perfect storm, particularly since it occurred during a hectic political campaign season. The people infected were high-contact hubs. They all had important political or media positions and came within close physical proximity to dozens of people every day. The Rose Garden event put them all together in one place. These hubs connected to hubs immediately prior to and during the ceremony, often in interactions that did not follow recommended precautions such as mask wearing and social distancing. Any one of those people becoming infected could have led to a super-spreading event on its own even without the Rose Garden event happening. All of those people together in one room, at one time, without masks and huddled together, was a recipe for disaster. One spark here and many piles of kindling go up in flames.

After the event, President Trump attended political rallies over the next week, politicians returned to Congress, and the press staff interacted with hundreds of people. The president of Notre Dame returned to an office full of staff members and a campus full of thousands of students and hundreds of faculty members and facilities workers. The campus had already shut down in August due to a widespread COVID-19 outbreak at the onset of the semester. The situation was referred to as a "never event."[45] The term was coined by Ken Kizer to refer to egregious medical mistakes, such as performing surgery on the left arm when the right arm is injured. The Rose Garden ceremony, attended by many highly connected people all clustered together and not following recommended medical precautions such as masking and social distancing, should *never* have happened. We will never know how many people were infected and died as a result of this event.

In the weeks after the Biogen conference, only seventy cases were tied directly to the conference attendees. The hundreds of thousands of others were only found because of a quirk of evolution and genetics. If the unique mutation hadn't occurred, the world would never have known the scope of the outbreak that began at the conference. The attendees at Biogen had fewer social connections than the prominent people attending the Rose Garden ceremony, and yet the Biogen conference created 250,000 infections. At the time of the Biogen conference, we didn't know the danger of mass gatherings. In September 2020, we did. How many secondary infections did the Rose Garden ceremony create? How many hospitalizations, cases of long COVID, and deaths? We will never know the degree of devastation created by the recklessness of the people attending the Rose Garden ceremony.

These questions and the massive spread from the Biogen conference highlight the importance of secondary infections. The key to containing an epidemic isn't about keeping one particular individual safe; it is about stopping infectious people from infecting and harming others. From the reproduction number, we know that each infection creates a number of new infections that grow exponentially. To stop an epidemic, we need to stop this exponential growth. Even more importantly, we need to stop super-spreading from increasing this growth even more. A few infections in Boston, for example, can grow to 250,000 across the world. If we stop the process from originating in Boston, then we won't need to suffer the consequences of the hundreds of thousands of other infections that land disproportionately in homeless shelters, overcrowded neighborhoods, and other inwardly dense locations.

How do we control super-spreading? One avenue is easy to see: limit mass gatherings. In March 2020, sporting events, church services, indoor dining, and K–12 and university classes were quickly canceled or moved to remote online settings across the country. While this stops super-spreading at events, it doesn't address super-spreading of individuals who are hubs. When we begin to stop hubs, we find that epidemics are both resilient and fragile at the same time. This seems contradictory, but it isn't.

Airline networks are efficient at allowing people to travel far distances. We like this efficiency. Infectious disease networks spread in a similar manner. Obviously, this is an efficiency that we do not like! How can we disrupt this efficiency most effectively? Again, airline networks provide intuition. Imagine for a moment that we want to cause chaos for US flight travel. We have the power to shut down an airport somewhere in the United States, but we don't know which one to choose. We draw the name of one of the 500 US airports out of a hat, and shut it down without notice.

What happens? There are few hubs. Only twenty-eight airports carry more than ten million passengers per year. There is only about a 5 percent chance that the airport we choose randomly will be one of these twenty-eight hubs. Instead, the selected airport is much more likely to be one of the smaller, regional airports that vastly outnumber the hubs. For every Detroit Metro Airport, there are many more commercial airports in Michigan at places like Houghton, Kalamazoo, and Sault Ste. Marie. If service is interrupted at one of these smaller airports, only flights originating or terminating at this airport will be affected. If Houghton, Michigan, drops out of the network of airports, very few travelers in other parts of the United States will notice.

Alternatively, we could ask, what airport shutdown would wreak the most havoc for travelers? Atlanta would be a good choice. It connects to 150 domestic and 75 international airports and carries more passengers each day than any other airport in the United States. As flights in and out of Atlanta are canceled, flights and connections across the country and globe are affected. If you punch out the hub at the center of a wagon wheel, all the spokes fall with it.

Because the airline network depends so strongly on the hubs to work efficiently, any interruption of service in any one of the hubs creates a cascade of interruptions across the vast network of flights everywhere. A winter storm in Chicago, Minneapolis, or New York can strand thousands of travelers. The impact is felt everywhere, even across the country in San Diego! It is in this sense that the airline network is both resilient and fragile. If something happens to disrupt the airline network in a random place like Houghton, Michigan, then very little happens and few people are impacted. Airline networks are resilient when it comes to these random interruptions. Yet if a hub is interrupted, the network falls apart; it's fragile to interruptions at any one of the few hubs.[46]

This is what makes stopping super-spreading through hubs so important. Super-spreading sustains pandemics. We need to stop the most highly connected people and events from generating chains of mass infections. We can break the chain very quickly if we apply leverage in the correct places. When we think of the network of airlines, it is easy to identify these places. We simply look at the map in the on-flight magazine or, more easily, we can rattle off Hartsfield-Jackson in Atlanta, O'Hare in Chicago, JFK in New York, and LAX in Los Angeles without difficulty. When we think about infectious disease networks, it is difficult to identify the hubs. Who are the hubs for influenza, tuberculosis, or COVID-19? The answers are less obvious. We don't have the equivalent of an airline flight map for social networks that we can reference to identify super-spreaders. In some cases, we can hazard a good guess. The hubs are created by people who have a larger number of person-to-person contacts than most. A good place to start are people who have jobs at which they come into contact with large numbers of people. Many employees at retail establishments, like groceries, clothing stores, and banks, fit this description. Bus drivers and other public transit workers fit the description. Medical workers come into contact with large numbers of people, many of whom are already ill or vulnerable. Schoolteachers, especially those teaching ninth to twelfth grade, come into contact with a variety of students in a number of different classes throughout the day (in contrast, elementary schoolteachers spend the day with largely the same group of students). People in these jobs are all likely to play a role as hubs in the network of infectious disease.

If we want to break apart the network of infectious disease transmission, we need to offer protections to ensure that these people are not infected. We also need to test them more frequently than other populations so that they don't spread their infections widely if they come to be infected. However, many of these people are workers in essential services. We can't shut down hospitals, grocery stores, and public transit, and still expect society to function. Therefore, intervening in these locations by providing extra protections for these workers against infection and transmission is essential, especially if these stores and services cannot be shuttered.

Another place to look is inwardly dense neighborhoods. By definition, many of the people in these neighborhoods have higher-than-average numbers of contacts within their homes. They face more exposure risk themselves and share more exposure risk with others once infected. We need to identify these neighborhoods and provide avenues of protection for residents. Vacant hotel and college dorm rooms during a pandemic need to be made available to de-densify these homes when infections occur. Masks can be allocated to these areas free of charge. Testing resources can be over-provided within these neighborhoods in schools or other public and easily accessible areas. All the standard protocols used to fight a pandemic should be emphasized within these neighborhoods, and easy access to resources should be provided for all. We know the damage that occurs when these inwardly dense neighborhoods are shorted on safety measures such as tests. We saw this damage in inwardly dense neighborhoods of New York City in the spring of 2020.

Beyond these back-of-the-envelope calculations, things become more difficult. How do we identify people, like Bill Clinton, who know and interact with a vast number of people? I'm sure many of us know at least one person in our own social networks who is exceptionally well connected. It is the person who seems to know everyone in town, at our firm, or at our school. These people are the hubs. But from a public health perspective, these people are difficult to identify.

A group of physicists—Reuven Cohen, Shlomo Havlin, and Daniel ben-Avraham—provided a solution to the challenge of identifying these social network hubs.[47] Their strategy involves thinking about connections rather than people, flights rather than airports. Suppose the only information that we have about airports in the United States is a listing of the names. Like before, our goal is to break apart the network of airline connections. If our aim is to bring air travel to a grinding halt, we could choose one of the 500 airports at random and remove it from service. However, we know that we are unlikely to succeed in significantly disrupting the airline network—the probability of picking a hub is too small. Suppose instead that when we randomly choose an airport, such as Houghton, Michigan, we are also given information about the next flight arriving at that airport, including the airport from which this flight originated. The airport in Houghton, Michigan, is small. All the commercial flights arriving there come from one of two airports, Chicago or Milwaukee, which are both much larger airports. If we shut down the airport of origin of the first flight arriving at Houghton, then we shut down a much larger airport (Chicago or Milwaukee) than our original random choice.

If we don't pick Houghton, chances are that we will pick another small airport. Flights to small airports come from big airports. Therefore, the flight arriving at our airport likely came from a big airport—maybe even one of the mega-hubs, like Atlanta. If I pick Cedar Rapids, White Plains, Sault Ste. Marie, or one of the other hundreds of small commercial airports, there's a good chance that I find a hub by examining the flights arriving to it, and then I can intervene at that hub. The trick is concentrating on the interactions *between* the airports and not the airports themselves. This is also how you find the hubs in a pandemic.

The approach of Cohen and his colleagues may seem far removed from practice, but it has direct application to designing efficient contact-tracing protocols. In traditional contact tracing, a tracer identifies all the people who have been in close contact with a recently infected individual to determine if any of them have been infected. Those close contacts are then tested or placed in quarantine to try to forestall infections in the future. However, as we know from the 80/20 rule, most of these potential infections will not result in large numbers of new infections. Many of those placed in quarantine have not been infected at all. The vast majority are the end of spokes on the wagon wheel. The chain of infections ends with them.

However, we also know that this event is important because a few infected people will become the next hub of the wagon wheel (like Mary Mallon, Liu Jianlun, and the attendee of Andrew Mitchell's funeral) and result in a large number of new infections. Thus, of course, it is important to consider these subsequent contacts and make sure that they are sequestered so that super-spreading does not take place starting with them. While this preventive act of contact tracing going *forward* is important and necessary, it misses a key piece of stopping the epidemic: tracing *backward*.

Instead of looking forward, we can look backward to the newly infected person to try to find the source of their infection. By looking backward in time toward the source of the infection, we are much more likely to find a super-spreading person or event. Just like identifying the airport of origin of a random flight arriving in Houghton leads back to a larger airport, tracing the source of an infection leads to a super-spreader—a social-contact hub or a super-spreading event at which many other infections occurred. If we start with Kwan Sui-chu in Toronto, we can trace backward to find Liu Jianlun in Hong Kong. From Liu Jianlun we can find all of the other super-spreaders at the Metropole Hotel. This type of contact tracing is especially important if some of the Metropole guests were asymptomatic carriers, like Mary Mallon. We would never have known of their existence without backward contact tracing.

When some individuals create much higher numbers of new infections than others and continuing contagion depends upon super-spreading individuals and events, backward contact tracing has huge benefits.[48] A typical infected person is not likely to pass the infection on to large numbers of additional people. That is the lesson of the 80/20 rule. Because of this, most efforts at forward contact tracing will reach dead ends, with limited additional cases being found. As epidemiologist William Hanage told *Bloomberg News*, "If 80% of cases do not transmit [or only transmit to a few], then 80% of cases where you are forward tracing contacts are wasted effort. Because you know transmission occurred in the backward tracing, the marginal benefit is greater."[49] Of course, forward tracing has benefits when the occasional would-be super-spreader is found before they infect a multitude of others, but such cases are rare. Limited contact-tracing resources are better allocated to backward contact tracing, for which the payoff is larger. This is particularly important when contact-tracing resources are underfunded.[50]

Some countries, particularly those in Asia, have had success with backward contact tracing. Japan attempted to locate all contacts of an infected person up to fourteen days *prior* to a newly identified positive case. By going back two weeks, the government hoped to identify super-spreading events at which a large number of people were infected by the same source, often a gathering or event, but sometimes by a single person.[51] Such efforts were limited in the West except for a few instances. After watching a seminar from Japanese scientists on the benefits of backward contact tracing, KJ Seung, who helps to oversee contact tracing in the state of Massachusetts, implemented some of their methods. Using them he was able to uncover otherwise undetected clusters of infections at weddings, funerals, and bars. He told *Bloomberg News*, "It's been eye-opening. You can discover more cases, more efficiently."[52]

Backward contact tracing also breeds confidence in the contact-tracing process. Because most people will not spread the infection to many others, many people placed in quarantine from forward contact tracing may become frustrated. Most will turn out not to have been infected. They may begin to distrust the contact-tracing procedures. A malaise of indifference may develop. This indifference may result in a lack of cooperation with the process. For instance, more than 50 percent of people in some regions of the United States did not provide information on contacts after testing positive for COVID-19 and being interviewed by contact tracers. In the United Kingdom, 18 percent did not provide information.[53]

We can imagine several reasons for this refusal to provide contact information. If we know that the contacts named will be forced to quarantine, we may be reluctant to place that burden on our neighbors, friends, and relatives. This issue is even more important in low-income communities, where a quarantine may substantially affect household finances. Ten days out of work may cause the loss of a job. Missed wages may limit the ability to eat and pay rent. Thus, there are incentives for communities with populations balanced on the edge of poverty to withhold contact information. In addition, immigrant populations may be reluctant if their communities contain undocumented residents. Again, this leads to disproportionate effects on vulnerable and marginalized populations. When contact tracing is less effective in these populations, the pandemic grows larger in these communities and elsewhere throughout society.

To overcome these negative incentives, contact tracing needs to be combined with robust public health social programs. We need to provide assistance to the general population in the same way that the BHCHP provided assistance to people experiencing housing insecurity. Many cities attempted to do this, at least in part. Hotel rooms left vacant by the pandemic were rented by municipalities to provide shelter for those that could not isolate at home because of overcrowded housing. New York City, among other cities, provided food delivery. However, many of these programs were not well advertised, nor were they available in locations outside of large metropolitan areas that had large and well-funded public health departments to coordinate them. Those living in rural areas and municipalities with more limited finances did not receive the same assistance as those living in large cities, such as London or San Francisco.

In addition to providing housing for isolation, mandatory paid leave for illness, isolation, and quarantine will help to encourage compliance with recommendations during pandemics. Childcare and eldercare assistance is needed too. There are mental health and physical health issues impacted by quarantine as well. All of these issues need to be met robustly and particularly targeted to low-income communities to engender faith in, and compliance with, contact tracing and quarantine procedures. Too often the populations most vulnerable could not access the needed assistance or did not know the range of services that existed. As with super-spreading, the effects across a population experiencing an epidemic are not uniform. Some are harmed more than others. Some need more help than others. Some are more vulnerable than others. Our policy makers need to recognize these inequities and not assume that a one-size-fits-all approach will address the most pressing needs.

While applying these methods of targeted help, we need to keep an appreciation of super-spreading at the forefront. Like airport hubs sustain air traffic throughout the world, super-spreading sustains an epidemic. Because financially and socially vulnerable populations are most commonly afflicted in epidemics, directing help to them benefits society as a whole. Assisting inwardly dense locations limits the possibility of a super-spreading event occurring within an inwardly dense home or community. Helping to protect essential workers at their place of work limits the possibility of an essential worker becoming a hub of infectious disease. In this sense, targeting vulnerable populations for assistance during times of epidemics helps everyone in society because it is likely to have the largest impact on decreasing the intensity of an epidemic for all.

Chapter 4

BRIDGES OF DISEASE

In late August of 1665, a parcel of cloth arrived in the small English village of Eyam. Tailor Alexander Hadfield had ordered the cloth for use in preparation for the upcoming Wakes Week religious festival. Because it was damp when it arrived, Hadfield's assistant, George Vicars, hung the cloth to dry by the fire. Within days, on September 7, 1665, Vicars was dead.

The cloth sent from London carried fleas that transported the plague. At this time, London was under siege during "The Great Plague of London," which, upon its abatement in 1666, was the last major incidence of the Black Death in England.

What happened next in Eyam is one of the great instances of folklore in the history of infectious disease.

Following Vicars' death, the plague began to spread slowly within the small village. By the end of the year, 42 of the 800 villagers had perished. When the plague didn't disappear over the cold winter months, as was customary, villagers became nervous. A smattering of cases persisted into the spring and early summer. With deaths mounting in late June, village reverend William Mompesson took an extraordinary step—he encouraged a quarantine for the village. The quarantine wasn't designed to prevent entry, as was common for the time, but instead, was meant to have the villagers remain within Eyam to prevent spread outward to surrounding villages in Derbyshire. The reverend asked the villagers to make the ultimate sacrifice, knowing many would die, to spare neighbors in nearby villages.

Mompesson was not alone in making this request. As a young and newly appointed reverend within the community, he called upon Thomas Stanley, the former reverend whom the community trusted despite his dismissal for failing to take the Oath of Conformity. Mompesson tasked Stanley with convincing the population of the benefits of the quarantine. The Earl of Devonshire stepped forward as well. Eyam was not self-sufficient. They needed to trade goods and money for food and other supplies. The Earl promised these necessities if the self-enforced quarantine held. The supplies were delivered to the southern edge of the village. The villagers left coins in vessels containing a mixture of vinegar and water intended to prevent contagion of those collecting the money.

At this point, the mixing of history and folklore makes the events slightly unclear. Did the Earl offer the support because he admired such self-sacrifice? Or was his offer of support tantamount to a bribe in order to keep the villagers within and to protect the health and economic functioning of the surrounding communities? Historians disagree on the answer.[1] Cynics note that Mompesson sent his two young children away prior to the quarantine. He may not have been as selfless as the folktales claim. The romantic writing of novelists and poets in the years following describes the death of Mompesson's wife, Catherine, employing the tale of heartbreak as evidence to the contrary.

Whatever the motives and whoever truly devised the plan are lost to history. In the end, the village paid a hefty toll. Out of the 800 residents, 260 died across 76 families during the 14 months of the epidemic. One woman, Elizabeth Hancock, lost six of her children and her husband within the span of eight days. She buried them herself in a grave on the family's farm. Still, the quarantine succeeded in preventing any other large outbreaks in the region.[2]

The strategy of a quarantine seems obvious at first glance. If you restrict infections from spreading to other areas, you stop the epidemic. However clear this logic may seem, though, there is a deeper reason to consider this further. Quarantines, self-imposed or otherwise, entail a more nuanced picture of how an infectious disease spreads across social and commercial bridges within our society. These bridges enable us to remain close to each other. At the same time, they allow infectious disease to spread more easily.

How do bridges do this, and how do we take advantage of them in our quest to stifle the spread of an infectious disease? The answer comes, in part, from social psychologist Stanley Milgram and his research during the 1960s. In the mid-twentieth century, there was a feeling that the world was shrinking. Far more people had ventured outside their country's borders than ever before. For some, this was due to participation in the conflicts of the World Wars. For others, travel by airplane and ship to other countries and continents became increasingly common as transit speed quickened. Milgram was interested in this shrinking world and the closeness of people within it.

To better understand how small the world had become, Milgram designed an experiment to measure the social distance between people in the United States. He sent postcards to a random set of recipients in Wichita, Kansas, and Omaha, Nebraska. Each postcard was accompanied by a set of instructions to return the postcard to a target contact who was a banker in Massachusetts. Upon receiving the packet, the recipients were able to read the name and profession of the target and were asked if they knew this person on a first-name basis. If they did, they were asked to address an envelope and mail the postcard back to the target. If not, the recipient was asked to place their name on a roster and mail the postcard, instructions, and roster to someone they personally knew who they deemed to be socially "closer" to the target. Through this series of mailings and subsequent guesses as to who a closer contact may be, letters wound paths across the country. Eventually, about 20 percent of the original letters reached the target in Massachusetts. While the number of intervening steps to reach the target varied, the returned postcards needed an average of five mailings to reach the target.[3] Combining this result with previous writing on social connectedness and a bit of fictional license, somewhere in the 1970s the "six degrees of separation" and "small world" memes were born.

The result surprised many. Friends tend to be linked within small social groups in the same cities, towns, schools, and churches. If most people list their ten best friends, many times, these ten people all know each other. If most of one's friends know each other, it is difficult to link people across the world because the friends of friends keep circling back to the same set of people in the same city. Social-network scientists call this phenomenon *clustering*. If all of our friendships were clustered like this, then all of Milgram's letters would have remained in Kansas and Nebraska and never reached Massachusetts. The world would be big, not small. How do our worlds become small, in the sense of Milgram's experiment, when there is so much clustering in our social networks?

Two mathematicians, Duncan Watts and Steven Strogatz, discovered the answer. If you have social networks that are tightly clustered but you have just a few acquaintances who connect to others outside of your main cluster of friends, then the world can become small. Those few random acquaintances create bridges that take our social network to new places. As in the Milgram experiment, we can connect a random person in the United Kingdom to another random person in Indonesia by following paths created by these few acquaintances that span our social networks across the world.

Yet we remain surprised when we learn that the mother of the yoga instructor at the local gym happens to know our middle school art teacher from twenty years ago when we lived in a different state. Who hasn't had an experience like this at a party where you uncover some hidden link with a random person? We've all had this happen, and we all say, "Wow, it's a small world."

Because most people have a few acquaintances who connect to others outside of our main social network, getting a letter from a random person in Nebraska to a banker in Massachusetts isn't as difficult as people in Milgram's time imagined. The subjects who received a letter from Milgram probably knew a banker or a family member or a friend who took a job on the East Coast. That person probably knew someone in Massachusetts, who knew a banker, who addressed the letter to Milgram's target recipient. These loose connections that are outside of our mainstream social networks are the lynchpins that keep our social network from falling apart and also create the bridges that keep us all a short distance from each other.

This small-world phenomenon is intriguing and fun. At the same time, it is dangerous. A virus circulating on a continent in another part of the world is but a few short steps from reaching your home. The bonds that keep us close together also put us in danger. Viruses and bacteria hop aboard hosts who travel on busses, planes, trains, and ships to arrive at the funerals and biology conferences that create super-spreading events and wreak havoc on our lives. That is the bad news.

The good news is that, by understanding how connections create bridges to make the world small, we can break apart this web of connections and make it more difficult for an infectious disease to spread. Because these bridges are few, we may be able to disrupt an epidemic if we can identify these bridges and eliminate their connections.

What could a brilliant mathematician and a co-star of the movie *Animal House* have in common? (No, this isn't the start of a bad joke.) They each live near the center of their respective professional networks because of bridges.

Paul Erdős was one of the great eccentrics of mathematics. Born in Budapest in 1913 to two mathematics teachers, he displayed his mathematical mind early. At the age of four, he was famous for asking a person's birthdate and quickly calculating the number of seconds that the person had lived. He never married or had children. In adulthood, he referred to young children of friends and relatives as *epsilons,* the Greek letter commonly used by mathematicians to refer to an arbitrarily small constant added to a number or expression.[4] He was a quintessential academic eccentric. Over his career in mathematics, he published an astounding 1,500 scientific articles. However, he is best known for his nomadic existence and the production of something called an *Erdős number.*

Erdős would travel the world and arrive, unexpected, at a mathematical colleague's office and simply state, "My brain is open." The colleague was expected to state a challenging problem that was the subject of their research at the moment. Erdős, with his uncanny ability to distill problems to their essence, would assist in solving the problem over the course of days or weeks, contribute to the writing of academic papers, and move on to the next stop on his life's mathematical journey.[5]

Over the course of these meetings, Erdős published research with over 500 colleagues scattered across the world, unlike most scientists of his time who wrote with nearby colleagues. He created bridges upon bridges. Because of his fame, it became a badge of honor to co-author an article with Erdős. He didn't spend time with those he considered unworthy. Even being two or three steps removed from Erdős's co-authors was noteworthy. Over time, this distance from Erdős became known in academic circles as one's "Erdős number." It works like this: the 500-plus people who co-authored with Erdős have an Erdős number of one. Those who didn't publish with Erdős, but published with one of his co-authors, have an Erdős number of two. The next step results in an Erdős number of three, and so on.

A clever tool on the American Mathematical Society webpage lets you calculate a scientist's Erdős number.[6] For instance, Albert Einstein has an Erdős number of two. He published an article with Ernst Gabor Straus, who is one of Erdős's direct co-authors. I have an Erdős number of five. I have published articles with Scott E. Page, who published with economist Lu Hong. I know Scott well and have met Lu on occasion. Lu has published with Jerry Stewart Kelly (another economist), who has published with Peter C. Fishburn (a mathematician). Peter is a direct co-author with Erdős on a paper they wrote in 1996, the year Erdős died. In my chain of contacts, Scott is a friend; Lu is a bridge. To the best of my knowledge, I have not met Jerry or Peter. Lu is the person whom I have met, but do not know well, who connects me to Jerry and Peter, two people whom I would not reach in my chain of academic connections if not for her bridge.

Kevin Bacon is the Paul Erdős of film. He is a full-time actor and part-time musician. He is well known for appearances in a variety of Hollywood blockbusters such as *Footloose* and *Animal House*. He is equally well known for the

Kevin Bacon party game. The game works like the calculation of an Erdős number: a member of the game names a random actor. Another participant in the game must then name a chain of actors who appeared in movies together that connect the random actor to Kevin Bacon. For instance, start with Charlie Chaplin. He appeared in *A King in New York* with George Woodbridge. George Woodbridge appeared in *Alligator Named Daisy* with Donald Sinden. Donald Sinden appeared in *Balto* with Kevin Bacon. It takes three steps to get from Chaplin to Bacon.

Before I lead you to believe that I have an encyclopedic knowledge of films (or if you would like to try this yourself), there is a fun website called the "Oracle of Bacon" that was developed by computer scientists affiliated with the University of Virginia.[7] It uses data from the Internet Movie Database (IMDb) and allows you to find paths between Kevin Bacon and any other actor in the database.[8]

Frequently, I have students play the game on the website when I teach courses on social network analysis. Students find it amazing that it is difficult to name an actor who has a path longer than three or four connections to Kevin Bacon. Once, I even had a student with a film credit in the IMDb for a role as an extra in a small independent film. He was shocked to find that his one movie appearance gave him a Bacon number of four! As long as an actor can reach another actor who is a hub, it is easy to get to anywhere else in the network of actors. Bridges get us to the hubs. Hubs get us everywhere else in movie networks just like they do in airline and social networks.

The longest distance between Kevin Bacon and any of the other 400,000 actors linkable to Bacon in the database is 10. Of those 400,000 actors, there are only about 11,000 who have a distance greater than 4.

Kevin Bacon appeared in many movies, some of them huge blockbusters. However, there are many actors other than Kevin Bacon who could have been central to the game. To some extent, the reason the game has appeal is that there isn't anything unique about Bacon compared to other famous Hollywood actors. From interviews, he seems like a nice, likable person. He turned his six-degrees fame into a non-profit that supports many charitable causes by connecting people across the world.[9] In terms of movie roles, he is a star, not a mega-star, yet we still move relatively easily from Kevin Bacon to almost any other actor in the film universe.

The average distance between Kevin Bacon and the other 400,000 actors who are reachable from him is about 3.2. However, there are other actors with an even smaller average—not greatly smaller, but slightly. The numbers change a bit every time a new movie is released and added to the IMDb, but as of this writing, Christopher Lee, of *Star Wars* and *Lord of the Rings* fame, has the shortest average distance to other actors in the network at about 2.9. Kevin Bacon currently sits just outside of the top 500 on the list of shortest average distance. Other actors in the top ten are household names such as Michael Caine, Martin Sheen, and Robert De Niro.

One name of interest sits just outside the top ten: Max von Sydow, who passed away in 2020. Von Sydow's film career took off in the 1950s with significant and leading roles in many of Ingmar Bergman's films, such as *The Seventh Seal, Wild Strawberries,* and *Through a Glass Darkly.* He remained productive in these smaller European films throughout the 1960s before playing Father Merrin in the classic horror film *The Exorcist* in 1973. He continued his acting career in a variety of roles in Europe and the United

States. He acted in blockbusters such as the Tom Cruise movie *Minority Report*. He also appeared in the *Game of Thrones* TV series and *Star Wars: The Force Awakens*.

Despite his successful career, he seems out of place listed next to Anthony Hopkins and Samuel L. Jackson. He appeared in fewer films and fewer blockbusters, and he never held the same level of fame. What he did have, however, were appearances in a diversity of film types at a variety of times, which linked him across genres and decades and tied him near the center of the acting universe. By connecting these genres together, von Sydow acted as a bridge that helped to make the film world small.

In the same way that bridges like von Sydow connect actors, bridges also connect the social networks across which infectious diseases spread. It takes only one bridge to get COVID-19 from one recent traveler to Europe into the Jackson Heights neighborhood of New York. Perhaps an airport employee brings the disease home after working a shift at LaGuardia Airport. Once there, the opportunities provided by inward density and super-spreading take over. One spark, brought by one bridge, and the fire erupts.

Super-spreading can be created by events and highly connected individuals. The networks these connections create can be fragile and robust at the same time. When we think about how these hubs of super-spreading connect to each other, we sometimes find individuals who are essential to those connections. These are people who connect disparate groups—bridges between different parts of society. Max von Sydow was this kind of a bridge. His roles in European art house films, Hollywood blockbusters, and smaller independent movies bridged the gaps between these different and frequently unattached film worlds. When bridges like these connect different and diverse groups, they build the web of connections that hold networks together. These bridges make the world small.

Sociologist Ronald Burt recognized that sometimes unconnected groups lack a bridge that connects them.[10] He referred to these gaps between groups as *structural holes*. For instance, engineers with new inventions may not have access to the capital needed to make those inventions a market success. Middle men and women who connect the inventors to the venture capitalists fill these structural holes and connect these groups together. Even before the television show *Shark Tank* existed, people like Barbara Corcoran, Mark Cuban, and Lori Greiner provided bridges between inventions and money. Their role in filling these structural holes was valuable to society because they brought new inventions to the marketplace. Without them or others like them, the connections would not have been made, and society would have lost out on novel ideas that improved our lives.

Filling structural holes in investment networks can benefit society. Filling structural holes in infectious disease networks can be deadly. Truck drivers played a key role in spreading HIV and other sexually transmitted diseases across Africa.[11] Their sexual interactions along their driving routes connected communities and cities that would not have been connected otherwise. They were bridges who filled structural holes with disease and death.

In the United States, people living in long-term care facilities make up less than 1 percent of the country's population, yet this same population accounted for at least 35 percent of COVID-19 deaths.[12] About 8 percent of people—one out of every twelve—in long-term care facilities in the United States died from COVID-19 in the first year of the pandemic.[13] Think about this for a moment. Note that this is not one death out of every twelve people who were infected; rather, it is *one death out of every twelve people who lived in long-term care.* If similar rates of mortality had occurred across the entire United States population, 25 million people would have died in the first year of the pandemic in the United States.

COVID-19 mortality rates of the elderly were much more severe than for any other group, yet eldercare facility deaths stand out. How did infections and deaths become that bad, despite most facilities restricting access to visitors? It was largely due to unintentional bridges that were formed between long-term care centers by part-time employees.

Researchers M. Keith Chen, Judith Chevalier, and Elisa Long used wireless phone IDs to identify workers at nursing homes during the lockdown period of the pandemic, when visitors were not allowed within these facilities. The researchers were able to identify half a million wireless devices within eldercare facilities; 5 percent of these devices were present for more than one hour in *two or more* facilities. Because visitors were not allowed during this time period, it is easy to infer that these devices belonged to workers or contractors who moved between facilities.

The researchers then used these multiple facility device locations to create a network of connections between the nursing homes in order to investigate whether these connected facilities had higher numbers of infections and deaths. Their estimates revealed that "forty-nine percent of nursing home cases [were] attributable to cross-facility staff movement . . ."[14]

These multi-facility workers provided the bridges across which the pandemic spread in eldercare facilities. These bridges were not numerous, but they did not need to be. A few bridges allowed this world to be small. Here, those few links—less than 5 percent of workers—connected facility to facility and allowed the pandemic to spread wildly in the homes of our most vulnerable citizens. Eldercare residents had the greatest health risk. The bridges that these workers provided created the exposure risk. The bridges weren't many, but they were enough.

This pattern of bridging was seen outside of the United States as well. Another study found that 11 percent of staff in four London nursing homes worked in multiple homes.[15] A 2012 survey found that 19 percent of nursing assistants and 13 percent of registered nurses worked multiple jobs.[16] This practice of holding multiple positions is common because of the low wages paid to most nurse aids, caregivers, food service workers, and cleaning personnel within these facilities. Hourly wages for a certified nurse aid ranges from $12–$15 an hour according to the *Washington Post*.[17] About 15 percent live below the poverty line, and 38 percent receive some type of public assistance. Three-fifths are people of color.[18] These workers need a second job to survive. In addition, because of low wages, it is likely that many of these workers reside in inwardly dense neighborhoods. They have more exposure risk at home, and this elevated exposure risk is shared at work. This exposure risk combined with the formation of bridges put long-term care residents in more peril than the rest of the population.

A second set of bridges, this time in multigenerational homes, attacked a second set of vulnerable victims. Eighteen percent of households within the United States classify as multigenerational (holding three generations or more). The rate is much higher among Latinx (30 percent), Asian (25 percent), and Black (24 percent) households than among non-Hispanic white households (15 percent). Multigenerational housing has many advantages for families. Elderly parents can be cared for by their adult children.

Grandparents living in the same home provide childcare options for dual-career parents. Multigenerational housing acts as a buffer against poverty when adult children who are unemployed move in with their parents, perhaps bringing grandchildren with them. Sometimes, multiple adult children live in the same household. It provides a safety net against unemployment and poverty. It also creates a connection across generations in which grandparents can live in harmony with their grandchildren and pass on cultural and familial traditions.

While the social, familial, and economic safety net aspects of multigenerational housing offer benefits, they also create the cost of increased exposure risk during a pandemic. There are multiple characteristics of this increased exposure risk in mutigenerational homes. First, multigenerational homes tend to be inwardly dense. These households contain more residents but typically contain less living space per resident.[19] They tend to be overcrowded. It can be difficult to isolate infected individuals within a multigenerational home. Combined, these effects lead to increased exposure risk, particularly for Latinx homes, which were found to have especially high rates of in-home coronavirus transmission.[20] Second, multigenerational homes create bridges to different parts of the community. Each member of a household has an individual contact network. The network includes the members of the household and also members outside the household. When the ages of the household members are more varied, less overlap exists in the networks outside the household. Young children go to schools, after-school activities, and clubs with classmates and friends their same age. Parents go to work and interact with other parents and adults. Grandparents interact with friends their own age and the family friends of the others within the household.

The household network of a multigenerational home provides bridges that connect to all of these different age groups and different parts of the community that each hold different areas of exposure. If a contagious disease enters into one part of a community, it is likely that some member of a multigenerational household has a network that exists within that realm. Whether infections pop up in a school or a local factory does not matter. The infections quickly enter a multigenerational home because of the bridges between the home and many areas of the community. Once in the home, it spreads within this inwardly dense home environment.

Ana Corrales lives with her in-laws, Jose and Ramona, in Southern California near Los Angeles. She runs a business catering Mexican *paletas* (popsicles) and frequently visits different work sites. When her work schedule conflicts with childcare, her children often are watched by Ms. Corrales's mother. Her mother's home includes four siblings of Ms. Corrales, all of whom hold jobs outside the home.[21] One can readily see the various avenues of exposure that exist. Infections could enter either of these homes through Ms. Corrales, her children, the siblings, or any of the workplaces of the siblings. Each of them provides bridges to different locations in the Los Angeles area. An outbreak in any one of them exposes the elders in either of these homes. Ms. Corrales's mother has heightened health risk as a cancer survivor.

Some public health agencies recognized the danger of multigenerational homes. In the state of Washington, after giving vaccine priority to essential health care workers and first responders, it next gave priority to those seventy and older as well as those fifty and older living in multigenerational homes. Other states, such as Alaska, Minnesota, and Oregon, created specific plans for multigenerational homes.[22]

Inward density is a second concern of multigenerational homes. While not as dire as the cramped conditions of Naples, many multigenerational families do not have the space to isolate an infected family member. Betty Rivera lives in a one-bedroom apartment in an inwardly dense neighborhood of Los Angeles. She shares the apartment with her daughter, her son-in-law, and her grandchildren. When she was infected, she locked herself in the bedroom that she normally shares with her grandson. The rest of her family slept in the living room while she isolated.[23] Despite best efforts, they could not contain the spread within the home. Ms. Rivera's daughter, son-in-law, and two of her grandchildren became infected.[24]

This situation was not different than the infections that ran through the inwardly dense and low-income areas in New York City in the spring 2020 pandemic wave. This story repeated throughout the country. The overcrowding within the Rivera household was not unique. When these inwardly dense homes are multigenerational, they are at greater risk because of the bridges that are created to different parts of society. These bridges are points of leverage in our networks as well. If we remove one bridge, we disconnect the network and break apart the web of connections.

Many of the nonpharmaceutical interventions meant to address the COVID-19 pandemic involved breaking apart the network of contacts in society. They reduced density and eliminated bridges. Stay-at-home orders, limits on mass gatherings, and reduced-density schools and office buildings all eliminated hubs and severed the bridges that link disparate and otherwise unconnected groups. These interventions made the network of contacts more sparse. There were fewer paths for the infectious disease to travel. In statistical terms, this pruning of the contact network made the average distance between individuals in the network longer.

The equivalent of our Erdős or Bacon number for infectious disease transmission gets larger for everyone in society as we break these networks apart. We create greater distance from the infected person whose virus may eventually reach us and make us ill.

When we closed schools, churches, public transportation, and sporting events, we stopped people who normally would not interact outside of these events from infecting each other. As a resident of a small town north of New York City, if I am not at a New York Jets game with my family, I won't come in contact with the family from Staten Island who has seats next to me. We cannot infect the Staten Island family and they can't infect us because we won't come in contact outside of the hypothetical Jets game that was canceled. If I were to become infected, my infection would have a much longer chain of subsequent infections to travel prior to reaching anyone on Staten Island.

We often think that we limit mass gatherings because we are worried about a super-spreader event infecting many people at the specific event. We are. However, equally important is stopping a handful of people from being infected at the event and taking the infection home to their everyday networks in different parts of society that are otherwise not connected. One SARS case from a single hotel floor traveled across bridges to Singapore, Canada, and Vietnam. We cancel the Jets game to stop a super-spreader event from occurring, but we also cancel the game to prevent huge numbers of bridges from forming between communities that otherwise would not come in contact with each other.

The Biogen conference was a super-spreading event. However, there were only a couple hundred people at the conference as attendees and probably a couple hundred more people who came in direct contact with the attendees in hotel lobbies, elevators, and restaurants. There were not

250,000 people infected at the conference. However, 250,000 people across the world were infected by the chain of events that unfolded beginning at the conference. A few people were directly infected, and those infections then percolated through populations across Massachusetts, the northeast United States, and eventually the world as people traveled from the conference back to their homes. The conference brought together many people who would not have otherwise been in contact. It gave the virus a chance to cross the bridges that were temporarily formed between interactions of attendees at the conference, and the virus took the express train across other bridges to neighborhoods that it would have taken much longer to reach had the conference not occurred.

If we sever these bridges, we contain the virus to a localized area. There, it will eventually run out of susceptible people to infect, just like a campfire will eventually run out of wood to burn. We want to stop bridges from leading the fire to new piles of wood, where a flare-up will occur in a new area. Eventually, one bridge leads to a super-spreader and a firestorm erupts. With this firestorm, more piles of wood are found across more bridges, and more fires start to burn. This is the way that epidemics spread across geography. By eliminating bridges, we can stop the epidemic from reaching new piles of wood.

The history of the spread of infectious disease is littered with examples where people and their travels formed bridges and allowed pestilence to spread between otherwise unconnected communities and continents. The people of Northern Africa and Piraeus were separated by a vast sea, yet in 430 BC, passengers on trading ships connected these distant lands. One of these passengers was infected in Africa and brought disease back to Piraeus. This disease almost destroyed Athens. Other travelers on other ships provided the bridges between groups of people on other routes of trade and conquest.

Procopius, a mid-sixth-century historian, wrote that the plague arrived at the port of Pelusium, an Egyptian city on the easternmost mouth of the Nile River, in 541. From there it spread throughout Egypt as well as east to Palestine before reaching Constantinople in 542 through one or many of the numerous military and commercial voyages between these otherwise unconnected areas.[25] This infectious disease bridge sparked the Justinian plague, which was the first instance of plague in Europe. Plague massacred the population of Constantinople. Procopius claimed there were 10,000 deaths per day; modern historians put the number at about 5,000. In total, this initial wave of plague is believed to have killed between 20 and 40 percent of the population of Constantinople and around 25 percent of the Byzantine Empire. Total mortality estimates range from 25 million to 50 million people in the initial two-century-long bout with plague. After this, the plague disappeared for six centuries.

In the mid-fourteenth century, it reemerged in Mongolia.[26] The city of Caffa sits in Crimea on the northern shore of the Black Sea in present-day Ukraine and is now called Feodosiya. It was established by Genoa in the mid-thirteenth century by agreement with the Mongols, who controlled the area. The city became the primary port for Genoese merchant ships connecting to the Don River and then to overland trade routes of the far east. Throughout its early history, tensions were high between the Mongols and the Italian traders and merchants. Military conflicts were frequent.

In 1343, the Mongol king Jani Beg laid siege to Caffa after a skirmish that included a group of Italian merchants, who retreated to the Italian outpost. After an initial defeat, the Mongols returned to Caffa in 1346. Writing in 1348 or 1349, Gabriele de' Mussi, an Italian notary, described the events that took place during these battles:

> In 1346, in the countries of the East, countless numbers of Tartars and Saracens were struck down by a mysterious illness which brought sudden death. Within these countries, broad regions, far spreading provinces, magnificent kingdoms, cities, towns and settlements, ground down by illness and devoured by dreadful death, were soon stripped of their own inhabitants.[27]

We now know that the mysterious illness was the plague that came to be known as the Black Death. De' Mussi goes on to describe the retreat of "Christian merchants" to Caffa and the subsequent attack by the "heathen Tartar [Mongols]."[28] He described a three-year besiegement of Caffa by land and how the Genoese survived by receiving shipments of food and supplies by sea. He continued:

> The dying Tartars, stunned and stupefied by the immensity of the disaster brought about by disease . . . lost interest in the siege. But they ordered corpses to be placed in catapults and lobbed into the city in the hope that the intolerable stench would kill everyone inside. What seemed like mountains of dead were thrown into the city . . . one infected man could carry the poison to others. . . . Thus almost everyone . . . fell victim to sudden death . . . as if struck by lethal arrow. . . .[29]

De' Mussi continued:

> As it happened, among those who escaped from Caffa by boat, were a few sailors who had been infected with the

poisonous disease. Some boats were bound for Genoa, others went to Venice, and to other Christian areas. When the sailors reached these places and mixed with the people there, it was as if they had brought evil spirits with them: every city, every settlement, every place was poisoned by contagious pestilence, and their inhabitants . . . died suddenly.[30]

The spread of the plague in the west began in earnest immediately after the events described by de' Mussi. Those who escaped Caffa and returned to Italy formed the bridges that brought plague to Europe. One ship arrived in Constantinople, which lost up to 90 percent of its population to the plague. Other ships from Caffa landed in Marseille, Sicily, and Venice. Plague erupted in these ports and moved inland and throughout Europe. Over the next few years, up to 50 percent of Europe's population died.[31] The siege of Caffa and the ships of people who fled were the most infamous examples of people acting as bridges and bringing infectious disease to a new land.

Despite the drama within Caffa, other bridges existed at the same time across overland trade routes and, notably, the Silk Road. The primary outbreaks of the Black Death traced along major shipping ports, overground trade routes, and rivers where trade frequently occurred.[32] All of these routes brought otherwise-unconnected people into contact with each other. These interactions provided the bridges that allowed infectious disease to travel to new populations.

Over time, technology created more bridges. Infectious disease historian William McNeill argued in *Plagues and Peoples* that the invention of ever-faster modes of travel greatly enabled people to travel more quickly and contributed to the spread of new infectious diseases from Asia into Europe. Early on, the travel between ports by ship was too slow and took too long to introduce infectious disease with a significant rate of mortality. A deadly infectious disease aboard a slow ship killed everyone who had been infected before arrival at a new port. If anyone who was infected managed to survive, he or she likely had recovered and was no longer infectious by the time of arrival in a new land. It was more difficult for infectious disease to spread too far too quickly. Unconnected populations were safer from one another than they were prior to the increase of rapid travel between lands. The lands were disconnected—the bridges that would connect them later in history did not yet exist.

Once steam ships arrived in the nineteenth century, it was much easier for an infectious disease to remain virulent onboard the ship for the duration of a journey because the journey took less time to complete. This was when new infectious diseases, such as cholera, arrived in the Americas in a matter of months after first spreading to Ireland and England from Asia.

Today we see this same effect at hyper-speed. One can fly to the other side of the world in a matter of hours. Many people do so every hour of the day. With each journey comes the possibility that an infectious disease makes a trip with a traveler.

The novel coronavirus, SARS-CoV-2, likely made many such trips in a short span of time. It took only weeks for it to travel from Asia to all populated continents. In earlier centuries, those same journeys took months or years.

Once we recognize the danger of bridges, we can work to remove them. At an intuitive level, we have tried to do so for centuries. It was the purpose of the Eyam self-isolation in 1665. In times of the Black Death in Europe and the yellow fever outbreaks in nineteenth-century North America, we used a similar form of intervention—forced quarantine of ships. Venice was one of the first cities to try to insulate itself from bridges of disease by using quarantine stations at major ports called lazarettos. In 1423, Venice built the *Lazzaretto Vecchio* ("old lazaretto") at the site of a monastery on the Island of Santa Maria of Nazareth.[33] The location of the original lazaretto near the Lido made it convenient yet far enough away to provide safety from the city. In their book *Until Proven Safe*, Geoff Manaugh and Nicola Twilley argue that the nearness also brought peace of mind to Venetians, who saw proactive steps being taken to maintain safety within the city. Originally, the lazaretto isolated and treated those already afflicted with plague. However, as the number of cases grew, they constructed a second *Lazzaretto Nuovo* ("new lazaretto") in 1468.[34] The second lazaretto was closer to the entry of the Venetian Lagoon.

Over time, Venice used the lazarettos within a system designed to isolate itself from infection by sea. Ships approaching Venice through the narrow opening to the lagoon were directed to the nearby Lazzaretto Nuovo with a strategically chosen location that made it easy to control entry to the port. There, goods, passengers, and crew members were inspected. People and cargo considered questionable were confined to the lazaretto for a period of forty days. The length of the term was taken from Christian scripture where forty was a common number.[35] The term "quarantine" developed from the Italian word *quaranta*, meaning forty. When illness was found, those infected were transported to the original Lazzaretto Vecchio. The system proved effective. Historian Frank Snowden reports that plague only evaded the system twice—once in 1575 and once in 1630. Otherwise, the system held off large-scale epidemics from shipping bridges that connected Venice to the world. Following Venice's example, other ports in Italy and throughout Europe from Marseille to Amsterdam copied the practice of lazarettos and quarantine. Lazarettos were an effective means to safeguard against the formation of bridges.

Despite their effectiveness at protecting Venice, the lazarettos were far from safe. Snowden reports that up to two-thirds of their patients died while confined and hospitalized. He states, "Confinement was therefore widely regarded as a death sentence to be served alone and forcibly cut off from friends and family."[36] Still lazarettos and other methods of quarantine offered protection to cities, and their use became more common.

As the use of quarantine increased debates about the balance of public health and commercial interests arose. These tensions led to New Orleans hiding the initial periods of yellow fever outbreaks in the nineteenth century. Precautions such as quarantines caused delays in shipping. This cost firms and merchants money. Some saw these precautions to protect a population from infectious disease as being given too much importance compared to their city's or their nation's commercial interests. Others believed that for commerce to thrive a strong stance had to be taken to control infectious disease. When cholera escaped Bengal in the early nineteenth century, the English position in these debates became clear.

Beginning in 1817, cholera spread widely across bridges in seven major epidemics that resulted in millions of deaths.[37] These outbreaks, combined with faster modes of transport, forced the nations of Europe to more seriously consider standardized quarantine procedures. England was opposed. A writer in the English medical journal the *Lancet* described the threat of cholera as a "humbug got up for the destruction of commerce."[38] One can imagine the same idea was held about COVID-19 by those opposed to stay-at-home orders and business closures in 2020. In the nineteenth century, other nations recognized that the bridges formed by global trade aided the spread of infectious disease and needed to be controlled. To better control contagion, France stepped forward and organized the first International Sanitary Conference in Paris in 1851.[39]

At the Paris conference, one center of discussion concerned adding suspicion of cholera to quarantine requirements. At the time the germ theory of disease was in its infancy and many of the conference debates centered around whether cholera was communicable. England played a pivotal role in the arguments against quarantine for cholera. Their motives were thinly veiled attempts to encourage free trade even at the expense of enabling the spread of infectious disease. In response to the English complaint that quarantine cost time and "time is money," the Spanish medical delegate, Pedro F. Monlau, intervened. He retorted, but "public health is gold."[40] In the end England and its free trade allies would not relent. The conference ended without agreement. England considered the routes of trade from India and throughout the colonial system too valuable a bridge to tear down. For three decades England obstructed international efforts to impose quarantine restrictions that would interrupt and restrict the free flow of trade between India and Europe.[41]

Commerce won out—England's economic interests trumped public health and more stringent control of infectious disease bridges in that round of debate. However, thirteen additional International Sanitary Conferences would follow, with the last occurring in 1938.[42] These conferences and the international cooperation and dialogue that they engendered around the topic of international public health led to the formation of the World Health Organization in 1948.[43]

In the summer of 2020, the refrains from these nineteenth-century debates returned and highlighted the tension for some between public health and commerce. How do we return toward normalcy within business, education, and society but also do so safely? Many people thought deeply about this question. Schools were put in a position of rethinking how they educated students at the same time that they limited interactions within the school. Retail stores, gyms, and restaurants had to think about how to serve customers but also keep the customers and employees safe. Continually, the methods of social distancing and curtailing bridges of contacts became central to the conversations.

We no longer wanted a middle school math teacher seeing both sixth and seventh grade students in the same day. A teacher doing so would act as a bridge between otherwise unconnected students in different grades. We wanted students separated into pods that traveled together between classes or, even better, remained in the same classrooms with teachers shuffling carts of instructional materials down hallways between classes so that students didn't interact with other pods of students in hallways. Those interactions would have created even more bridges than the one teacher. In commerce, we no longer wanted two people touching the fast-food burger, two others touching the fries, and a fifth touching the soft drink container before it reached the customer. We didn't even want the water cooler and coffee machine to be shared by coworkers.

As the initial wave of the COVID-19 pandemic receded, economist Scott E. Page provided advice about how to reopen businesses safely.[44] Many of his suggestions focused on eliminating bridges. Bridges that unnecessarily connected too many workers to customers, too many customers to workers, or too many workers to other workers needed to be eliminated. He emphasized the different layers of networks in which we live. Our traditional business world was enmeshed in networks of different types. We had worker-to-worker networks, worker-to-customer networks, and worker-to-object-to-worker networks. This last group encompassed shared resources like coffee machines, whiteboards, and bathrooms. Our social networks also contained a multitude of levels across friendships, work, education, and entertainment.

Within these various types of business and personal contact networks, we had evolved efficiency over a great number of years. Henry Ford was credited with inventing the assembly line for producing automobiles, and we saw this organizational structure replicated throughout our economy, even down to a fast-food sandwich shop. The local Subway sandwich franchise perfected an assembly line of tasks that provided sandwiches to customers in as little time as possible. Customers appreciated this speed and efficiency on short lunch breaks, and the franchise made higher profits because it served more customers in a shorter amount of time.

Our firms, government institutions, and even our social fabric had evolved to create these great efficiencies over decades. The complex interactions that wove throughout our economic and social lives resulted after being tried and tested, and we arrived at efficient solutions to the problems that we encounter *daily*. This was not just within economics and business. The social support networks that we held and our network of friendships evolved in this manner as well. If all of our friends were identical, life wouldn't be much fun. Instead, we grew to cater to a diverse collection of characters in our lives. Some we depended upon for emotional support, while others were entertaining. We wanted multigenerational homes to buffer us against job loss and poverty and to provide options for childcare and cultural connections between generations of family members. With all of these efficient solutions in our lives that provided everything from entertainment to mental health, we had created social networks with broad reach that spanned many bridges. These bridges kept the world small. They held our society together and made life fun.

These contact patterns also made the economic engine of our society hum. They allowed us to reach out at great distances for information. They gave us an economic advantage. At the same time, they put us in harm's way of an infectious disease. These diverse contacts that led us to greater economic opportunity and more diverse and exciting lives also provided the efficient opportunities for disease to spread. Because the network of contacts that we lived in daily were not tested with consistent evolutionary pressure from infectious disease, we hadn't evolved our contact networks to be robust against this infrequent but sometimes deadly challenge. When confronted with a pandemic, our networks across the layers in our lives were efficient in an unwanted way.

This was a cost of our social and economic efficiency. It was a cost that we haven't faced in large part since the 1918 influenza epidemic. It seemed unnatural to distance ourselves from what seemed normal and what had given us advantages as a society for so long. When confronted with a pandemic, we needed to unravel and tear holes in this fabric that previously bound our economic and social lives together. Undoing the efficient structure of our social and business networks was the great challenge that we faced as we confronted a return to a new normal amidst the COVID-19 pandemic.

Chapter 5

SAFER THAN
THE CITY

"I left my troubled city behind. Now I feel guilty."

George Blecher titled his May 16, 2020, *New York Times* column with these words.[1] Like many New Yorkers, Mr. Blecher, then seventy years old, left the city when the COVID-19 pandemic began. His son had pleaded with him to leave Manhattan and the Upper West Side apartment that he loved.

Eventually, he relented.

One of the porters in his building joked with him as he left, saying, "Don't desert us." Mr. Blecher displayed his wisdom in recounting this comment. He recognized that the Bronx neighborhood where his porter lived would face more severe pandemic outcomes than more affluent locations. He knew the pandemic would not be a great equalizer.

He recognized his privilege. He knew that affluence and luck provided him a means to escape heightened exposure risk within the city. He held plague insurance that allowed him a means to escape. He did not want to leave even though he knew it to be a wise choice. At the same time, he knew that others would not be as privileged nor as lucky.

Although not all recognized their luck and privilege as Mr. Blecher did, stories like his were common in the opening weeks of the COVID-19 pandemic. Those with the means to do so left behind familiar urban dwellings and patterns of life. They retreated to less risky environments.

Sometimes the retreat was obvious—like a move to a country home or remote beachfront property.

For others the retreat was more subtle. Office-based work was moved to the home and these workers avoided crowded office space and densely packed commuter trains or buses. Grocery delivery or Instacart services replaced common everyday shopping habits.

Of course, not everyone could afford these luxuries. Those without the means to do so continued life in much the same way as they previously had. Their financial circumstances did not allow them to do otherwise. Commutes, shopping trips, and life in inwardly dense environments continued. Limited financial resources left many exposed. Those with the ability to flee pandemics have always done so and left the less fortunate behind.

The Indigenous population was nearly destroyed by infectious disease when Europeans arrived in North America. Yet this did not mean that Europeans and other settlers were fully immune to all disease. Epidemic outbreaks routinely afflicted cities and towns throughout the continent. Yellow fever, in particular, posed a serious threat for Europeans entering the New World.

The arrival of yellow fever in the Americas is not a simple story. Multiple introductions occurred through ships traversing routes connecting Europe, Africa, and the New World. One particularly lethal strain was traced to a British ship and its travels that began on the eve of George Washington's second election as president.

In November 1792, the British merchant ship *Hankey* set forth to the island of Bolama, just off the west coast of Africa. The ship carried 300 abolitionists who hoped to hire, rather than enslave, Africans and set up a colony. Unfortunately, upon arrival, the group was swarmed by pestilence and many were infected with yellow fever. Surrendering their ill-fated plans, those still alive set sail in early 1793 for Grenada.[2] Upon arrival, the epidemic spilled outside the ship and invaded settlers, Indigenous people, and ship crews throughout the West Indies. Subsequent travels out of the area spread this particularly harmful strain of yellow fever far and wide.

Early in August 1793, yellow fever arrived in the United States capital of Philadelphia. At the time of the outbreak, Philadelphia was a vibrant port city with a continuous flow of ship traffic. With the steady mix of people entering and exiting the port, and their subsequent connections to the rest of the city through dockworkers and their families, a widespread epidemic erupted. One of the first afflicted was Elizabeth Hodge, the daughter of physician and Revolutionary War hero, Hugh Hodge. Unable to cure his daughter, he called upon another physician and friend, Benjamin Rush—one of the youngest signatories of the Declaration of Independence—for aid. Rush was unable to help, and Elizabeth soon died. Within weeks dozens of others were dead, shops were shuttered, and panic overtook the city. In the coming months, Rush would play the most prominent role of any person during this epidemic. When cases skyrocketed, Rush treated up to 150 cases per day.

President George Washington, in the first year of his second term as president, attempted to keep the seat of government established within the city. By September the risks were too great. Washington left with his family for their estate in Mount Vernon. He later returned to reassemble his cabinet near Philadelphia, but he did so in more rural Germantown. Other dignitaries and almost anyone with the means to do so fled the city as well. As Secretary of State Thomas Jefferson wrote to James Madison on September 1, 1793, "Every body, who can, is flying from the city, and the panic of the country people is likely to add famine to disease."[3] Contemporary historian William Kashatus described the plight of those remaining in the city: "Only poor whites, free blacks, and a few of the courageous affluent remains."[4] Philadelphia, with a population of fifty thousand at the time, was reduced to fewer than thirty-five thousand inhabitants. About half of those who remained were infected with yellow fever and five thousand died. Much of the labor of caring for the sick in the city was left to the Black population who were believed by prominent doctors of the time, such as Rush, to be immune because of their African roots and potential previous exposure.[5] This belief was false. Black workers who were thrust into labor caring for the sick and burying the dead succumbed to even higher rates of mortality than the general population.

As devastating as this yellow fever outbreak in Philadelphia had been, the 1830s saw the arrival in North America of a new and even more terrifying foe. Cholera was like no infectious disease to come before it. The vicious disease posed an unparalleled threat to safety. Until 1817 the disease had not been seen outside of India, but it was feared before it even arrived.[6] Reports of its travel through India and its arrival in England in 1831 were well known before any cases appeared in the New World. Its ghastly symptoms inspired dread in even the most stoic. As described by medical historian Charles Rosenberg:

> The symptoms of Cholera are spectacular; they could not be ignored or romanticized. . . . The onset . . . is marked by diarrhea, acute spasmodic vomiting and painful cramps. Consequent dehydration, often accompanied by cyanosis, gives to the sufferer a characteristic and disquieting appearance: his face blue and pinched, his extremities cold and darkened, the skin of hands and feet drawn and puckered.[7]

The disease set in fast and death arrived swiftly. As Rosenberg quotes from a diary written during the 1832 New York City cholera epidemic, "To see individuals well in the morning & buried before night, retiringly apparently well [in the evening] and dead in the morning, is something which is appalling [even] to the boldest heart."[8]

The gruesome nature with which it afflicted its victims and the sudden arresting time-frame frightened even the bravest souls. The lack of understanding of its cause—which wasn't discovered until 1883 by Robert Koch—made the disease seem all the more sinister to the wealthy and poor alike. In 1831 it sat in England on the doorstep of America. Quarantine restrictions were broadened across ports in the New World. Concern quickened in June when cholera was reported in Montreal, Quebec.

Cholera had reached North America, and it would soon hit New York.

On July 2, 1832, the first infection in the city occurred. The citizens of Manhattan, however, had responded in advance. Rosenberg notes, "A hyperbolic and sarcastic observer remarked later that Sunday 'fifty thousand stout-hearted . . . New Yorkers scampered away in steamboats, stages, carts, and wheel barrows.' Farmhouses and country homes within a thirty-mile radius of the city were filled. Yet the exodus continued . . ."[9] To those who were able to do so, escape was the only sensible option. Yet fleeing the city was not available to all.

As Rosenberg laments, "The poor having no choice, remained."[10]

Nearly 200 years later, the pattern repeated. Similar feelings of anxiety struck when, instead of cholera, COVID-19 sat on the doorstep of New York City in early 2020. News reports from China and Italy had the city on edge. By watching other countries, New Yorkers knew what was coming.

In February, Italian hospitals had been overrun with cases. There were not enough resources to treat all patients. Supplies such as breathing tubes were rationed. Beds in the intensive care units (ICU) of hospitals were triaged. Only those most likely to survive were given these precious commodities. Physicians tried to maximize the number of lives they could save, acting as "soft utilitarians," as one Italian doctor phrased it.[11] For some there was nothing that could be done with the limited resources available.

Ill family members were kept apart from their loved ones, except in unique circumstances. One emergency room doctor at Papa Giovanni XXIII Hospital, 50 kilometers from Milan, recalled a particular episode to the *New York Times*: A sixty-eight-year-old former lung transplant patient arrived to the hospital with low oxygen levels and rapid breathing. All of the ICU beds were filled with younger, healthier patients who were more likely to survive. The physician received special permission for the patient's wife and daughter to see him for a few minutes. The doctor told the *New York Times*, "'I saw his face when he saw his wife coming inside the room. . . . He had this wonderful smile. . . . Then I saw that he was looking at me. He realized that there was something wrong if only *his* relatives were coming inside.' The man knew in that instant that he was going to die."[12] Twelve hours later, he was gone.

As New Yorkers watched from afar, they were afraid that they were destined for these same tragedies.

Soon after, when infections grew in number within New York, Governor Andrew Cuomo and New York City Mayor Bill DeBlasio recommended that residents should only leave home for essential purposes. In response, those who could afford to do so ordered groceries to be delivered, worked from home, and avoided congregating with others. This influx of new behavior stressed the systems of the economic marketplace.

Just months before, only the wealthy or time-stressed parents purchased grocery delivery services. That changed when the pandemic hit. In New York, acquiring a coveted delivery time became so competitive that people stayed up into the wee hours of the morning to try to secure a time slot and hoped that the essential goods they desired were still available to order.[13] Grocery store delivery services in the United States, like Peapod and FreshDirect, and more general personal shopping companies, like Instacart, hired thousands of workers to meet the new demand. In the United Kingdom, the London-based food delivery company, Deliveroo, had a large enough increase in customers during the early months of the pandemic that it led to an initial public offering of its stock in March 2021.

In the early days of the pandemic, people chose to isolate, not because of a known exposure to someone afflicted, but to prevent such an exposure from happening. Like in centuries past, financial means dictated how much exposure risk one could avoid. Finances played an even larger role in the coming weeks. In March 2020, whether by wealth or by luck, a great flight from New York City occurred just as had been done for centuries. In some cases, the flight was to a relative's home—perhaps a parent, child, or cousin—who lived in a more rural location nearby. For the even more wealthy, an earlier than normal move to a summer vacation home in the Hamptons or in more rural parts of New England was common. Such moves were made even easier for parents when schools shifted to online, remote forms of education. Prices for housing rentals in the Hamptons, Catskills, and other nearby secluded areas skyrocketed.

As you might expect, the well-off population drove this process. How do we know this? It appears in the mobile phone data that tracks people as they move. According to the Pew Research Center, 81 percent of people in the United States own a smart phone. This percentage is even larger for the relatively affluent and for younger adults.[14] Nearly all smart phones contain global positioning system (GPS) features. As we know, GPS is what allows our Waze and Tom-Tom apps to give us turn-by-turn driving directions.

Less widely known is the fact that companies like Facebook and Google can locate a user's position when they post content or search for information on the internet. While it is possible to turn this feature off, many users find it inconvenient to do so. After all, allowing Google permission to track one's location makes it more convenient to find a nearby restaurant, gas station, or other point of interest. Many other third-party apps also track our location unless we specifically take steps to stop them.

Companies that provide applications on mobile phones collect this data, aggregate it into batches by geographic location (in order to preserve individual anonymity), and sell it for profit. It is big business. Companies collected $21 billion in revenue in 2018 by selling this type of data.[15] The data is used in a multitude of ways, primarily for targeted advertising.[16] Firms also use this data to locate new franchises of brick-and-mortar stores based on demographic and traffic data. With this data, researchers also can examine how people change their behavior during a pandemic by comparing typical behavior before, during, and after a pandemic strikes.

In May of 2020, the *New York Times* partnered with Descartes Labs, a geospatial analysis company, to use smart phone data to look at how the behavior of New Yorkers changed between March and April 2020. The most obvious change: 420,000 New Yorkers—about 5 percent of the population—left the city.[17]

This was not a behavior that was equally chosen across all neighborhoods. In some of the wealthiest neighborhoods of Manhattan, such as the East Village, Gramercy, and the Upper East Side/Carnegie Hill, more than 40 percent of the residents left during a brief two-week period in mid-March. Mass exodus from the city was largely contained to Manhattan except for a few unique neighborhoods. In fact, there were only six neighborhoods outside of Manhattan that saw more than 20 percent of residents leave. Three of these were affluent neighborhoods in Brooklyn: Brooklyn Heights, Cobble Hill, and Clinton Hill.

There were three more in the Bronx. Two of these were upscale neighborhoods that sit along the Hudson River, Fieldston and Riverdale. In addition, Riverdale is home to Manhattan College. The third neighborhood was Belmont, which contains the Bronx Little Italy district along Arthur Avenue, as well as a campus of Fordham University. Like most colleges, Fordham and Manhattan closed their campuses in mid-March and thousands of their students returned home. Other than these neighborhoods, no other area in New York City outside of Manhattan saw more than a 20 percent decline in residents. The majority of neighborhoods outside of Manhattan saw less than a 10 percent decline.[18]

Some who left did so almost by accident. These people took a short weekend trip to a bed and breakfast or to a relative or friend's home partly for fun, partly out of trepidation. Once the pandemic struck with full force, many of these people simply never came back until the first wave of the New York City pandemic was over. The flight of others was more intentional: SUVs with hastily purchased extra rooftop carriers were packed to the brim with clothes, school supplies, passports, laptops, and all the food and water that would fit. These people wanted to get out of town, and quick! For these people, it wasn't a lush vacation. A feeling of necessity and the luxury of opportunity led them to escape the pandemic wave that they saw cresting on the horizon.

For many others, leaving simply wasn't an option.

Low-income, inwardly dense neighborhoods like Jackson Heights, Corona, and Elmhurst saw minimal change. Residents of these areas were tied to home by jobs that could not be performed remotely and limited budgets that would not allow for flight. They rode out the pandemic with few changes in behavior. They had no choice—their financial constraints were too rigid.

Many of the residents fled to traditional summer vacation homes in places like the Hamptons and New England. They simply arrived a couple of months earlier than normal. Others were quick, spur-of-the-moment renters. These impulsive moves led to local bidding wars for prime housing. One realtor in the Hamptons described a landowner who had never rented his home before. He asked a price of $750,000 for an eight-week rental of a waterfront house; the listing was immediately taken.[19] This was just one of numerous six-figure, short-term rentals.[20]

These exorbitant prices harken back to the experience of the eighteenth-century yellow fever epidemics in Philadelphia. In his diary, Edward Garrigues described a yellow fever outbreak in 1798 when up to 80 percent of Philadelphians left the city. He notes: "Affluent Philadelphians rented, often at outrageous prices, rooms in homes in nearby villages."[21] In 2020, New York City replicated the experience of wealthy urban flight once again.

The northeast United States wasn't the only area of the world to use flight to escape epidemics. For centuries, evacuation of urban areas was a common strategy whenever populations were confronted with the bubonic plague. Set in 1348, Giovanni Boccaccio's collection of novellas, *The Decameron*, tells the fictional tale of ten affluent residents of Florence who flee to a countryside villa in order to escape the plague.[22] Despite it being a work of fiction, the setting of the story was likely common practice in the early days of the plague by those who could afford to do so. The ability to flee outside of cities was a form of plague insurance that only the wealthy could afford to buy.

A less well-known illness, the sweating sickness, tormented Europe over the course of five epidemics, beginning in 1485, and killed between 30 and 50 percent of those infected.[23] During one of these epidemics in 1517, Thomas More wrote to Erasmus and described the conditions in England: "If ever we were in trouble before, our distress and danger are at their greatest now, with many deaths on all sides and almost everyone at Oxford and Cambridge and London taking to their beds . . ." He further noted, "One is safer on the battlefield than in the city."[24] Faced with such danger in the density of the city, residents fled.

Epidemics of various diseases ravaged England, and beginning in 1518 King Henry VIII mandated that the Church of England begin printing weekly statements on mortality across parishes. These were known as the "Bills of Mortality." They were sold weekly by the Clerk of London to those who could afford to purchase the warning of the arrival of plague and other pestilence.[25] When the plague began to infect nearby parishes, the wealthy, who could afford to receive notice from the bills, fled the city. They used the bills as a warning of coming danger and escaped with haste.

Historian Kira Newman describes the experience of bubonic plague by noting that "the popular recommendations were simple: 'flie far . . . flie speedily . . . and returne slowly.'"[26] Of course this advice depended upon the ability to do so. She continues: "The monetary barrier was significant for the lower middling sort and the poor, who often lacked transportation options, places they could stay, and money to finance a journey."[27] As the wealthy left cities, the poor were left behind.

Even the wealthy who stayed behind enjoyed some comforts of safety. The financial means to self-isolate allowed the wealthy an insurance not available to all. They could afford to send staff to shop for them. They didn't cook meals, and therefore avoided the places where food was stored. These were the same places where vermin congregated searching for crumbs. The wealthy could avoid these conditions that the poor could not. Their homes were more safe than other residences in the city. Isolation by the wealthy provided a second form of plague insurance. For the poor and working-class citizens of the time, remaining isolated was simply not an option because of the lack of financial resources to do so.[28]

Like George Washington centuries later, national leaders had even more flexibility. Henry VIII is said to have slept in a different location every night during the summer of 1528 in order to escape a sweating sickness epidemic.[29] In July of 1665 Charles II escaped London to Oxford during the Great Plague. At the time of the king's departure, the plague was taking about one thousand lives per week in London. By September the total peaked at over seven thousand deaths per week.[30] During this same epidemic, Parliament was also moved out of London to Oxford.[31] The elite and powerful escaped the city for safety.

Their wealth and power allowed them to escape exposure and afforded them a level of insurance against epidemics. The poor remained stuck in their homes and were unable to access the freedom of movement away from outbreaks that, in some cases, could have saved their lives. They couldn't afford the buffer in space or time that wealthier people could afford.

When writing about the plague in Vienna in 1678, historian Mary Wilson reports, "For each 1,000 of the poor who died, scarcely 10 of the wealthy died." As such, it came to be known as the "beggars' disease."[32] This nomenclature conflates cause and consequence. The poor didn't cause the epidemic and did not deserve the blame indicated by the name. Instead, the poor's lack of financial resources left them more exposed to the risks of the plague. It was a beggars' disease only because the poor were unable to buy their safety through flight or isolation.

Flight occurred during New World epidemics too. It was so widespread that we see its lasting legacy in the fabric of modern metropolises. New York City experienced a series of four yellow fever epidemics between 1798 and 1822. During these epidemics, the well-off fled from the bustling port and financial district at the southern tip of Manhattan to the northern countryside in what is now known as Greenwich Village. Of course, it seems odd that the bustling village of today was once the countryside. But that was the reality of the time. The flight to Greenwich Village during these epidemics was so strong that it led to a reorganization of the city's financial center, at least temporarily. During the 1798 outbreak, a clerk of the Bank of Manhattan, which was founded by Alexander Hamilton, became infected.[33] The bank executives worried that a larger outbreak could force the bank to close. In order to insure against the potential lost earnings, they opened a second location for the bank in Greenwich Village near where many of their customers had fled in previous epidemics. Subsequent outbreaks led additional banks to do the same. One particular street that became populated with these relocated banks became known as "Bank Street." This small street is still present in Greenwich Village.[34] Despite its name, it exists today as a quaint residential street.

Again, exodus was common whenever epidemics arrived. In the midst of New York City's 1822 yellow fever epidemic, one resident wrote to his father: "Thousands have left, and other thousands panic stricken, are daily leaving. Stores and dwellings are closed and deserted. The custom house, post-office, all the banks, insurance offices, and public places of business have been removed to the upper part of Broadway and the Greenwich Village."[35] Many other instances of flight from cholera and yellow fever occurred during the nineteenth century in the United States. The evacuation from Memphis as a result of yellow fever in 1878 was another example.

In each historical epidemic, we can imagine the differences in the plight of the poor and the rich. Wealth consistently allowed people with more means the ability to escape. They waited out waves of epidemics by sheltering in safety. The poor did not have these luxuries. They had to work or go hungry. They could not retire to country estates or to remote second homes.

The world today exists in a different time than that of bubonic plague, cholera, and yellow fever. Yet we can see these same patterns in behavior during our own time. In the past, there were servants to shop and cook. Today we have Instacart, Ocado, and Blue Apron. Further, the wealthy can often afford the luxuries of working from home, remote shopping, and isolated commutes in personal automobiles. All are forms of plague insurance.

In modern times, we can measure these differences in behavior even more exactly using mobile phone data. Data from Google measures various categories of behavior across many parts of the world, such as the amount of time spent in grocery stores, retail establishments (restaurants, stores other than grocery, etc.), public transit stations, and workplaces, along with the amount of time spent away from one's home and the amount of time spent in parks.[36] The data categories can be compared to a baseline prior to the pandemic and then presented as percentage changes from this baseline.

In normal times, someone may spend an average of ten hours per day at a location other than their home. Once the pandemic started, that time may have dropped to three hours per day. This would be recorded in the data as a 70 percent decrease in time spent outside the home.

This type of data tracks the general experience and movements of people throughout our days. We all remember the days and weeks in late February and early March 2020 when we heard stories of the pandemic emergence in China. During this time, grocery store shelves were ransacked. Pasta, beans, chicken, milk, and bread disappeared almost overnight from stores. Hand sanitizer, toilet paper, and Clorox wipes existed only in stockpiled basements or garages or were held to be sold at exorbitant prices on websites like eBay. Early in the pandemic, large bundles of toilet paper and small containers of hand sanitizer listed for over $100.

After mass shortages began to develop, stores started limiting purchases to one package of essential items like toilet paper, milk, and cleaning supplies. Yet by mid-March many of these items were unavailable regardless of price or purchase limits. In this frenzy, stores were packed with shoppers waiting, in some cases, for over an hour in checkout lines after waiting two or three hours just to get into a store.

In Los Angeles, on March 17, 2020, the first shopper arrived in the dark. He stood in line at 2:55 a.m., waiting for

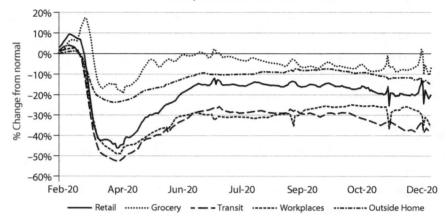

Mobility Patterns in the United States

Legend: Retail ········ Grocery – – – Transit ······· Workplaces ·–·–··· Outside Home

Change in the movement of United States residents during 2020. *Data are provided by Opportunity Insights (https://opportunityinsights.org), based on information from Google, and aggregated by a team of academic researchers at Brown University and Harvard University. More information is available at https://tracktherecovery.org.*

the local Costco store to open. Three days earlier, this same person had arrived at 4:00 a.m. only to find that the baby wipes that he needed for his two-year-old child were out of stock.[37] He now returned an hour earlier before opening, hoping to have better luck.

We see behavior of this time in the mobile phone data. During the days when people lined up with shopping carts full of chicken, pasta, beans, and toilet paper, the time spent in retail stores shot up by 10 percent and the time spent in grocery stores went up by 18 percent across the United States. Shoppers stockpiled in preparation for an uncertain future.

Simultaneous to this spike in grocery and dry good purchases, people responded in another way. They curtailed all other forms of mobility. The time spent in places outside the home, other than grocery stores, dropped rapidly prior to widespread outbreaks in the United States. New York City's use of public transit dropped by 28 percent before the March 15 school closure announcement. The decrease was already 47 percent by the time the shelter-in-place order was given about a week later.

At its low point, time in public transit stations hit levels 70 percent below normal. About two-fifths of the overall decrease happened before the school closures occurred and two-thirds of the decrease occurred prior to the shelter-in-place order. The same pattern occurred in London where transit station visits were already about half of the normal levels when the United Kingdom stay-at-home order was given. The lowest level of transit station visits in London was about 80 percent below normal levels in mid-April.[38]

In both London and New York City, people were responding to concern about the pandemic prior to any government orders and prior to any massive outbreaks in their cities. Residents of the cities acted with caution in much the same way that nineteenth-century New Yorkers acted in anticipation of cholera. This behavior prior to a widespread outbreak underscores the agency of people in responding to potential exposure risk. Citizens across the world were not waiting for a government to tell them what to do. Instead, they were responding to the uncertainty that they perceived in their environment. They saw the pandemic approaching and responded by stockpiling groceries and curtailing their exposure risk. Others were only able to respond to the extent that their financial circumstances would allow.

Stockpiling groceries depends on the financial means and transportation options to do so. Pamela Brown, a retired courtroom clerk in North Carolina, told the *Washington Post*, "Of course I would've like to stock up on groceries sooner, but I'm only getting checks once a month. Once that one's gone, I'm broke until the next one comes."[39]

People who live paycheck to paycheck could not afford to stock up on groceries to wait out the pandemic. Another North Carolina resident noted that without a car "it's hard to even get to the store."[40] Without private transportation, stockpiling groceries is even more difficult. One needs to make more trips using public transit or risk a non-socially distanced ride with a friend. Many also did not have space to store canned goods and pasta in bulk. Most inwardly dense housing does not have large pantries or basements to store such goods.

Perhaps even worse, for the people who were not able to stock up early, an arrival to the grocery store left them staring at empty shelves. Sixty-year-old Sandra Lotz, a former medical transcriptionist from the Chicago suburbs, had to stop working due to cancer. After retirement her reduced income left her to rely on food banks that were frequently without food early in the pandemic. Without food and without a vehicle to aid her trips to the store, she told the *Washington Post* that she "went to the supermarket with $2, hoping to pick up a loaf of bread or a box of pasta for a few days' worth of meals. . . . 'It was like the apocalypse was coming . . . I needed cheap bread . . . and all they had was $4 and $5 loaves of Pepperidge Farm. If coronavirus doesn't get us, starvation will.'"[41]

When the pandemic did arrive, people responded even more strongly. Overall, residents of Europe and North America spent less time outside their homes in all facets of life in late March and early April 2020. This was particularly noticeable in the drops of time spent in retail stores, public transit centers, and places of employment. In the United States, time spent in all of these categories decreased to a range between 40 to 50 percent below normal levels by mid-April. The response in the United Kingdom was even stronger. Time spent in all of these locations decreased to levels 65 to 75 percent below normal in the United Kingdom.

People had stocked up on groceries and other essentials. Those who could do so were working from home or had fled to environments they considered to be safer. Many governments had placed stay-at-home orders or equivalent mandates across their jurisdictions. Restaurants, gyms, and many other non-essential businesses were shuttered. By law and by choice, people across the world were not leaving home unless they had to do so. They had prepared for the pandemic tsunami and sat waiting for it to recede.

It did not take long before things began to change once US President Donald Trump vocalized his eagerness for states to begin relaxing restrictions. Like the English in colonial times, he saw too much weight being placed on the public health side of the scale and not enough on the commercial side. One might say that President Trump saw COVID-19 in much the same way as some English saw cholera in the nineteenth century, "a humbug got up for the destruction of commerce."[42] On March 23, 2020, Trump stated, "Our country wasn't built to be shut down. America will, again, and soon, be open for business. Very soon. A lot sooner than three or four months that somebody was suggesting. Lot sooner. We cannot let the cure be worse than the problem itself."[43] He saw the upcoming April 12 Easter holiday as a potential inflection point for the country.

Likely due to his comments, along with the general restlessness and feelings of isolation, people's mobility across the nation began to rebound the week after Easter. By early June, the time spent in grocery stores was back to near prepandemic levels before slightly receding again in July when the next wave of the pandemic arrived. Other facets of life bounced back to a lesser degree. Time spent in public transit stations increased somewhat but still remained far below normal levels.

This was the time period when feelings and actions began to diverge and polarize across the United States. Those hit the hardest in terms of economics, such as small business owners and workers who had lost jobs, were ready to loosen restrictions on movement and behavior. They wanted their earnings and jobs back. Those facing larger exposure risk wanted business activity to remain muted. Opinions on the topic were dictated partly by politics and partly by economic necessity.

In late March 2020, Mercedes Addington lost her job working for a trucking parts and supply company. Even though the company was considered an essential service, the Kansas City, Kansas–based company laid off most of its employees due to the pandemic. Ms. Addington told the *Washington Post*, "I am very frustrated and scared. I have bills to pay soon. . . . If I don't risk it and go back to work somewhere, I'm not sure that I'll still have a home to come back to."[44] Economic necessity of people across the world dictated choices that had to be made about confronting the risks of the pandemic.

In the United States, all major cities hit low points in mobility in the early to mid-April timeframe and then returned to more normal behavior as the summer approached. However, the magnitudes of these decreases and the following increases were very different. Major cities that were hurt the most in the early wave of the pandemic had larger decreases in mobility than areas hurt less. People in New York City and New Orleans both decreased time spent in retail establishments by more than 70 percent. Southwestern cities such as Houston and Phoenix, with their smaller caseloads in spring of 2020, bottomed out at levels only 40 percent below normal. They quickly bounced back toward normal behavior. They would pay with their health for doing so.

These higher levels of time spent in retail stores, restaurants, and other congested spaces during the early summer fueled another wave of the pandemic. Cities that maintained large decreases in mobility had fewer new cases per capita on average than those that returned to normal more quickly. On average, a 10 percent reduction in mobility within a metro area was associated with 18 percent fewer cases per capita over the months from July to October 2020. For example, New York City residents continued to limit mobility and had an increase of just under 500 cases per 100,000 residents between July and October. Miami went back to normal more quickly and suffered an increase in cases per capita that was about ten times higher than NYC during this same time. Miami had the largest per capita increase in cases of any metropolitan area of the country during this period. Other studies of United States cities found similar relationships between mobility and the spread of COVID-19.[45]

Part of these increases resulted from the expected movement of the pandemic from early cities toward more interior parts of the country that had not yet been visited by the virus. Because we were unable to stop the pandemic when it first invaded port cities in March and April 2020, it would eventually move inward to the heart of the country. Other parts of the summer spread were due to changes in behavior. In Miami, a medical resident told *NBC News* that he "continued to socialize and attend parties until he fell ill."[46] He admitted that he should have known better, but he felt "invincible" as a healthy twenty-seven-year-old.

He was not alone. Similar stories were reported across the country. Tony Green, a resident of Dallas, Texas, initially referred to the pandemic as a "scamdemic." Frustrated with the limits placed on social gatherings, he hosted a small family gathering in June. "We just felt the worst was behind the country because everything was easy, things were re-opening and none of us were experiencing any symptoms," Green told *NBC News*. He and his partner did not wear masks at the gathering and neither did their parents.[47] Within days, fourteen members of his and his partner's family were suffering from COVID-19. His partner's grand-mother would die. Green was hospitalized along with his father-in-law. To Green's credit he wrote a letter to the *Dallas Voice* describing what had happened and encouraging skeptics to take the pandemic more seriously.[48] These episodes were not isolated. As mobility picked up in parts of the country, COVID-19 cases and deaths followed.

While patterns of mobility returned to normal, they didn't match pre-pandemic levels. Part of the continued decrease in mobility occurred because of changes in the work experience of adults in 2020 and beyond. Unemployment soared in the early months of the pandemic. Many who retained their jobs were able to work from home. Researchers at the University of Birmingham and University of Kent found that four out of five workers in the United Kingdom worked from home during the spring pandemic wave. This was up from about one out of three workers prior to the pandemic.[49]

Similar patterns were found in the United States where about 70 percent of employed adults worked from home in October 2020. Prior to the pandemic only 20 percent of employed United States adults worked from home. As in the times of the bubonic plague, those with the opportunity to isolate did so.

This work-from-home experience was not shared equally across all spectrums of the workforce. In the United States, 76 percent of lower income workers reported that their jobs could not be done from home.[50] This disparity extended to those with lower levels of education.[51] This pattern of socio-economic status and ability to work from home was replicated in the United Kingdom. Neighborhoods that had the highest Index of Multiple Deprivation (a measure associated with poverty that considers income, employment, education, health, crimes, barriers to housing, and living environment) had fewer than 25 percent of residents with the ability to work from home.[52]

This change in behavior not only had an effect on working life, but it also affected other aspects of the economy. Areas of London with the largest percentage of workers who vacated offices to work from home had the largest drops in retail and hospitality activity. The City of London (which houses London's financial district) and neighborhoods like Westminster (home to Parliament) and Camden had between 60 to 80 percent lower rates of retail and hospitality activity in the summer during the stay-at-home orders. With many workers staying closer to home, they simply weren't buying the same number of lunches, cups of coffee, and other day-to-day items traditionally purchased during work breaks and commutes. Residential areas outside of these commercial districts such as Waltham, Enfield, and Redbridge had decreases only about 20 percent below normal.[53]

This decrease in workplace activity greatly changed commuting patterns too. Public transit ridership was lower by over 60 percent across the United States in fall of 2020 compared to the year prior.[54] The effect on car commutes was somewhat more complicated. Fewer commuters took to the road, and those who remained enjoyed less stressful and faster commutes.[55] At the same time that the streets emptied, some individuals shifted toward commuting by car and away from public transit for reasons of safety. The transition to automobiles for this segment of the commuting population drove the price of used cars up by 9 percent.[56]

Not everyone could afford an automobile. The poorest one-fifth of American households spend 36 percent of their budgets on transportation; most people with these stringent budget constraints could not afford a car to avoid public transit and exposure risk.[57] This left many workers no choice but to ride to work by bus and train and they did so with trepidation.

A Los Angeles resident reported to the *Associated Press*, "I get on the bus, I just pray."[58] Another rider from the Bronx notes, "It's stressful in the sense that you don't know who's going to be next to you. I try to keep my distance, and keep my mask on at all times. There's nothing else I can do. I just hope I don't get sick."[59]

During the early pandemic, riders like these boarded buses that were still crowded and congested. They were forced into proximity with some riders who ignored mask mandates. In parts of the United States and in the United Kingdom it was common to see masks not fully covering faces and creeping below the nose. Social distancing guidelines of 6 feet (2 meters) were frequently ignored. When London loosened mobility restrictions in May 2020, one rider noted, "people were sitting close together on the Jubilee line and others were having to stand. There was no two-metre spacing."[60] Confrontations were common between mask wearers and those refusing to wear them.

Congestion and commuting times became even more problematic as transit authorities cut back on services due to a lack of funding from reduced revenues that forced staff layoffs. As an example, Atlanta cut 69 of their 110 bus routes in April.[61] Fewer remaining routes resulted in longer commuting times on average and greater levels of mixing across riders from different neighborhoods on the routes that remained. These newly combined routes created new social bridges between neighborhoods that were normally separated and increased the chance that local outbreaks would spread to new areas.

As decreased routes became more common, riders reported waiting as buses that had reached capacity passed them by. This caused unexpected commuting delays. When a bus did arrive, cautious riders boarded, noting who was wearing a mask and the location of the most socially distant seat. As one frequent rider of the usually congested 729 Rapid Los Angeles Metro bus stated to *Los Angeles Magazine*, "We're just communicating with our eyes. . . . Right now, the eyes are saying, 'Please don't sit next to me.'"[62]

At the same time that these public transit riders were facing crowding and congestion on buses, those able to flee cities or isolate at home were safer. Their neighborhoods had de-densified. Even those who did not flee affluent neighborhoods found that their streets and stores had emptied. Stay-at-home orders and non-essential business closures were not meant to provide an advantage for the most affluent, but they did. Even though the affluent leaving cities reduced exposure risk for everyone by reducing overall density, the effects were not equal. The poor were left to face the brunt of the pandemic while still crowded together in inwardly dense environments that had not changed. The next challenge they faced would be financial.

Imagine for a moment that your household income doubled. How would you use this extra money? A lavish vacation? A new automobile? A larger house? Extra savings for college? The answer is different for everyone. Now imagine that your answer was more peanut butter and bread. This is the reality for some.

The median household income for a family in the United States is a little over $60,000 per year. In the United Kingdom it is slightly under £30,000. Most families with income near these levels do not struggle to afford food or shelter, but also do not live an extravagant lifestyle. If the income of a family like this were to suddenly double, they likely would not double their spending on food cooked within their home. Instead, they might double their spending on any or several of the other options listed above.

This distinction defines what economists call necessities and luxuries. Necessities are goods whose consumption increases by a small percentage when income rises and luxuries are goods whose consumption increases by a large percentage when income rises. In the typical median-income family in an affluent country such as the United States or the United Kingdom, food cooked within the home is a necessity. Items like restaurant meals, vacations, and other more extravagant purchases are luxuries.

Sandra Lotz only had $2 to spend in the supermarket and hoped to buy some bread or pasta. If she had $4 instead of $2 in her budget that day, it is hard to imagine that she would have spent that money on anything but food. Extra money wasn't going to be used on a vacation nor on a lavish meal at a restaurant. It would have been used to buy the $4 Pepperidge Farm bread that was her only option on the grocery store shelf. For Ms. Lotz, even things that many families would consider a necessity were a luxury. Without a large increase of income, she could not even consider purchasing a $4 loaf of bread. That expensive loaf was an extravagant luxury to her—one that, in this case, she could not afford. If her income doubled, she still could not have afforded a vehicle so that she could avoid congested public transportation. For her, a car was a luxury far beyond her means. A move to a $750,000 beach-front safehouse was impossible even if it could save her from a deadly infectious disease.

We can also apply this concept of luxuries and necessities to changes in the patterns of movement that occur

during pandemics. In the United States, residents of affluent counties had larger decreases in mobility than residents
of impoverished counties.[63] Affluent counties had a 5 to
16 percent larger decrease of time spent in grocery stores,
retail establishments, public transit stations, and time spent
in the workplace. These people decreased their time in places
that created exposure risk far more than residents of poorer
counties. People living in more affluent areas were able to
better shelter themselves from exposure risk. For the wealthy
decreased exposure risk was a luxury that they were able to
afford that the poor could not.

Those of lower socioeconomic classes were consistently confronted with more exposure risk because of their
economic circumstance. They could not afford to decrease
their time spent shopping, in public transit, or outside the
home to the same degree as those who were more affluent.
Further, because everyone around them faced more exposure risk, this increased their exposure risk all the more.

Exposure risk is shared. If everyone around me acts less
safely they create more exposure risk for themselves. They
are more likely to be infected. Because they are more likely
to be infected, I too face more exposure risk from them. In
addition, these communities that couldn't decrease exposure
risk also contained more inward density. Exposure risk was
being added to areas that were already the riskiest.

Let's contrast the work-from-home experience with one
of the more unsafe and controversial professions during the
early pandemic—meat processing. Over a period of forty
days approximately one out of four workers at a Smithfield
meat processing plant in South Dakota tested positive for
coronavirus. This wasn't a small plant where a handful of
infected workers skewed a statistical result. At Smithfield,
over 900 workers were infected in a plant that employed
about 3,600 people.[64]

To put this in perspective, the states that had the worst number of coronavirus cases per capita within the United States had less than 15 percent of their population test positive in one *year*. This meat processing plant had 25 percent of their workforce test positive in just over one *month*!

How did this happen? It was a mixture of poor working conditions and a corporation providing misaligned economic incentives.

Many of the workers on the meat processing line work shoulder to shoulder. Wielding large knives with skill, the workers carve cuts of meat by hand. This assembly line was part of the economic efficiency that was dangerous during the pandemic. As one can imagine, it was not the most hygienic of jobs. Cutting oneself was not an uncommon occurrence. The workers on the processing line stand so close together that sometimes one is even cut by a neighbor.[65] This is not a description out of Upton Sinclair's *The Jungle* circa 1906. This is present-day, mainstream, meat processing in the United States in 2020. These close working conditions were primed for the spread of infectious disease. It was everything COVID-19 could want—unsanitary and inwardly dense.

As one might expect, the workers who performed these jobs were not wealthy. Many were recent immigrants. Some were refugees. It was estimated that eighty different languages were spoken in this Smithfield plant.[66] These workers earned about $15 per hour. It was a job that paid relatively well but it wasn't safe in normal times and became even less safe when COVID-19 arrived.

Once outbreaks occurred in parts of the United States, Smithfield became concerned that workers would take days off instead of facing exposure risk on the cut floor. The workers themselves were on edge. One worker at Smithfield told BBC, "I have a lot of bills. My baby's coming soon—I have to work."[67] Workers like this faced crucial decisions between food and health, earnings and safety.

Smithfield tried to tip the balance in favor of finances. In early April, they offered their plant workers a $500 bonus. It was termed a "responsibility bonus" in a video featuring the company CEO, Kevin Sullivan. To earn the bonus, workers had to attend every single scheduled shift during the month of April 2020.[68] When the bonus plan was announced there were already known cases in Smithfield plants. The fact that Smithfield called it a responsibility bonus dripped with irony. Worker responsibility to the company and to the food security of the nation was at the forefront of the message. There was no mention of company responsibility to the workers. At a time when we should have provided targeted financial security to workers facing the most danger and exposure risk, Smithfield was doing the opposite. They were providing financial incentives to encourage high-risk workers to take on even more exposure risk.

To these employees, $500 was not a trivial amount. For most it amounted to the pay for one week of work. Forgoing this bonus was a luxury that many could not afford. They could not afford to take time off as it was. The quandary stared them in the face. The only way to gain this bonus was to put their lives at risk. The incentives worked against safety. All it took was one ill person, who hoped to avoid losing the bonus, to arrive in the workplace. That was all that was needed to provide the spark and set the fire.

The obvious result occurred. Many workers showed up every day whether they felt well or not. Once the virus entered the packed and inwardly dense factory, it spread like wildfire. At the height of the outbreak in the factory, employees at the Smithfield plant in Sioux Falls and people connected to them accounted for half of the coronavirus cases in the entire state of South Dakota. Smithfield eventually closed some of its factories temporarily. They implemented some nominal safety providing improvements once they reopened. They also agreed to pay workers the bonus if they missed shifts because of a positive test for coronavirus, or if they were forced to quarantine because of exposure. It was too little too late. The damage was already done. Nine hundred workers were infected, 25 percent of the plant, in only forty days.

One can better understand the difficult choices these workers faced if we consider other aspects of the economy at the same time. The workers were forced to choose between food and shelter or health. They couldn't stay home and still pay rent and buy food. Employment rates were plunging throughout the country. There were no other jobs to be had if they quit working at Smithfield. Unemployment benefits would not be paid to them if they voluntarily chose to stay home. The essence of their choice was exposure to the pandemic or financial ruin.

To make matters worse, because of supply disruptions, such as the closure of meat processing plants like Smithfield, and the lack of available items due to the forementioned stockpiling, food prices grew at rapid rates. In the month of April 2020 alone, food prices increased by 2.6 percent in the United States. At the time, this was the largest one-month increase in food prices since the 1974 OPEC oil crisis.[69] By August the price of beef was 20 percent greater than when the pandemic began and eggs, poultry, and pork were all at least 8 percent higher in price.[70]

Overall, the consumer food price index grew by 3.9 percent across the United States in 2020. This was over twice the increase for 2019 and the largest one-year increase since 2011.[71] To put this in a broader context, the average American household spends just under 10 percent of before-tax income on food. So the median household with a $60,0000 income spends about $6,000 per year on food. An increase of 3.9 percent in food prices means that the median family would spend an extra $240 per year on food because of inflation (assuming that they bought the same items after inflation).

A family in the lowest 20 percent of income earners in the United States spends about 30 percent of income on food. The twentieth percentile is a little less than $20,000 per year. So, these families spend $6,000 per year on food just like the median-income family. They also experience the same $240 increase. Note that the amount of money spent on food indicates that it is a necessity. A family earning $20,000 spends about the same amount of money on food as a family earning $60,000. The problem for the poorer family is that this extra $240 is over 1 percent of their before-tax income for the year. At the Smithfield plant it is the equivalent of about two days' wages. It was also about half of the bonus that Smithfield offered workers. This made the need to attain that bonus even more necessary.

The family making $60,000 per year felt the increase in food prices far less than the financially poor family. This occurred for two reasons: First, the increase is a smaller part of their budget overall. Second, because the $60,000 family can consume more luxuries in normal times, they can more easily cut back on those luxuries in more difficult times. The wealthier family can give up a weekend vacation or a few restaurant meals and recover the $240. The poorer family is consuming primarily food, shelter, and transportation. There is no place to find an extra $240 to spend on food without giving up a different necessity. This is the dilemma that meat processing workers and other workers like them faced. It was a choice of giving up necessities while they also faced increasing exposure to the pandemic.

Some lower-income workers were lucky and found alternatives to balance out the dilemma. One Costco shopper told the *Washington Post* that his six-week grocery shopping bill increased from $600 to over $1,000. Coupled with the loss of a job, the increase in grocery prices was so extreme that he and his family had to move into his in-laws' home.[72] This person was able to use the shelter at a relative's home to compensate for the necessity that he could no longer afford—food. Yet even though this person was lucky enough to find shelter, he and his extended family created a new multigenerational home. The move created more bridges and more exposure risk for the family and for the in-laws. What was gained in terms of finance was lost in terms of safety.

Even further down the line of income distribution, in 2020, forty-four million Americans received support for food purchases through the Supplemental Nutrition Assistance Program (SNAP), sometimes referred to as food stamps. This was an increase from thirty-six million in 2019. Despite the early-pandemic increase in buying groceries online, 15 states did not allow SNAP recipients the ability to use benefits for online purchases. In these states, grocery delivery payment with SNAP funds was not an option in any circumstance. Even in states where SNAP benefits could be used for online purchases, many major grocery delivery services were not set up to accept SNAP payments online. In these situations, SNAP recipients had no choice but to resort to less safe means to put food on the table. They had to shop in person.

The changes in mobility patterns over the course of the early pandemic revealed how different the circumstances were for different groups within our society. People at the lower end of income distribution faced constraints that were not present for the more affluent. These additional constraints depended upon the economic resources at one's disposal, such as the type of job they held, the amount of money in their bank account, and even their budget for groceries that increased in price each week. These additional constraints forced the most vulnerable members of our society into greater exposure risk throughout the pandemic.

Financial means have provided safety during pandemics throughout history. Luxuries of safety available to the rich are frequently unavailable to the poor. Returning to Philadelphia in 1793 makes this all the more clear.

Dr. Benjamin Rush was a physician by training who signed the United States Declaration of Independence. Enlightened for his time, he was a staunch abolitionist and critic of capital punishment. He promoted the founding of the Young Ladies' Academy of Philadelphia, which was the first chartered institute of higher education for women in the United States. He founded Dickinson College in 1783.[73] It was one decade later that he played an instrumental role in Philadelphia's yellow fever epidemic that brought together his profession of medicine and his abolitionist beliefs.

When one-third of the city's population fled at the start of the outbreak, including most affluent members of society and most physicians, Rush stayed behind. He was the most prominent physician in the city to treat the ill. He was infected but survived. Unfortunately, his sister wasn't as lucky and died as a victim of the epidemic.[74]

As infections escalated in late summer and early fall of 1793, care for the sick became an immense burden for those who remained in the city. Those who fell ill had few options for care. Nurses were in short supply. Many had already left the city and others who remained behind refused to treat the ill out of concern for personal safety. Gravediggers and transporters existed only in limited supply. Most people simply saw the risks of performing these tasks to be too great, despite a lack of other employment opportunities during the epidemic.

To meet this lack of labor supply, Rush and other city leaders turned to the community of free Black citizens. As an abolitionist, Rush promoted the formation of separate Black churches in years prior to the epidemic. When the epidemic came to be too dire, Rush approached two local Black ministers, Richard Allen and Absalom Jones, to encourage them to employ members of Philadelphia's Black population to assist the sick and to bury bodies.[75]

Rush's plea included a claim that Black citizens were immune from infection. Perhaps this was from confusion over the observation of Black men and women who arrived in Philadelphia with some immunity from time in the West Indies, an area consistently afflicted with yellow fever. Or, perhaps, it was a convenient excuse to encourage the population to take on essential work in order to keep the city functioning.

As further inducement, Rush suggested the possibility that Black assistance in a time of need may stem some of the racism that existed within the city and perhaps garner favor for the Black churches, whose presence within the city was consistently opposed by white residents. Whatever the reason, Rush's dubious promises and pleas proved convincing. Allen and Jones encouraged their congregation to take on tasks that many white laborers would not.

At the height of the pandemic, Rush wrote to his wife Julia, "Parents desert their children as soon as they are infected, and in every room you enter you see no person but a solitary black man or woman near the sick."[76] Following the epidemic, Allen and Jones published a pamphlet that detailed the work of the Black community.[77] The pamphlet was written in response to accusations made by a prominent local writer and publisher, Mathew Carey, who claimed that Black caregivers stole from the sick and dying. Allen and Jones described work taken on by the Black population that included bloodletting, digging graves, and transporting dead bodies.

Within the pamphlet there are heartbreaking descriptions of experiences: a white woman was thrust into the street by her husband who was afraid to be infected by her; a white man threatened to murder an infected white woman if she did not die by morning—she perished in the night so it is unknown whether the threat would have been carried out. Perhaps most harrowing:

> A woman died, we were sent for to bury her, on our going into the house and taking the coffin in, a dear little innocent accosted us, with, mamma is asleep, don't wake her; but when she saw us put her in a coffin the distress of the child was so great, that it almost overcame us; when she demanded why we put her mamma in the box?[78]

This was the circumstance that faced the Black community doing the work that few would consider. In the end, and contrary to Rush's claims, they were not immune. Allen and Jones note, "In 1792, there were 67 of our colour buried, and in 1793, it amounted to 305; . . . was not this in a great degree the effects of the services of the unjustly vilified black people?"[79] The census of 1790 listed only 1,630 Black residents of Philadelphia.[80] If this is a reasonable approximation of the Black population three years later, slightly more than one in six Black Philadelphians died in the 1793 yellow fever epidemic, many of whom performed essential tasks that white residents would not. They maintained the society that most fled in fear.

The experience of the Black population in Philadelphia during the 1793 epidemic foreshadowed the experience that Black essential and key workers would face when the COVID-19 pandemic arrived in 2020. While many of these workers were employed in the medical profession, others faced similar risks, but in much lower-profile jobs.

Early in the COVID-19 pandemic transit workers, such as bus drivers in cities or ticket takers on New York City commuter trains, faced continual exposure risk. Further, when considering their role within the network of potential infections, these types of workers were both hubs and bridges. They came into contact with large numbers of people every day. The people they met originated their daily commutes from a wide variety of places. If a cluster of infections broke out anywhere within their city, it was likely to enter a public transit route, and once there it could spread to any neighborhood within the city in only a few subsequent infections. Transit workers sat at the nexus of these infections as they spread throughout the city.

In the early days of the COVID-19 pandemic in the United Kingdom and the United States, these types of workers faced higher rates of infection and death. Researchers at University College London found that the rate of death due to COVID-19 was almost three times higher for men who were London bus drivers than for men of similar age across England and Wales. These bus drivers were also more often members of Black, Asian, and minority ethnic (BAME) groups.[81]

The story was similar in the United States. In the first six weeks of the pandemic in New York City, over 2,500 Metropolitan Transit Authority (MTA) workers had been infected and 68 had died. Another 4,000 had been quarantined due to exposure.[82]

These grim population statistics were met with even more grim personal tales. In March 2020, Jason Hargrove, a bus driver in Detroit, posted a video protesting the recklessness of a woman who was coughing on his bus "without covering her mouth." Within two weeks, Mr. Hargrove had died from COVID-19.[83] Perhaps the most egregious incident occurred in London when two transit workers were spat upon at Victoria Station by a man who claimed to have been infected with coronavirus. Two weeks later Belly Mujinga, one of these two transit workers and the mother of an eleven-year-old girl, died from the disease.[84]

The disproportionate effects on essential and key workers extended beyond transportation. A study of deaths in California documented that line cooks in restaurants had the largest increase in mortality rate during the early weeks of the pandemic. People in this profession died at rates 60 percent greater than normal.[85] The list of workers who were most at risk was littered with people who held low-paying jobs, many of which involved essential tasks. Agricultural workers, construction laborers, sewing machine operators, maintenance workers, maids and cleaners, and security guards all died at rates at least 30 percent above normal.[86] More general categories of essential workers also had high rates of mortality: food and agricultural workers died at rates 39 percent above normal. Transportation and logistics workers died at rates 28 percent above normal. Health and emergency workers died at rates 19 percent above normal. All of these rates compare to non-essential workers with rates 11 percent above normal.[87] Not surprisingly, the rates for people of color within these sub-groups was often even higher. Just like in centuries before, essential tasks performed by people of color placed these citizens on the front lines of the pandemic.

Repeatedly we see the cost of a pandemic to society paid by those in lower income groups. We see that we all pay either with our wealth or with our health. Either you can afford plague insurance, or you can't. Some aspects of this insurance change over time and others don't. Throughout history, the course of pandemics was determined by the movement and the behavior of people as much as by medicine and biology. The pattern repeated again when the COVID-19 pandemic arrived.

When we consider the varied circumstances across the economic spectrum and the choices and constraints that people have faced, we should not be surprised that the COVID-19 pandemic has not been a great equalizer. Pandemics have never been great equalizers. The idea of the great equalizer was a fallacy from the beginning. It was a fallacy during the Black Death and it is a fallacy today. It will be so again in the future unless we change our institutions and the circumstances of the poor and the vulnerable. While viruses and bacteria don't discriminate—economic circumstance does. As much as medicine and science, it determines who lives and who dies when we face pandemics.

After the experiences of 2020, people of the twenty-first century now understand better.

We can vividly imagine the cries to flee cities during the bubonic plague in Europe or during a yellow fever epidemic in Philadelphia. We can envision the wealthy buying Bills of Mortality and reading them, ever on edge, ready to escape should numbers begin to rise in a nearby parish. At the same time, we can imagine children in poverty-stricken slums watching the exodus with wonder as the carts and wheelbarrows roll out of the city, leaving them behind. And we can imagine the little girl watching the strange men entering her home, and leaving with her mamma in a box.

They, without the means to escape, pay their debt to the pandemic, not with money, but with their health and with their lives.

Chapter 6

BELOW THE MARGIN

For twenty years Maria Hernandez worked for Ralphs grocery, a large chain in Los Angeles. Bouncing between stores over her career, she worked the night shift stocking shelves and cleaning. Shortly after a busy holiday shopping period in 2020 she left work early. Exhausted, she slept all day. A positive test confirmed her fear. She was suffering from COVID-19. She can't pinpoint with certainty when she was infected nor who infected her. However, she suspects that the infection happened at work.

Ms. Hernandez wrote about her experience in the *Los Angeles Times*.[1] She told of a rushed trip to the emergency room with a fever and difficulty breathing. She lived in a multigenerational home that she shared with her husband, four daughters, a granddaughter, and her eighty-five-year-old mother. She spent seven weeks isolated in a bedroom of her home. Throughout this time, her long-held daily ritual of breakfast with her mother was replaced by a greeting of "good morning" passed through a window. For seven weeks she didn't hug her children out of fear that she would infect them.

After her recovery, she was set to return to work. She arrived for her first shift and stood outside the store for five minutes. Did she really want to go back? Eventually she eased inside. She encountered a world that seemed uncaring, from the customers to the management. Policies were in place to maintain social distancing and mask wearing. Yet the policies were only as good their enforcement. Rules did no good when not followed in practice. The stores were too crowded. Customers wore their masks as "chin straps." Managers tasked with enforcing the rules were not always available on the late-night shifts when she worked. Ralphs didn't hire enough workers to maintain the rules. When the managers were there and tried to enforce policies, some customers accosted them. One was struck by a shopping cart. Ms. Hernandez was cursed at when she asked a customer to wear a mask.

Her article ends with a plea to her employer to take a leadership role in curbing the pandemic. Ralphs is owned by Kroger, which is second only to Walmart on the list of largest grocers in the United States. Ms. Hernandez believed her large corporate employer, with its vast resources, could do more than turn a blind eye after stating vacuous policies that had little effect. She wanted executives to listen to their workers and to recognize their plight. She says in the end, "By including its enormous workforce, Kroger could do a better job of protecting the lives of its employees and customers—and help stop the spread of this deadly virus."[2]

Many people across the globe were placed in circumstances similar to Ms. Hernandez during the COVID-19 pandemic. Essential workers often faced indifferent customers and a distant corporate governance structure. They felt abandoned and unheard. Many of the essential jobs that continued throughout the pandemic were front-facing roles that paid low wages. These workers faced an economic and health dilemma. With modest earnings and savings and reduced opportunity for other work in a crashing economy, they had nowhere to turn. They faced a choice between a job with significant exposure risk or forgoing work and having no money to buy food and pay bills. Many felt that their corporate employers didn't do enough to protect them. With little economic opportunity elsewhere, the workers had little choice but to don a mask and hope for the best. Many who faced this tension between finance and health were the economically disadvantaged and vulnerable members of society.

These workers faced traditional exposure that risked their health within the pandemic. Many also were concerned about the possibility of financial ruin or hunger. These additional types of exposure lived alongside exposure to the virus and were most prominent for the working poor of the country.

People of color and women are over-represented in what have come to be termed frontline and essential workers.[3] Not only did these workers face more exposure risk, but they also had less choice to avoid the pandemic. Many essential occupations are low paying.[4] They include store and grocery clerks, bus and transport drivers, cashiers, and warehouse packing and shipping workers, among many others. Jobs such as these require a physical presence in the workplace. Many of these jobs do not provide health care benefits or paid sick leave. Many of these jobs create bridges between different groups in society and thereby increase exposure risk for these workers and the public all the more.

At the same time that these essential workers faced exposure to the virus, many other service sector jobs disappeared. Leading up to the pandemic, unemployment rates in the United States were at a fifty-year low after steadily decreasing during the Obama and Trump presidencies. In late March 2020, the economic world changed. Initial unemployment claims exploded to over 6.8 million, *10 times* greater than at the height of the Great Recession in 2009 and almost 10 times greater than the largest total on record.[5] To economists, this number was unthinkable.

These job losses were not distributed uniformly across the economy. Three out of eight workers in the bottom quartile of income earners (those below about $27,000) lost their jobs during March and April 2020. These lost jobs did not return quickly. Even as late as August 1, 2021, this group had employment rates that were still 25 percent lower than levels in January 2020.[6] Economic opportunity had fully stalled for this group, which lost over eight million jobs during 2020.[7]

The top quartile of workers (those with income greater than $60,000) also struggled, though they fared much better than the bottom quartile. One out of eight of these workers lost their job at the start of the pandemic. However, this group bounced back more quickly. By August 1, 2021, this group had employment rates that were greater than on January 1, 2020. In total they *gained*, not lost, nearly one million jobs during 2020.[8]

There was a racial and ethnic component within these numbers as well.[9] Black and Latinx workers more often became unemployed in the early months of the pandemic and their jobs returned more slowly. Further, women, younger workers, and workers with lower levels of education across all ethnic and racial groups experienced worse labor market circumstances.[10]

Job loss was especially difficult for single-income families. Erin Bailey, a single mother with four children from Greenacres, Florida, lost her lawn care business due to a lack of customers when the pandemic began. She was crestfallen. She told CNN, "I was so excited to finally have my own business and it was going so well, then all of a sudden everything just stopped. I was so happy and proud, and now I feel like a failure."[11] With her young children staying at home during the pandemic school closures, she couldn't leave her home to search for work. Without other options, she and her children turned to an old-school approach to making money—a family lemonade stand. Standing on their sidewalk in the hot sun, they typically earned about $30 per day. Ms. Bailey reported, "We use the lemonade stand money to stock up, but there were days when I would barely eat in case one of them gets hungry later. It's just a fear I can't make go away."[12] Ms. Bailey fell behind on rent and other bills. Her children offered to help by contributing their share of lemonade proceeds to pay family bills. Imagine for a moment the desperation felt by a mother who could only feed her children and pay rent and bills through lemonade stand revenues. For families like this, food security became the primary issue in their lives.

Food insecurity is measured through a household's physical and economic access to food and considers levels of food nutrition as well. Families with food insecurity face "limited or uncertain availability of nutritionally adequate and safe foods or limited or uncertain ability to acquire acceptable foods in socially acceptable ways."[13] Overall, 23 percent of United States households and 30 percent of households with children experienced food insecurity in the early months of the pandemic. This was an increase from a projection of 8.5 percent prior to the onset of the pandemic.[14] Black and Latinx households experienced much higher rates of food insecurity than average. For households with children, 41 percent of Black households and 36 percent of Latinx households experienced food insecurity once the pandemic began.[15]

Kimi Ceridon wrote about her experience growing up with food insecurity for *Bon Appetit*.[16] She recounted her memories of standing in line at the grocery store checkout. She watched her mother handling "coupons like a blackjack dealer" as the items from the shopping cart were rung up. With a necessity of staying within the budget, her mother had calculated the total bill prior to checkout in a small notebook that she carried about the store. Still, "she always loaded the conveyor belt with the most essential items first." These included, "sandwich fixings, eggs, milk, log-shaped rolls of fatty ground beef, canned tuna, canned and frozen vegetables, soups, and pasta. If the budget allowed, she'd add chicken, fresh fruit, snacks . . ."[17] These last items were luxuries in her family—they couldn't afford them every week. Her mother worked full time as an airline reservation agent. Her father ran a janitorial franchise. They had consistent full-time work, but the budget was always tight. "Mom preferred to divvy our food among plates rather than watch my brother, my sister, and I argue over who got more. Mom got what was left . . ."[18] As a child Ms. Ceridon didn't always leave dinner without hunger. Her "stomach seemed to always volley between growling for more and overflowing."[19]

Despite living a more comfortable financial life as an adult after attaining a master's degree in engineering, Ms. Ceridon still carries the emotions of her childhood food insecurity with her. She writes, "Shared appetizer platters beckon me like a siren: 'Eat me before someone else does.' I go bonkers over food waste, wanting to save it from the trash by eating it."[20] To this day, the sight of canned green peas brings her to audibly mutter, "I hate green peas."[21]

As job losses mounted in the pandemic, so too did food insecurity. The non-profit group Feeding South Florida helped to combat food insecurity. Prior to the pandemic, they provided sixty million pounds of food per year to families throughout southern Florida. From March to June 2020, they matched this yearly total in only four months. In their first food distribution event in Miami after the pandemic began, they expected to serve 500 to 700 families. Instead, three thousand families arrived seeking food. They ran out of food at most food distribution events.[22] In

April a line of cars stretched for over 1.5 miles at one of their distribution centers that provides 2.5 million meals per week.[23]

Lauren Bell, a resident of this southern Florida area in 2020, worked in data entry before losing her job early in the pandemic. As a single mother of two girls under the age of two, when her steady job disappeared, she suddenly faced difficulties that she never expected. Meat and fish became unaffordable luxuries that were replaced with plain pasta from the local dollar store. There were days when she didn't have money for even these paltry meals to feed her children. Her children were too young to qualify for the Pandemic Electronic Benefit Transfer (P-EBT) program designed to replace food from free and reduced-price school lunches. At the worst of times, she had to resort to stealing food to feed her family. "There's been multiple times where I had to steal food, no matter how bad that sounds, just to make sure my kids can eat. Sometimes there's just nothing else I can do."[24] Three out of ten households with children confronted dilemmas of food insecurity early in the pandemic. Organizations like Feeding South Florida could not keep up with demand to help all of these families. People began lining up at 11 p.m. the night before distributions began in order to increase their chances of receiving food.[25]

With limited savings and minimal job opportunities once unemployed, low-wage workers felt less financially secure than ever before. Some lost jobs, while others had to take pay cuts or make do with reduced working hours, or both. This increased financial stress created emotional stress. Aaron Crawford, a thirty-seven-year-old Navy veteran, resided in Apple Valley, Minnesota. He searched for work early in the pandemic, but he couldn't find a job. His family's economic stress mounted. His wife, Sheyla, had her hours cut at the daycare center where she worked. The family was running out of food to feed their five- and ten-year-old boys. Mr. Crawford was uncomfortable seeking help. He told a reporter from the *Associated Press*, "I felt like I was a failure. It's this whole stigma . . . this mindset that you're this guy who can't provide for his family, that you're a deadbeat."[26] Sheyla insisted that they seek help from a local food bank, where they received boxes of fresh produce, dairy, deli meat, and enough food staples to fill two grocery carts.[27] While there Mr. Crawford met others like him, and he learned to see his situation differently: "It didn't make me a bad man or a terrible husband or father. On the contrary, I was actually doing something to make sure that my wife and kids had something to eat."[28] There were millions across the country that had to overcome these stigmas and seek help for the first time.

Overall, 25 percent of adults in the United States reported that they had "trouble paying bills."[29] This was particularly common for Black and Latinx individuals, with 43 and 37 percent of respondents affirming this difficulty. Another necessity, medical care, posed a problem, too. According to a Pew Research survey, 19 percent of lower income respondents had trouble paying for medical care. This compared to just 2 percent of upper income respondents.[30]

Due to the threat of extreme financial strain, many low-income workers could not afford to forgo an employment opportunity when other job prospects were virtually nonexistent. Many workers in 2020 had little choice but to face exposure—a story that had played out similarly a century earlier.

The 1918 influenza pandemic arrived in the midst of World War I. By the end of the pandemic fifty million people had died. This was more than double the number of people killed in the war and also more than the number of people killed or wounded combined. As influenza spread, factory workers and miners saw more and more of their coworkers become infected and die.

The war effort was in full force, and the government desperately needed workers to produce munitions and ships. Other forms of heavy industry needed for the war effort employed vast numbers of men and women. In 1918 coal production in the United States reached levels that, except for the years of World War II, would not be seen again until the 1970s.[31] Industry at home was vital to the war effort. In a 1918 article titled "Health at Home to Help the Army," Frank Stockbridge wrote, "It is just as much the Government's duty to keep the industrial army fit as it is to sustain the fighting forces in the field. It is just as much our war—this war on diseases that threaten our efficiency in the greater war on the Mad Dog of Europe—as is the conflict raging overseas."[32] The call to patriotism rang loud from shore to shore amongst the working women and men. This work often put them at great peril.

When recounting his research on the 1918 pandemic to *Smithsonian Magazine*, author of *The Great Influenza* John Barry wrote, "Shipbuilding workers throughout the Northeast [United States] were told they were as important to the war effort as soldiers at the front. Yet at the L. H. Shattuck Co. only 54 percent of its workers showed up; at the George A. Gilchrist yard only 45 percent did; at Freeport Shipbuilding only 43 percent; at Groton Iron Works, 41 percent."[33] Whether the absent workers were ill or afraid is not known; it was likely some of each.

Miners, too, heard the call to the domestic front. Yet like the shipbuilders, absences added up here, also. Mines were forced to close when pandemic infections and deaths became too large. Teamus Bartley was a coal miner in Kentucky during the 1918 pandemic. At the age of 95 he recounted his memories to the University of Kentucky Library Oral History Project.

> It was the saddest lookin' time then that ever you saw in your life. . . . That epidemic broke out and people went to dyin' and there just four or five dyin' every night dyin' right there in the camps, every night. . . . My brother and all his family took down with it. . . . I'd stay with my brother about three hours and do what I could to help 'em. And every one of them was in the bed and sometimes Doctor Preston would come while I was there. . . . And he said "I'm a tryin' to save their lives but I'm afraid I'm not going to." . . . Nearly every porch I'd look at . . . would have a casket box a sittin' on it. And men a diggin' graves just as hard as they could and the mines had to shut there wasn't nary a man, there wasn't a mine a runnin' a lump of coal or runnin' no work. Stayed that way for about six weeks.[34]

Across the country workers feared that influenza would invade their mine or factory. Residents felt similar fears in crowded cities too. Barry recounts how city health officials made calls for aid. "In Philadelphia, the head of Emergency Aid pleaded, 'All who are free from the care of the sick at home . . . report as early as possible . . . on emergency work.' But volunteers did not come."[35] Pleas to house children of dying and dead parents received only scant reply.[36]

The fear was justified. Barry reports that a study by the Metropolitan Life Insurance Company estimated that 3 percent of industrial workers between the ages of twenty-five and forty-five died of influenza. Six percent of coal workers in this age group succumbed to the illness.[37] These rates were five and ten times higher than the 0.6 percent that died across the country from the pandemic.

The factories and mines contained dense working conditions without adequate ventilation in 1918. These working conditions were similar to the meat packing facilities in the early months of the COVID-19 pandemic. In both locations nearly invisible viruses circulated and infected workers who could not protect themselves in the congested working quarters. Reverend John McDowell wrote of the life of a coal miner from the age of "nine years until death" in 1902. Even at a coal miner's highest possible earnings as a senior miner, he would earn only $1.60 per day. This equated to about $55 in 2020. This was the highest wage in the mines. Others made much less doing work that could crush them at any time from a collapsed shaft, exploding gas, or mine blast gone wrong. Even if they managed to avoid these sudden disasters, many would die slowly from black lung disease. It was work so dangerous that life insurance was not available.[38] These workers faced some of the highest rates of mortality from the pandemic—yet, with no savings or wealth, they had little choice but to continue.

What option did they have? Unemployment benefits and social security did not begin until 1935. The government didn't provide pandemic relief checks in 1918. As economist and public policy expert Karen Clay writes, "In 1918 the safety net was close to nonexistent. . . . One implication is that almost all workers . . . had to work unless they were absolutely physically unable. . . . If workers did not work, they and their families might not be able to eat."[39] Factories had to stay open in order to support the military. Laborers in these factories were forced into exposure.

Conditions were similar in the United Kingdom. Historian Simon Heffer writes that "[by] July 1 the flu was scything through London, notably in the East End textile trade. People working in enclosed, overcrowded premises with poor air quality . . . were especially vulnerable . . .

with around a quarter of the (mostly female) workforce of London's textile workshops affected."[40] Of course, London was not the only area affected. Laborer after laborer confronted the pandemic in factories throughout the United Kingdom. Heffer reports that "70 percent of men were absent from heavy industry in Newcastle."[41] Like in the United States, factories supplying the military were struck with absenteeism. Coal production dropped. A second wave arose in September striking these same occupations, as well as "capital firemen, police officers and nurses."[42]

The 1918 influenza pandemic hit manufacturing the hardest, but a century later a broad range of industries were affected by the COVID-19 pandemic. In some industries, workers faced exposure risk, and in others they faced financial risk as jobs disappeared. Restaurants contained both. In 2020, 110,000 restaurants closed temporarily or permanently. These closures, along with other restaurant layoffs, resulted in the loss of 2.5 million jobs and nearly a quarter of a trillion dollars in sales.[43] We don't often think of the restaurant industry as a driving force of our economy, yet it provides around 10 percent of all jobs in the United States.[44] Restaurant work is difficult in normal times. It is physically and mentally exhausting. In times of pandemics, it places workers directly in the path of danger. It is not surprising that line cooks registered the largest increase in mortality rates in all of California during the early pandemic. In restaurants, poorly ventilated workspace is often congested. People crowd together, shoulder to shoulder, and continually intermix throughout kitchens, prep areas, and serving areas. Servers act as hubs and interact with dozens of customers who create bridges across neighborhoods, cities, and sometimes even countries. In turn these servers act as microbridges to other workers within the restaurant and onward to other customers throughout their work shifts. For all of this exposure risk, most restaurant workers receive low pay. Median wages in the restaurant industry are about $22,500 per year with cooks earning $26,000 per year.[45] These wage levels represent the most conflicted type of worker. These workers have minimal, if any, cash reserves to fall back upon when out of work. Like the Smithfield meat processing workers, they don't have the financial ability to decline a work shift over concern for safety. At the same time their work puts them directly at risk.

When the restaurant industry began to recall unemployed workers, many faced difficult decisions that pitted finances against health. Chef Aaron Verzosa co-owns the Archipelago restaurant in Seattle with his spouse, Amber Manuguid. In describing the challenges of the pandemic, he told the blog *Eater*, "Work through the pain, work long hours. It's the mentality of the industry, and one of the most difficult ingredients to the pandemic, especially if this is your sole income."[46] The situation was even more difficult for the couple because of their multigenerational living situation. Ms. Manuguid's mother, sister, and her sister's child lived with them. Because of these complications the couple decided to sacrifice income in order to maintain the safety of their family. They ran their restaurant as a takeout and delivery-only establishment in the winter of 2021. They had the good fortune and financial resources to allow themselves this luxury of choice.

For others, financial pressure dictated a lack of choice. Restaurant server Kimberly Anderson told *Eater* that her husband was in a high health risk category for COVID-19. "The doctor at the V.A. told me, 'Don't go back.' But I'm the sole income."[47] Ms. Anderson was in a no-win situation. Her choice was exposure and health risk for her husband or no income. She had no good option.

Many restaurant owners did their best to limit the danger faced by their employees. Some voluntarily lowered capacity and rearranged working shifts and duties to limit exposure risk to their employees who faced heightened health risk within their households. Yet even in the best circumstances, restaurant work enhances the exposure risk of employees. Customers must go maskless to consume food and drink. Further, with a diversity of opinion as to the danger posed by the pandemic, restaurant workers were forced to face many customers who were not as careful as the workers would like. They were trapped in a service industry where the "customer is always right," except when they aren't, such as when they put the health of low-wage workers at risk. As one chef from Los Angeles put it, "We need you to know that we are here with you, not for you, and ask that you don't think of us as disposable as the boxes your food is packaged in."[48]

The sense of entitlement among customers and divisiveness over rules heightened tensions in already tense situations. The same chef noted, "On top of living in constant fear of losing their jobs . . . they are also dealing with some of the poorest treatment from guests that I have witnessed in my 15-year career as a restaurant worker."[49] A bartender stated, "We're making less money, either getting lower tips or no tips. . . . We also feel like babysitters, taking care of belligerent brats; I'm the mask police and social distance police."[50] While disputes about masks in grocery stores did not cost a grocery worker a wage, in restaurants they did. Employees who rely upon the generosity of customers' gratuity for the majority of their income knew they were risking their livelihood any time they had to enforce rules.

Many decided that enough was enough. When Jim Conway started working in restaurants in 1982, he was paid $2.13 an hour plus tips. Nearly four decades later, at a restaurant near Pittsburgh, Pennsylvania, his base wage was only $0.70 higher. With concerns over the danger of the pandemic after a four-month furlough, he decided to retire at age 64.[51] Many felt the same way. The *Washington Post* reports that almost one million restaurant and hotel job ads were posted in March of 2021 across the United States. Limited applications for these jobs led to a small increase in wages of $0.58 per hour in the first three months of 2021.[52] Even with a small wage increase, few wanted to work in an exposed industry paying low wages in the midst of a pandemic.

The city of Memphis voted Allan Creasy the best bartender three times, yet the pandemic proved too big of a burden for him to continue in the industry. He made $2.13 an hour plus tips. When he returned after the shutdown, he told the *Washington Post*, "I didn't come back to the same job I left previously. . . . It was difficult to have to constantly police people about mask-wearing . . . while making significantly less money than I'd been making previously." With a bachelor's degree, Creasy moved on to a new less-exposed career in social media.[53]

It wasn't just the combination of increased exposure and health risks compared to low wages that drove workers away. The behavior of patrons grew increasingly worse as customers returned to restaurants. This was a particular flash point for servers who derive a majority of their income from tips. Servers were often in the awkward position of cajoling customers into compliance with protocols at the risk of losing tip-income if they upset customers. A survey of 1,600 food service workers by the One Fair Wage advocacy group found that two-thirds of service workers claimed to receive smaller tips after enforcing mask-wearing and social distancing policies. Three-quarters of these workers reported hostile behavior from customers over enforcement of these policies.[54]

Partly because of this erosion of power, female servers often found themselves in situations of increased sexual harassment. Sexual harassment has long been a part of restaurant work. Some customers took the pandemic as license to act even more obnoxiously and offensively toward women working in the industry. Examples included being asked to remove their masks in an implicit gesture to judge their appearance before a customer determined the amount of gratuity. Explicit jokes were made about not being able to "touch you anymore" because of social distancing regulations. Others made comparisons between condom use and mask wearing.[55] As Saru Jayaraman, executive director of One Fair Wage, stated in the press release, "Women are literally being asked to expose themselves to illness and death for the pleasure of male customers—and all for a subminimum wage."[56]

In addition to the sexual harassment, restaurant workers did not feel protected from the virus. Nearly 90 percent of food service workers claimed that their employers did not consistently follow COVID-19 protocols. Furthermore, 84 percent claimed to be near at least one maskless person on every shift and 33 percent claimed to be near thirty or more maskless people on every shift.[57] The balance of power between customer, employer, and service worker put these low wage employees in a vulnerable position. It was a position that put their lives at risk.

Like many restaurant workers, Sidney Ramos lost her job as a server at the beginning of the pandemic. By the summer of 2021 she was re-employed in a different industry. However, she recalls the last day of her job and her manager's comments as he expressed his opinion on the requirement that they close. "One thing he said, that I'll never forget, is that he thought we should be able to risk our lives to serve people during the pandemic. Looking back on it, it's not okay to risk your employees' lives over someone's cheeseburger."[58]

While the danger and controversary of restaurants were front and center, one of the most dangerous places of exposure existed almost hidden from view—nursing home and eldercare facilities. Raised in the Philippines, Imee Villavicencio came to New York in 2006. She is one of the numerous workers who cared for nursing home patients over the course of the pandemic. Early in the pandemic she kept a Facebook diary recounting her thoughts and experiences, which she shared with the *Washington Post*:

> The day-by-day work is hard both mentally and physically. I cried every day feeling so hopeless . . . Colleagues die, my co-workers get sick one by one . . . My patients die . . . body bag after body bag . . . Every time I go inside the room of a covid patient . . . I feel very scared . . . [59]

In addition to her physical danger, she paid a mental toll:

> Every time I FaceTime a family member to say their final goodbye to my dying patients . . . I'm crying silently and choking . . . I can't wipe my tears because of the face shield. . . . I remember vividly, one of my patients is dying . . . gasping for air while I'm adjusting her IV line . . . She opens her eyes . . . grabs my forearm and said, "I'm afraid! Don't leave me." At the back of my mind . . . I can't stay here . . . I'm exposing myself too long . . . I was telling myself don't be stupid . . . get out . . . you gave the [morphine] already . . . it will comfort her . . . but I can't. I can't let this woman die scared and alone . . . I can't do that as a human being. I stayed with her until she took her last breath . . .[60]

Her mental toll has not disappeared. As she wrote, "I have a phobia with ambulance sirens . . . that sound associated with crisis and death."[61]

It is difficult to imagine the horrors of the work in nursing homes that women and men like Ms. Villavicencio faced due to the pandemic. Most are anonymous except for occasional stories dotted through newspapers and magazines. Most had experiences similar to Ms. Villavicencio. Many were infected and many died. Ms. Villavicencio was among those infected. Her ailments included coughing and difficulty breathing for twenty days before she returned to work.[62]

Ruthie Fishman, a director of a group of homes for dementia patients in Maryland, noted how the lack of recognition hurt the morale of her workers. She told the *Washington Post*, "Nursing home workers are underpaid, overworked, they're often immigrants. They got no applause. We didn't have the support."

These workers faced a trying task for low wages. Adarra Benjamin, a home health and personal care aid in Chicago, summarized the year of the pandemic to the *Atlantic* with the phrase "panic, panic, suspense."[63] In those three words one can envision parallel worlds—one where time races forward in an effort to save lives and care for the infirm, and yet at the same moment time stands still in a breathless anticipation of what is to come, with a mind racing through scenarios to escape the present circumstance.

Workers in nursing homes saw some of the most severe circumstances of the pandemic in the United States. If you had a loved one in a nursing home in the United States, the probability of your loved one dying due to COVID-19 in the first year of the pandemic was 8 percent.[64] More than 170,000 lives were lost in nursing homes in the United States due to COVID-19 infections.

The stress within this environment resulted in significant mental health challenges. One study of nursing home staff in Ireland found that 45 percent experienced moderate to severe symptoms of post-traumatic stress disorder and one in seven reported thinking of ending their life.[65] Another study of nursing home staff documented findings of uncertainty, anxiety, helplessness, and work overload associated with the COVID-19 pandemic.[66] These workers struggled with their own mental health while trying to aid patients and residents who themselves were experiencing atypical mental health challenges of loneliness and anxiety from pandemic-induced isolation and fear of infection.[67]

Even in normal times, work in nursing homes is challenging and the pay is low. Almost one-quarter of aids in long-term care facilities work in multiple facilities. An additional 15 percent work a second job outside of long-term care. The majority work a second job for financial reasons.[68] A 2020 study found the median hourly wage to be $12.80 with a median income of about $21,000.[69]

This was not a living wage that provided basic necessities for a family without a second job. Given their experiences and the low wages, it is easy to understand the difficulty of filling these positions. By June 2021 one-third of nursing homes employed fewer nurses and aides than before the pandemic began. This resulted in an average of twenty-one fewer minutes of contact per day, and eleven fewer hours of contact per month for each nursing home resident in the United States.[70] Fewer hours resulted in fewer showers, less assistance at mealtime, and, in the worst case, less assistance in an emergency. Further, with stringent limits on visitors, there were minimal opportunities to advocate on behalf of loved ones living in these understaffed facilities.

Tamika Dalton's seventy-four-year-old mother suffered from multiple sclerosis. Her mother lived in a nursing and rehabilitation center in Greensboro, North Carolina. As rates of staffing fell, her mother's care worsened and her health deteriorated. "Her hair was often matted and her toenails grew long. A bedsore the size of a fist festered on her backside. . . . 'She would call out for help and no one would come.'"[71] She blames the staffing shortages on greed. "They did that for their own pockets," she told the *Associated Press*.[72] In February of 2021 her mother passed away from COVID-19.

Ms. Dalton's observations of staff shortages were not unique to the facility where her mother lived. At the beginning of the pandemic there were about 3.3 million staff workers at nursing homes across the United States. By August 1, 2021, there were under three million.[73]

During these times everyone worried about personal safety, finances, children in remote school, social isolation, and all the day-to-day struggles of living through a pandemic in our own homes. The lower-paid nursing home aids faced these struggles as well, but many had even more difficult financial constraints and then faced the pandemic onslaught at work seeing lives lost every day. It is not surprising that many left the nursing home industry later in the pandemic when staff shortages in other service sector industries made less stressful jobs available.

There were other times in history when labor shortages followed a pandemic. The Black Death, the second and most devastating of the major episodes of bubonic plague, arrived in England in 1348. The first instances in the country occurred in the ports on the southern shores of England. In a few short months it moved inland to London before spreading across the entirety of England by mid-year in 1349. In total, it killed between one-third and one-half of the population. During this time, England's economy revolved around feudal agriculture. Landholders laid claim to serfs who were required to cultivate a plot of land. Serfs were not fully enslaved, yet neither were they free. They were not owned as property themselves but they were bound to the land on which they toiled. They could not leave their land or village without permission of the landholder. Nor could they marry or dispose of property without permission. The serf earned a living at subsistence levels. After the majority of growth was turned over to the landholder, the serf was responsible for producing or obtaining food and clothing from what remained. Next up on the hierarchy were the free peasants. Some of these were sharecroppers who rented land from a landholder in return for payment in the form of a share of production. Other peasants worked as free laborers and were paid a paltry wage.

The massive decline in population from the Black Death created turmoil in labor markets. Landholders saw their labor sources dwindle as people died by the day. Some farms were struck more severely than others. Some had a full arsenal of labor to produce, while others were left with no one to cultivate the land. Those without labor faced a dilemma. Either let their fields go unused and substantially reduce output and profits or try to hire or claim workers on other farms. Serfs who were bound to their lords in normal times escaped to more lucrative terms on other farms. Others escaped to work as free laborers in London or a nearby village. When a portion of a nearby farm sat unused, the sharecroppers took advantage of labor scarcity to bargain with landholders for better terms. They bid down rents in order to increase the share of the production that they retained. Free laborers demanded higher wages as worker shortages developed. All of this competition for increasingly scarce labor dwindled the profits of the landholders and reduced their position of power over workers.

As wages rose and labor became scarce, serfs and free peasants used their new bargaining power to their advantage. Landholders resented this newly shifted balance of power. They saw those in the servant classes below them as greedy and lazy. John Gower, a Kent manor lord, poet, and friend of Geoffrey Chaucer, wrote of the labor market following the Black Death. Historian Allan Kulikoff summarized his writing: "Peasant workers, formerly pliant and agreeable, had become 'sluggish,' 'scarce,' and 'grasping.' For the very little they do they demand the highest pay. . . . Yet a short time ago one performed more service than three do now.' Not only did they refuse to work as servants or sign a yearly contract; they wanted 'the leisures of great men . . . he scorns all ordinary food . . . he grumbles and he will not return tomorrow unless you provide something better.'"[74] With this view of serfs and peasants, landowners grew frustrated as they saw their profits dissipate from unused land and growing wage bills.

King Edward III responded by issuing the Ordinance of Labourers on June 18, 1349. The ordinance contained three main stipulations: First, the king attempted to increase the supply of labor. All men and women sixty years or younger without land holdings, whether a serf or free laborer, were compelled to serve any landholder who required their labor. A landholder had preferential claim to labor of his own tenants. However, in order to make labor less scarce he could use only as much as he needed. He must release any excess laborers to serve on other farms. This was intended to more evenly distribute the remaining laborers across farms and to decrease competition between landholders. Any servant or laborer leaving their landholder to serve another without permission would be imprisoned. Limiting the mobility of workers and requiring labor of all working-age peasants was another intentional device to lower competition for workers. Second, all wages must not exceed those of 1346. The king placed a ceiling on the wages that servants could earn in order to return profits to the landholders. The king wanted the landowners to earn more so that he could receive larger profits passed up to him. The penalty for noncompliance in the form of payment or receipt of excess wages was double the amount of the excess. This not only eroded the power of the laborers to bargain, it decreased the ability of landholders to compete for labor by outbidding each other. Third, in order to limit inflation, all food and goods must be sold for reasonable prices. Excess prices were punished with fines of an amount double the excess. Parliament followed with the Statute of Labourers in 1351, which repeated many of the same rules but provided for more concrete methods of enforcement.[75]

The responses in 1349 and 1351 were the equivalent of a present-day executive order by a US president, followed by a legislative act of Congress, each requiring that the labor market return to 2019 levels of wages and that labor shortages be abolished. These actions would not have brought about a solution to labor market problems caused by the COVID-19 pandemic, and the new laws didn't solve the problems of the fourteenth century either. Supply and demand were at work in the past as they are today. The result was that the ordinance and statute were poorly enforced. Landholders and laborers circumvented the orders of the king and Parliament, and competition continued for the scarce labor. Wages for peasants continued to increase. Still, the lower classes grew hostile to the king's efforts to suppress them and to the feudal system in general. Their resentment planted the seeds that led to the Peasants' Revolt of 1381.[76]

Although to a lesser degree, similar labor market difficulties followed the early part of the COVID-19 pandemic.

These did not occur as a result of one-third of workers dying. Instead, they occurred because of frustrations about working conditions and constraints imposed upon workers by the pandemic. Companies couldn't find workers as job postings did not receive applications. In an effort to attract more employees, wages increased but only mildly. Many small businesses struggled financially in the early recovery and didn't have excess profits to pay higher wages. At the same time, workers flexed their muscles by demanding more power to control their careers and their lives. Like the peasants of the fourteenth century, they wanted better working conditions along with better wages.

The labor shortages that developed frustrated customers. Customers expected instant gratification and service, with next-day delivery and smooth, on-demand transactions at their convenience. Now they were met with signs stating "Please be patient, we're short-staffed."[77] Here, there was a mix of contradiction. Some laborers found it nearly impossible to find work; some businesses found it nearly impossible to find labor. Reminiscent of John Gower in the 1300s, many companies and customers blamed pandemic relief checks and extended unemployment benefits for creating entitled and lazy workers. Very few firms found concerns for safety in the workplace or the complications of childcare to be significant issues in the lack of response to job postings. Workers disagreed. Those who became unemployed and searched for new positions to no avail blamed companies for paying less than the jobs the workers held previously. They cited a poor match of their skills to available jobs, along with concerns of safety and lack of flexibility that was needed when families confronted the pandemic.[78] Throughout the economy there was a mismatch of firms and workers. Many on both sides had yet to find a match for worker or job as the pandemic moved into 2022. These mismatches of firm and worker desires and constraints fell most heavily on women, particularly women of color.

At the beginning of the pandemic, Alexis Lohse resided in St. Paul, Minnesota, with her husband and two children. She had a master's degree and a job with the state government. When the pandemic hit and schools closed, she cut her hours and declined to pursue a promotion at work so she could tend to her children. Her husband was a letter carrier and remained employed full-time in person. She was frustrated. In the summer of 2021 she told the *New York Times*, "I don't know how to get back on track, especially with questions out there—how schools reopen; when; variants; the way everybody else is behaving; having the schools open and close at bizarre random hours."[79] Earlier in her life as a single mother in poverty, she struggled to make ends meet before returning to school in her thirties. "It just feels so frustrating that the same brick walls I hit 16 years ago, I hit again in the pandemic."[80]

In the spring of 2020, women in the labor force lost jobs at rates that exceeded men in most countries around the world. Despite having nearly identical rates of unemployment before the pandemic, the US unemployment rate for women jumped to over 16 percent. This was 2.5 percent higher than the unemployment rate for men. This mismatch of women losing more jobs than men was unique for a recession. Commonly men tend to lose more jobs in recessions because male dominated industries, particularly manufacturing and construction, lose jobs most frequently. In the Great Recession 70 percent of jobs lost between December 2007 and June 2009 belonged to men.[81] In past recessions men's employment plummeted while women's employment remained more stable.

At the onset of the COVID-19 pandemic, the opposite occurred. Women lost more jobs than men. In the economic recovery from the pandemic another unusual thing occurred. The unemployment rate for women returned to near pre-pandemic levels. Yet this hid a reality not captured within unemployment rates. The unemployment rate only measures people who are actively looking for work but cannot find a job; it does not count people who have left the workforce and no longer seek employment. Missing from the unemployment rate were the 2.3 million women who left the labor market entirely in the first year of the pandemic.[82] This resulted in the lowest labor market participation rate for women since May of 1988.[83] About 3 percent of women who had been in the labor force disappeared from the labor market. These exits decreased the overall labor force (of women and men) by 1.4 percent.

One reason for the labor market exits included demands of increased childcare responsibilities and time spent helping their children with education in the new remote home-schooling environment. This combination took its toll physically and mentally. Sarah Joyce Wiley, from Sharon, Massachusetts, is the mother of three grade school–aged children and works as a chief client officer (CCO) for a health services company. She told the *New York Times,* "I feel like I have five jobs: mom, teacher, CCO, house cleaner, chef." She continued, noting with humor that her children call her "'principal mommy' and the 'lunch lady.' It's exhausting."[84]

All parents faced increased stress, but mothers in the labor market were hit especially hard. They found more severe conflicts between separating time for their families and time for their jobs than fathers did.[85] A survey by the Pew Research Center found that mothers in the United States were twice as likely as fathers to say that they had "a lot" of childcare duties while working and that childcare became more difficult as the pandemic lengthened. Mothers were also more likely to report that they could not give 100 percent effort and needed to reduce labor market hours early in the pandemic.[86] They also needed to recharge mentally, but the pandemic did not allow this luxury. An increased toll on their mental health grew as the pandemic continued. Dekeda Brown reported to the *New York Times*, "I feel like a ticking time bomb that is constantly being pushed to the breaking point, but then I am able to defuse myself. Goodness, this is taxing."[87] Further she stated, "With everything going on, I just don't have time to take care of my mental health right now. I have to keep it together for everyone else."[88] Mother of two preschool children, Elise Kelner of Gilbert, Arizona, called a *New York Times* phone line set up to record the impressions of mothers in early 2021. On her call she stated, "I don't know how to feel sane again. I'm just stuck in this position for God knows how much longer."[89]

C. Nicole Mason, president and chief executive of the Institute for Women's Policy Research, noted how the government response to the pandemic recession did not take substantial notice of the particular effect on women. "Even when presidential candidates were campaigning and talking about job creation, Joe Biden was in a factory, in a hard hat, talking about how we are going to get people back to work [presumably in factories]. . . . Donald Trump said, 'Don't worry women, we'll get jobs for your husbands,'" at a political rally in Michigan.[90] At the highest levels, policy makers seemed oblivious to who had lost their jobs and how to get them back. The roles of working mothers did not enter large-scale policy discussions to an extent that could solve the problem.

Women in low-income jobs that did not allow for remote work confronted even more difficult challenges.

According to the National Women's Law Center in 2018, women in the United States comprised nearly two-thirds of the workforce in the forty lowest paying jobs. The highest average hourly wage on this list is $11.82.[91] These include occupations (proportions of women given in parenthesis) such as servers (71 percent), childcare workers (93 percent), cashiers (71 percent), maids and cleaners (89 percent), home health aides (88 percent), and personal care aides (86 percent). Each of these jobs employ at least one million workers and are substantial categories among the roughly 150 million workers in the United States. According to the same study, 39 percent of all women with full-time labor market jobs lived in or near poverty.[92] For women of color the rate was 53 percent. Workers in this position are commonly termed the *working poor*. Even in the best of times, these women live near the margin of poverty, and two-thirds of mothers in these low-paid professions were the primary earners in their families.[93]

These job categories are all in-person positions. They are not jobs to be performed over teleconference. They are not salaried jobs. Many don't have benefits of health insurance or paid vacation. If you don't show up, you don't get paid. Yet when you show up during a pandemic, you face exposure risk. These women worked difficult jobs and made a steady but low income before the pandemic. It was an income that did not allow for savings and luxuries but was close to recession-proof before the pandemic. As single mother and waitress Ilanne Dubois told the *Washington Post*, "I had a good rhythm going. I wasn't rich, I couldn't complain saying I was poor. Now, all of that stability is gone. We're falling into a hole."[94]

When numerous businesses shut down at the onset of the pandemic, many of these steady jobs in service industries disappeared. Restaurants closed entirely or reduced their staff when only take-out dining was available. Tourism disappeared and vacant hotel rooms needed no servicing or cleaning. Non-essential retail stores closed, as did many childcare centers. With parents at home, many in-home childcare providers were let go. Not only were women of the working poor concentrated in the industries with the most severe job losses, but they were over-represented in the job losses within these professions.[95] Even if jobs weren't lost, many had hours cut back, pay reduced, or both. In April 2020, over 30 percent of women were forced to work part time even though they desired full-time work. Prior to the pandemic only 11 percent of women found themselves in this position.[96]

It wasn't just the direct effect of the labor market and the jobs lost. Women faced additional constraints and expectations at home, particularly from disproportionate shares of home childcare.[97] Economist Betsey Stevenson predicted what was to come in a comment to the *Washington Post* in May 2020, saying, "If summer camps don't open up, if schools don't open up in the fall, who goes back to work?"[98] In the fall of 2020, with many schools and day-care centers closed or only providing for part-time attendance, someone needed to care for young children. As Stevenson predicted, it wasn't men who gave up their jobs and careers to care for children, it was women. Coinciding with partial school openings in the early fall, more than 860,000 women left the workforce compared to just under 170,000 men. In total, over two million women left the US labor market in just the year 2020 alone. As Kate Ryder, CEO of Maven Clinic, noted in a December 2020 *CNBC* article, "What was a leaky bucket is now a waterfall of talent leaving the workforce."[99]

Single mothers felt the effects of labor market participation most strongly.[100] These women faced the most challenging situation and for many it combined food insecurity, exposure in the workplace, and childcare. After losing her job as a waitress at the onset of the pandemic, Ms. Dubois spoke further about the possibility of finding part-time work. She considered looking for a job as a delivery driver but did not know how she would handle the care of her six-year-old son. "I can't afford to pay the babysitter anymore." With no school or daycare options, "I haven't thought of what I could possibly do next."[101] Women like her, those in essential front-facing jobs with low pay and children, had nowhere to turn. There were multitudes in her situation. Many lost their jobs, and those who did not faced exposure risk in the workplace. If they had children, childcare options were limited and often unaffordable at the wages of the working poor. All of these factors together led back to food insecurity and choices between which necessity to cut or trim. These were the people that President Trump and future President Joseph R. Biden were not addressing on the campaign trail. Instead, they were in factories talking about jobs traditionally held by men. Addressing the needs of women like Ms. Dubois was not a serious, wide-ranging part of the political conversation.

Women, men, and families with jobs paying wages of the working poor whether in restaurants, nursing homes, or many other low-income industries, were already sitting at the margin of survival before the pandemic. The pandemic pushed them below this margin into dire need. Those without extended families or other support networks who could offer housing, food, childcare, or financial assistance to pay for rent or health care had nowhere to turn. Yes, an unexpected pandemic pushed them under, but they struggled at the financial margin of survival before the pandemic. Any one of a thousand potential incidents of illness, job loss, unplanned accidents, or health emergencies would have pushed them under. In large part, they are more noticed now because the pandemic caused so many to sink below the margin all at once. Their emergencies occurred simultaneously so that their plight became a collective emergency that forced more eyes to take notice. Now that we see the plight of low-income workers and their situations more clearly, we must ask how we can move beyond recognition and help to move the working poor above the margin with living wages, high quality health care, and affordable childcare. At the outset, we never should have allowed them to live so close to the margin in the first place.

Chapter 7

THE PANDEMIC DILEMMA

In the fall of 1918, the great influenza pandemic marched toward its apex. With the number of cases and deaths rising, public health officials began a series of campaigns that encouraged citizens to wear face coverings to protect against infection and transmission. Many of the campaigns called upon civic duty and responsibility to society.[1] One Red Cross poster stated, "The man or woman or child who will not wear a mask now is a dangerous slacker."[2] Oakland Mayor John Davie affirmed, "It is sensible and patriotic, no matter what our personal beliefs may be, to safeguard our fellow citizens."[3]

In 1918 the Red Cross poster and the words of civic leaders tried to encourage responsible behavior by shaming noncompliant individuals. In some places, such shaming worked for a time. As the pandemic continued, however, shame alone proved insufficient. Cities were forced to become more stringent. They converted from appeals and recommendations to mandates and requirements. San Francisco acted first with a mask ordinance that required face coverings to be four layers thick. When Mayor James Rolph enacted the ordinance on October 22, 1918, he asserted that "conscience, patriotism, and self-protection demand immediate and rigid compliance."[4] Soon six other major cities—Seattle, Oakland, Sacramento, Denver, Indianapolis, and Pasadena—enacted mask mandates.

To encourage compliance, some cities levied fines that ranged from $5 to $10 (the equivalent of $85 to $170 in 2020) and imposed jail sentences of eight hours to ten days.[5] On November 9, 1918, one thousand people were arrested in San Francisco for failure to comply with the mask mandate. So many were arrested that the jail cells approached capacity.[6]

Nevertheless, compliance was slack in some areas, and some individuals vehemently protested against the mandates. During a 1918 Portland public hearing about instituting a mask mandate, one attendee declared such a law to be "autocratic and unconstitutional . . . under no circumstances will I be muzzled like a . . . dog."[7] At a hearing in Oakland, another protester claimed that "if a cave man should appear . . . he would think the masked citizens all lunatics."[8]

As individual behaviors diverged and as protests became more common, scuffles broke out. On October 27, 1918, five days after the San Francisco mask ordinance became law, James Wisser, a blacksmith, stood at the corner of Market and Powell Streets and encouraged people to forgo their masks. "They are bunk,"[9] he screamed. City health inspector Henry D. Miller approached him and ordered him to don a mask. Wisser refused. An altercation ensued, and Wisser knocked the inspector to the ground with a bag of silver dollars. According to the *San Francisco Chronicle*, "While being pummeled, Miller drew his revolver, and four shots rang out."[10] One shot hit Wisser in the hand and leg. Two uninvolved bystanders were wounded. Everyone involved recovered from their injuries. Miller was charged with assault with a deadly weapon; and Wisser was charged with disturbing the peace, resisting an officer, and assault.[11]

In San Francisco the mandates lasted only one month. With only six cases reported on November 13, 1918, the city began relaxing restrictions. At noon on Thursday, November 21, a whistle rang across the city that signaled the end of the mask mandate.[12] The decision was premature. By mid-December cases escalated to levels above 1,500 per week. Debates within the city administration ensued. Dr. William Hassler, the San Francisco city health officer, strongly favored reimplementing restrictions. On December 17, 1918, in the midst of these debates, a bomb was placed on the steps of Hassler's office. He was not injured, nor was he intimidated. He continued arguing in favor of mask mandates along with other precautions. In the end, Hassler lost the debate to commercial interests that focused on lost revenues during the December holiday season.[13] The tensions between public health and commerce continued to be fierce.

As the new year began, cases and deaths continued to increase. On January 12, Mayor Rolph issued a statement requesting the voluntary use of face masks. This was followed by a flurry of letters from citizens and businesspeople. Some supported reinstituting a mask mandate, and others opposed it. The opposition questioned evidence of the cause of influenza and the efficacy of face masks in preventing infection. Others called the mandate an infringement on civil liberties. As infections climbed to over four thousand in the following week, Rolph could wait no longer. He implemented a new mandate on Friday, January 17, 1919.[14]

The very next day an announcement appeared in the *San Francisco Chronicle*. The Anti-Mask League, a citizen protest group created and run by a group of affluent and influential San Francisco women, were to hold a public meeting at the Dreamland Roller Rink. The event drew over 4,500 maskless attendees in protest of mask mandates.[15] Nearly 1 percent of the entire population of San Francisco gathered in one place at one time, maskless. They were there to protest a law intended to stave off a worldwide pandemic that would kill 650,000 people in the United States and fifty million people across the world. Large groups such as this one often create far more danger during a pandemic than we realize.

Each August, the population of Sturgis, South Dakota, swells from 7,000 people to nearly 500,000 for the Sturgis Motorcycle Rally. Originally called the Black Hills Classic, the event started in 1938 with a nine-participant motorcycle race. Today it includes a variety of group rides, concerts, and food vendors, along with a tattoo contest and a poker tournament. Other than a three-year hiatus during World War II, it has occurred every year since it began. In 2015 the seventy-fifth-anniversary rally drew a record attendance of 750,000 people.[16]

When the COVID-19 pandemic arrived in the United States, immediate concern developed about holding the 2020 rally. Such a large group congregating in such a small place was almost certain to spread the virus. Some on the city council recommended postponing the rally, as did 60 percent of respondents to a city survey.[17] However, once South Dakota Governor Kristi Noem supported holding the rally as planned, the holdouts relented. Even if Governor Noem had not spoken up, Sturgis Mayor Mark Carstensen expected it would have been impossible to stop the rally. He told the *New York Times*, "I said back in March, do you want me to build a wall around Sturgis or a wall around South Dakota, because that is the only way we could have stopped [the rally goers from arriving]."[18]

As planned the ten-day-long eightieth-anniversary Sturgis Motorcycle Rally took place in August 2020. Bikes rumbled into the Black Hills of South Dakota from across the country, and 450,000 people descended upon Sturgis.

Concerts and parties overtook the town. Visitors flooded restaurants, bars, campgrounds, and hotel lobbies. As the rally rolled on, Harleys were many and masks were few. One Associated Press reporter counted fewer than ten masks in a crowd of thousands at one event.[19] With a spirit of rebellion, some attendees purchased patches adorned with the words "Sturgis Motorcycle Corona Rally." Others bought T-shirts labeled with the slogan "Screw COVID I went to Sturgis."

Bikers are known for their spirit of freedom above all else. Yet even among the attendees the pandemic was of concern. One told the Associated Press, "I don't want to die, but I don't want to be cooped up all my life either. . . . I think we're all willing to take a chance." Another attendee told the *Washington Post*, "No one that I spoke to there wasn't aware of coronavirus, and wasn't aware that there was a risk of them being there. . . . It was just a risk that they accepted."[20]

When people use the word *risk* in this context, what do they mean?

Suppose that I offer you the following two options: Option 1 is $10 million in cash right now. Option 2 is a coin flip where a coin landing heads-up yields you nothing and a coin landing tails-up yields you $20 million. Which option would you choose?

When I offer this hypothetical choice to students, almost all respond that they prefer the guaranteed $10 million. They prefer to avoid the risk of potentially receiving nothing. Here the meaning of the word *risk* is clear. Risk is measured by the 50–50 coin-flip probability and the monetary difference between the two prizes. Economists call the phenomenon of a person preferring the sure thing to a gamble that has the same expected outcome *risk aversion*. Most people exhibit some amount of risk aversion.

Now, what if I offered you $5 million in cash or the same $0 versus $20 million coin flip? Would you take the $5 million, or would you risk it on the coin flip? What do you think others would do? What if the amount of cash was $1 million? $500,000? $100,000? How small must the certain prize be before you would take the coin flip? What would your friends do? You probably know someone who would take the coin flip instead of $5 million and someone who would take $100,000 instead of the coin flip. We are all different in our financial circumstances and our levels of risk aversion.

In the case of an infectious disease, this is true as well. Some individuals are willing to accept more exposure risk and more health risk than others. But what does the word *risk* mean in the context of a novel infectious disease pandemic? Risk of infection, illness, hospitalization, long-term debilitation, death? How is this risk being measured by each individual? The answers aren't clear.

Risks in a pandemic are fundamentally different from risks involved in the coin-flip examples. In the coin flip, we know the probability of the outcomes and the value of the outcomes. With pandemic risks, we don't have this knowledge. We can't look in a book and learn how likely it is that we will be infected on a particular trip to the grocery store or a trip to a mass gathering like the Sturgis Motorcycle Rally, nor can we look up the probability of any particular outcome of an infection that could range from an asymptomatic case to death.

In 1921, economist Frank Knight made a distinction between risk and uncertainty in his book *Risk, Uncertainty, and Profits*: "There is a fundamental distinction between the reward for taking a known risk and that for assuming a risk whose value itself is not known."[21] To Knight, true uncertainty was "not susceptible to measurement."[22] To him, *uncertainty* was different than *risk*. He explained that the key to understanding the difference lies in not being able to calculate with precision the probability that outcomes will occur in an uncertain environment. This may be due to the complexity of the environment, or it may be due to unforeseen events. This does not mean that we do not know the direction of a change in risk. It is clear that attending a large maskless gathering in the midst of a pandemic increases one's exposure risk—but we don't know the amount of the increase precisely.

The situation we faced in 2020 corresponds to uncertainty, and it also corresponds to the description of a *black swan event* from Nicholas Taleb, an author, option trader, and risk analyst. He describes these events as rare occurrences that are not predictable in advance.[23] In some cases these events are not predictable because they are novel and new, such as the start of the COVID-19 pandemic. In others they are not predictable because of the perspective of the observer. Taleb describes the perspective of a turkey prior to a holiday dinner. Throughout its life the turkey lives day to day, being fed by a farmer. It is fat and happy. All of its history leads the turkey to believe (assuming some rudimentary consciousness of the turkey!) that its life will continue indefinitely. The turkey never has occasion nor experience that leads it to believe that it will become a holiday dinner—until it does. However, from the perspective of the farmer, the world of the turkey is ordered. It is clear to the farmer exactly when a turkey dinner is coming.

From our perspective, a pandemic like COVID-19 leaves us closer to the situation of the turkey than the farmer. There is a true exposure risk and a true health risk that exists for each of us and a particular set of behaviors and interactions. However, these risks are too complex to pin down exactly. For us, the outbreak of COVID-19 was a black swan event that contained Knightian uncertainty. The true risk of such an event depends on our own behavior *and* on the behavior of others in our neighborhood, community, state, nation, and the world at large. It depends on the location of each one of us in the network of social interactions. Are we a hub? Are we connected to a hub? How close are we to a bridge, or are we a bridge ourselves? The true set of risks depends upon the behavior of people near us. Do our friends practice social distancing? Do they wear masks? Do they take public transit? How inwardly dense is the neighborhood where they live? How dense are the stores in which they shop? In order to truly calculate our exposure risk, we need to know all of these things and the behavior of everyone to whom we are connected throughout the world. At the beginning of the COVID-19 pandemic, this risk was impossible to know. We were living in a world filled with uncertainty.

When people attend a large gathering like the 2020 Sturgis Motorcycle Rally or the 1918 meeting of the Anti-Mask League and claim to accept the risk, they are not using the word *risk* in a meaningful way. This risk cannot be calculated for an individual attendee. Instead, the attendees are saying that they accept the *uncertainty* of an action. Such reasoning creates a problem that combines guesses, information, and behavior.

In the midst of the COVID-19 pandemic, each of us needed to make a *guess* as to the true risk. Here I use the word *guess* with a specific purpose; I mean it to refer to something much less precise than an estimation made with a good amount of knowledge, data, or history. The sudden appearance of the COVID-19 pandemic was a black swan event, and we had the perspective of a flock of turkeys before a holiday. We woke up one morning and one of our flock was gone. We didn't know precisely how or why. We didn't know when the next holiday dinner was coming, nor when another one of our flock would be chosen. At the beginning of the pandemic, we had minimal history and data to guide our actions. Yet each of us had to make some assessment of the danger in order to choose behavior that we deemed acceptable, and our choices increased or decreased exposure risk for others around us. This exposure risk was a shared risk.

To make decisions in the midst of a pandemic, we each had to create beliefs based on limited information. The information that we used came from a wide variety of sources. Some came from diverse personal experiences. Those of us who lived in areas with more deaths limited our mobility more than others with fewer deaths. Other information came from friends. Those of us with Facebook friends in areas with worse pandemic outcomes behaved more cautiously.[24] Whether based on science or fiction, we relied on a multitude of sources to guide us, including friends, family, newspapers, television channels, and social media.

The constant flow of scientifically invalid misinformation, and in some cases outright lies, made it difficult to gather the needed information accurately. We were bombarded with misinformation on the effectiveness of preventative measures, the dangers of being infected, and the benefits of fake cures. This misinformation affected behavior, including decisions on masking and social distancing. Later in the pandemic, it included misinformation on the use of vaccines.[25] The government leaders in various states and in various nations gave conflicting information, in part for political purposes. Scientifically invalid misinformation and lies created a disaster of echo chambers. Anyone could find a statement, credible or not, that supported the behavior that was consistent with their personal views and the views espoused by the political leaders that they supported. It didn't matter if this information was sound or not. In many cases it only mattered that the information was consistent with what they wanted to believe.

People across the world needed the government and media to act as arbiters of clarity in this black swan world of Knightian uncertainty. They needed the most accurate information possible to overcome our limitations of knowledge. Many didn't get it. The Trump administration embraced a world of "alternative facts" from its inauguration onward.[26] This didn't change once the pandemic started, as President Trump continually downplayed the danger of the virus early in the pandemic and admitted to doing so in a taped conversation with journalist Bob Woodward.[27] Rebekah Jones, a data scientist at the Florida Department of Health, claimed she was asked to manipulate data on the state's COVID-19 dashboard. When she refused, she was fired.[28] The effect of misinformation extended to the media.[29] As John Barry, noted historian of the 1918 influenza pandemic, has written, "Those in authority must retain the public's trust. The way to do that is to distort nothing, to put the best face on nothing, to try to manipulate no one." In an October 2020 interview he stated, "You do not want to use fear as a tool, but you want them to be able to judge the risk themselves, truthfully. And to understand the risk . . . because it is pretty clearly the best thing to do."[30]

The lack of truth cost lives. Veteran Joe Joyce was stationed at Chu Lai during the Vietnam War. After returning home from the war, he taught physical education for disabled students.[31] To make some extra money, he began tending bar on weekends and eventually opened his own bar, JJ Bubbles, in the Bay Ridge neighborhood of Brooklyn. Although Joyce was a supporter of President Trump and a Republican, all were welcome and at home inside JJ Bubbles. A *New York Times* article described how "he didn't want to hear how much you loved Hillary Clinton . . . but he was not going to make the Syrian immigrant who came in to play darts feel as if he belonged anywhere else."[32] Joyce was described by a longtime patron as someone who was "always ready to help someone."[33] On the topic of the pandemic, he was a skeptic. His daughter Kristen stated to the *New York Times*, "He watched Fox News and believed it [the pandemic] was under control."[34] Feeling that the pandemic was a hoax intended to "bludgeon Trump,"[35] he didn't take precautions seriously.

Against his daughter's objections, Joe and his wife Jane flew to Florida and took a cruise to Spain on March 1, 2020. Kristen stated that "if Trump had gone on TV with a mask on and said, 'Hey this is serious,' I don't think he would have gone."[36] In mid-March, Joe argued with his daughter. "He said, 'Don't you think this is fishy? . . . Do you know anyone who has died from it?'"[37] Kristen responded, "Dad, I don't know anyone now, but give me a week and I bet I will."[38] Shortly thereafter, Joe began to feel unwell. Yet he resisted getting tested. "'He didn't think he could have it,' Kristen said, 'because he wasn't 100 percent confident that it was a thing.'"[39] Seven days later, on March 27, 2020, Kristen spoke to her father on the phone. Joe was wheezing. Kristen called an ambulance. Joe's oxygen level had dropped to 70 percent. He was admitted to the hospital. On April 9, 2020, Joe died of COVID-19.

This wasn't the only case in which information cost lives. A study by a group of economists found a statistically higher number of cases and deaths in areas that had a higher viewership of a news show that discounted the danger of the pandemic.[40] The populations in these areas were not getting a full and honest portrayal of the pandemic, and transmission of this misinformation had life-and-death consequences.

Different sources of information created different beliefs about the pandemic. These beliefs combined with different amounts of risk aversion and led each of us to act in a different manner. Those who believed there to be significant danger present or who were most risk averse took precautions to avoid interacting with people and wore face coverings without being mandated to do so. Those who believed there to be minimal risk or who were less risk averse acted in accordance with patterns of pre-pandemic behavior. This second group resisted wearing face coverings, attended social gatherings, ate in restaurants, and took cruises until the cruise industry shut down. This group also moved about less cautiously and made minimal changes in their lives.

The impact of those acting less cautiously was not the same as the impact of those acting more cautiously. The pandemic thrived because of the behavior of the less cautious group. As this group continued with pre-pandemic shopping and commuting patterns as well as patterns of maskless socialization, they faced more exposure risk and were more likely to become infected. If their increased exposure risk was their risk alone, then we wouldn't have needed to worry about it. But it wasn't their risk alone. Their behavior created extra exposure risk for everyone around them—including those who were more cautious. They attended gatherings like the Rose Garden reception and created super-spreading events. They moved about the country without masks and without getting tested, and they created pandemic bridges throughout their travels. They made the pandemic much larger than it would have been otherwise.

This seems horrendous, yet it was even worse. People with similar beliefs who acted with less caution interacted with others who also were less cautious. Those who discounted the danger of the pandemic went to restaurants, shopping malls, and large gatherings. While at these locations, they interacted with others who also discounted the danger of the pandemic. Birds of a risky feather flocked together. Through this process, society was sorted so that the risky interacted with the risky. Hubs met hubs each time that risky met risky, and exposure risk amplified even more. This sorting and the resulting amplification put even the most cautious in more danger.

The people who went to the 2020 Sturgis Motorcycle Rally did not interact with an arbitrary collection of people while they were there. The attendees were not drawn at random from across the population like ping-pong balls at a bingo parlor. Instead, they were part of a group of people who, on average, were just as likely to ignore the dangers of the pandemic in their daily lives in their hometowns. While at the rally, they proudly donned T-shirts that read "Screw COVID" and adorned their leather jackets with patches stating "Sturgis Motorcycle Corona Rally." They acted with less caution both before and after they attended the motorcycle rally. They were more likely to shun masks and more likely to ignore social distancing recommendations. We know this simply from the fact that they were in Sturgis for the rally. These were the people most likely to be infected prior to arriving in Sturgis—and then they all mixed together.

In 2020 Donn Hougham lived in Redmond, Oregon, with his wife Marni. They traveled to Sturgis along with a group of friends. In discussing his decision to attend the motorcycle rally and describing the group of friends with whom he planned to travel, he told the *Central Oregon Daily News*, "We pretty much live life. We're not afraid, we're cautious but we're not afraid." Mr. Hougham was not denying the existence of the pandemic. He felt that they were being cautious. However, *cautious* has a different meaning for everyone. He explained, "The flu virus is out there every year. People have died from that. Yes be careful, if you're worried . . . then wear a mask . . . don't stand next to your buddy . . . that's your personal choice and your personal fears. We as a group [the people he is travelling with] don't have those [fears] like others do, so we're going."[41]

Mr. Hougham's statement ignored the fact that his behavior increased the exposure risk faced by those around him. It ignored the fact that those who were worried could not protect themselves completely from the actions of people who, like him, acted less cautiously. We were all connected, and we all shared in the collective exposure risk that the least cautious created and contributed to increasing. We did not live in a vacuum. It wasn't his risk and his friends' risk alone. One couldn't simply cut off exposure risk by simply making a personal choice to wear a mask or to not stand next to a buddy.

In pandemics, each personal choice affects others because we share our exposure risk.

The attitude of Mr. Hougham and his friends was shared by the people who flocked to Sturgis. They recognized the pandemic and were willing to accept the exposure and health risk that they believed they faced. However, their actions increased the likelihood that others, even those who were cautious, would be infected, and that some would die. They all congregated in one place at one time. They arrived from across the country. They mixed and matched at events during the rally. Everything that was most dangerous about the pandemic was present in one place at one time.

The Sturgis attendees had engaged in a large number of risky interactions before they arrived. They weren't risk-averse and faced more exposure risk in their hometowns. During their travel to Sturgis, they created even more exposure risk. They ate in restaurants and stopped at hotels and gas stations. Their travels created a set of bridges across which their exposure risk was shared. These bridges all converged at Sturgis in August 2020. When the attendees arrived, some had asymptomatic or pre-symptomatic infections—maybe some even had symptomatic infections but did not believe that COVID-19 was "a thing," as Mr. Joyce had not. The mass gatherings at events over the course of ten days created uber density. They packed restaurants, hotels, and pubs, mostly maskless.

This wasn't just density. It was inward density. All the attendees at Sturgis had a large number of contacts, and each person there was a hub. During their time at the rally, many of the attendees' contacts changed from day to day. This created additional micro-bridges between attendees at the rally. Then they all returned home. When they did so, they created 450,000 additional dangerous bridges that spanned across the country. Every element that allows a virus to spread was present in Sturgis to the utmost degree.

The people who attended the rally claimed to have accepted the risk. However, the risk that they accepted wasn't just the risk for themselves. Through their actions they were accepting risk for everyone around them in Sturgis, everyone around them on their travels home, and everyone around them in their home communities when they returned.

Fifty-year-old Kenny Cervantes attended the Sturgis rally. His girlfriend, Angie Balcom, did not. She stayed home out of concern about getting infected at the rally. As Mr. Cervantes rode his Harley 400 miles from Sturgis back to Nebraska, he began to experience an ache in his throat. Eleven days later he was in the hospital, where he would stay for eight days. His girlfriend and sister became infected also. He had brought exposure risk to them, even though they were more cautious. He will never know for sure whether he was infected at Sturgis, but he believes that he was.[42] He will never know if he was infected before he arrived at the rally or during the rally. He knows that he infected his more cautious girlfriend, but he will he never know how many additional people he infected on his return trip home, nor how many more people he infected once he was home. He will never know how many additional infections occurred in the chain that he started. He wasn't the only one.

As attendees returned home from Sturgis, it didn't take long to see the effects of the 450,000 new bridges that had been created. By September 8, the South Dakota Department of Health identified 124 South Dakota residents who had tested positive after attending the rally. The Associated Press cast a wider geographic net and identified 290 cases associated with the rally across twelve states.[43] These were cases directly traced to specific transmission events. They were just the start. Many more resulted through second-, third-, and fourth-level (and higher) transmissions.

The difficulty of determining the true effect of events like Sturgis becomes more difficult when these chains of transmission grow long. Because of a lack of a concrete link showing that his infection occurred in Sturgis, Kenny Cervantes was not included in the official infection count connected to the rally. Neither were others like him. Kris Ehresmann, director of infectious disease epidemiology at the Minnesota Department of Health, discussed a group of infections from a fall 2020 Minnesota wedding with the *Washington Post*. The infections were linked back to someone who had gone to Sturgis but was not tallied in the official Sturgis case count because, she explained, "The web [of interactions] just gets too complicated."[44]

This is one of the problems with pandemic statistics: We can't directly observe infections. We have to infer the chains of transmission that occur across our communities. To try to identify the effects of the Sturgis rally more concretely, the Centers for Disease Control and Prevention (CDC) began requesting data from states that reported positive test results from people who had traveled to South Dakota during the time of the rally. Through this method, they were able to identify 463 primary cases and an additional 186 secondary cases in people who had contact with someone who had traveled to South Dakota in late August 2020.[45]

From each of these cases, one becomes two, two becomes four, four becomes eight, and so on. The important effects of events like Sturgis don't happen in Sturgis; they happen when Sturgis attendees go home and infections spread far and wide. It is the opposite of the television commercials for Las Vegas that state, "What happens in Vegas, stays in Vegas." With epidemics, what happens in places like Sturgis goes home with you and creates an epidemic in your neighborhood.

A group of researchers at the Center for Health Economics and Policy Studies at San Diego State University attempted to quantify the magnitude of the COVID-19 infections that could be attributed to the Sturgis rally. Using mobile phone data, they identified the home county of people in Sturgis during the rally.[46] Using data from these counties, the researchers compared the growth in cases in counties where some residents had attended the Sturgis rally to similar counties where no residents had attended the rally (along with various data to control for differences between these counties). What the researchers found shocked many. They attributed 115,000 to 260,000 cases to the Sturgis rally after just one month. This was between 10 and 20 percent of all cases within the United States during this time period.[47]

When we compare these results to the results of the Biogen super-spreading conference, their greater magnitude is not surprising. The individuals attending the Biogen conference and staying in the hotel where the conference took place numbered in the hundreds. The individuals attending the Sturgis rally numbered in the hundreds of thousands. The Sturgis attendees almost certainly sparked many additional super-spreading events in their home counties in subsequent weeks. The rally was bound to be a firestorm, especially in a world where vaccines were not yet available to temper the fire. Further, after Sturgis, the attendees continued risky interactions with other people who took risks. Just like in Sturgis, when the attendees went back to their hometowns and patronized restaurants and visited public places, they interacted with others who were also cavalier about exposure risk. Risky mixed with risky back home, and infections cascaded outward there as well. This was all for the personal right to, as the T-shirts stated, "Screw COVID I went to Sturgis."

Risk sharing of this unwanted nature has occurred before but among those much less aware of its damage.

Mecca is the holiest place in the Islamic religion. It was the birthplace of Muhammad and the location where Allah revealed the Qur'an to him through the archangel Gabriel. The Hajj is an annual pilgrimage to Mecca on which pilgrims perform a series of rituals that recall those performed by Muhammad and 1,400 of his followers in 628 AD. The pilgrimage is a central ritual of Muslim faith and is one of the five pillars of Islam, along with the profession of faith (*shahada*), prayer (*salat*), alms (*zakat*), and fasting (*sawm*). All Muslims who are physically and financially able must participate in at least one Hajj in their lifetime.

In contrast to the Sturgis rally, the number of attendees at the Hajj in the early years of the COVID-19 pandemic was purposely limited to promote safety. In 2020, fewer than one thousand Saudi citizens and residents were allowed to take part. In 2021, the event was limited to sixty thousand fully vaccinated Saudi citizens and residents. When limits like these are not in place, the Hajj attracts one to two million people to Mecca each year. Even centuries ago, when the world population was much smaller, the pilgrimage still attracted vast numbers of people.

Between 1500 and 1800 AD, the Ottoman Empire was a large sponsor of the Hajj. The empire created large caravans escorted by the military and built roads, fortifications, and other infrastructure linking Damascus to Mecca.[48] By the 1800s these caravans included pilgrims numbering in the tens of thousands. The British colonies in Southeast Asia and India were another large source of pilgrims. Prior to the nineteenth century, most Muslim people from within these areas were unable to afford passage to Mecca in terms of either money or time. As such, the pilgrims from this area tended to be wealthy merchants or elite officials.[49]

In the nineteenth century, the introduction of railroads and steamships converted the Hajj from a pilgrimage of elites to a mass event dominated by the rural poor. People now packed aboard steamships on inexpensive third- and fourth-class tickets to make their once-in-a-lifetime journey.[50] Such a ship provided a setting in Joseph Conrad's *Lord Jim*. With this easy and fast transport, more and more Muslims were able to participate in the Hajj, which created larger and larger gatherings. This massive growth of Hajj attendance occurred at the height of the Columbian Exchange, when expanding markets allowed microbes to travel the world. With the influx of pilgrims from poorer geographies, particularly those who inhabited areas with endemic cholera, the risk of widespread epidemics increased.

The Hajj led to at least forty outbreaks of cholera in the area surrounding Mecca between 1831 and 1912.[51] Estimates place thirty thousand cholera deaths at the Hajj in 1831.[52] From there, cholera spread across Europe, reaching England and Ireland, and then crossed the Atlantic Ocean to

North America for the first time. As epidemic disease historian William McNeill writes, "Thereafter [1831] until 1912 . . . epidemics of this dreaded disease were a common accompaniment of the Moslem pilgrimage."[53] Mecca became an intense breeding ground for cholera. The Hajj brought together people from across Asia, Europe, and northern Africa. They all mixed together in one place at one time. Once cholera took root among the pilgrims, a wildfire of infectious disease was set off that burned hot and bright throughout Mecca. From Mecca, cholera spread widely throughout the world. McNeill writes that the "inevitable result was the re-enactment of the patterns of epidemic dispersion long familiar within India, but this time on a much expanded geographic scale as followers of Muhammad headed homeward, whether west to Morocco or east to Mindanao, or to points between."

As it did in Sturgis in 2020, infectious disease was unknowingly carried to a mass gathering. There it festered among the participants. Afterward, they carried it homeward, depositing disease along the way. In Mecca, the pattern of cholera arrival and dissemination continued for decades. An 1852 epidemic is estimated to have killed over a million people in Russia.[54] In 1865, at least 15,000 pilgrims died. Then the epidemic spread widely within Egypt, leading to another 60,000 deaths, and then to Marseille and the rest of Europe. By the end of this epidemic, at least 200,000 people had died from cholera in major world cities.[55] Another outbreak at the turn to the twentieth century may have killed up to ten million people in India alone and another 500,000 in Russia.[56]

Tensions among liberty, religion, freedom, and commerce abounded in the circumstances surrounding the Hajj. First, the Hajj came to be a pilgrimage of the poor. As such, when nations of Asia, Europe, and North Africa stepped in to enact preventative measures such as quarantines, they had a disproportionate impact on the underprivileged. Wealthy pilgrims had the financial wherewithal to undergo a long period of quarantine, or perhaps several such quarantines, during a return trip home. They could afford private staterooms and more luxurious ships with fewer passengers packed aboard. The less wealthy traveled aboard more congested ships; and, when cholera was found, dead bodies were tossed overboard to hide the infestation at inspection points. One story described one hundred bodies being discarded from a single ship so that the presence of cholera was not detected at a Suez inspection station during a return trip from the 1865 Hajj.[57] The ship could not afford to be delayed on its return.

Second, particularly for the British, interfering in the religious sanctity of the Hajj was dangerous for maintaining political control of India. As historian Michael Low writes, the British "feared that direct interference with this fundamental Islamic practice would incite a backlash in India. . . . Britain worried that restricting access to the Hajj would agitate its Muslim subjects."[58] We can compare this tension to the tensions that mounted between some religious organizations and governments during the time of mass gathering limits of the COVID-19 pandemic. When government authorities enacted mass gathering limits, some religious organizations pushed back on grounds of religious freedom. Some even held ceremonies in spite of bans on large gatherings. Clandestine religious services were held in bookshops, cafes, and basements. As one minister of a London church declared, "I don't believe the government has the authority to tell the church of Jesus Christ that it can't gather for worship. They just classed us as non-essential. But we believe worship is the most essential thing in life."[59] This church continued to hold services twice each Sunday with about 160 people attending.

Third, colonial rule of India was vastly profitable for the British. Anything that inhibited the free flow of goods and trade between India and Europe was bad for business. Britain continually found itself trying to balance the competing incentives of maintaining control of the Indian subcontinent and encouraging free trade and commerce on one side and controlling the dangers of epidemic spread on the other. This balancing act brought it into disagreement with other nations that wanted greater attention paid to public health than profits. These nations wanted to control the Hajj and its routes to and from Mecca more forcefully. In contrast Britain went as far as denying that Indian pilgrims were the source of the outbreak to maintain control.

Within India the largest public health concern was the spread of cholera from pilgrims to the general population. In much the same way that the poor were blamed for the "beggar's disease" in seventeenth-century Vienna, the poor were blamed for cholera's spread across the world. If cholera had remained within the population of the "pauper pilgrims," few among the upper classes and colonial authorities would have cared about the outbreaks.[60] However, they did care when people of their social standing were affected. Quoting W. W. Hunter, English director of general statistics to the government of India, Low writes, "Although India's pilgrim masses might 'care little for life or death,' their 'carelessness imperils lives far more valuable than their own.'"[61] The British colonialists only cared about cholera if it affected those of their rank and class within society, or if it affected their trade. If they had been able to protect themselves, and if cholera had only affected the poor, they likely would have ignored the issue altogether.

Although less extreme, class concerns like this became an underreported issue of the COVID-19 pandemic. Life-saving vaccines and therapeutics became available but these technologies were neither equally available nor equally used across the US population. As journalist Ed Yong of the *Atlantic* frequently stated and wrote, new medical technologies frequently flow up to the wealthy while disease flows down to the impoverished.[62] When arguments over mask and vaccine mandates heightened in 2022, and those with limited financial means continued to struggle with the pandemic, many politicians, along with many civic and education leaders, no longer wished to expend the political capital necessary to continue efforts to enforce mask and vaccine mandates.[63] They relented. They removed mask mandates or let them expire while the Omicron wave was still near its peak and thousands were still dying every week. Politically, they moved to appease those calling for individual liberty. They gave up the fight, and we were left to wonder if they would have done so had members of their own social classes and communities been dying at rates similar to those of the financially less fortunate.[64]

The argument that individual liberty should prevail and enable large-scale attendance at the Sturgis rally led to a local super-spreading event at a minimum and a national super-spreading event at a maximum. The statements the attendees gave to the press only affirmed their individual preference for risk and their own level of risk aversion. Their statements did not express concern about the mass infections and deaths that their behavior would create in the rest of society for those who did not choose to accept this risk. The attendees at Sturgis created an externality just like that created when a firm pollutes a river.

When Sturgis attendees became infected, they infected others. Some of the newly infected were people like Kenny Cervantes's girlfriend, who explicitly tried to avoid exposure at Sturgis. Some were people who did not have the same choice as those who had created the externality. Some who faced the increased exposure risk created by Sturgis attendees were restaurant workers in Sturgis and convenience store workers on the routes that the attendees used to travel home. Some were essential workers, like bus drivers and medical staff, who came in contact with attendees in their hometowns. The exposure risk that Sturgis attendees created reached people on the margin of poverty who had little income, who may have lacked paid sick leave, or who may have lacked medical insurance and easy access to health care. Perhaps some worked in nearby South Dakota meatpacking plants and could not afford to take a week off of work to avoid exposure when cases spiked within their plant. Some of these people took infections back to multigenerational homes and put grandparents at risk.

The behavior of those who accepted their own risk created costs for others in society. In some cases, those costs were the loss of life. The most obstinate of the people calling for individual liberty created harm for others, just like F. Scott Fitzgerald's fictional characters in *The Great Gatsby*. They "were careless people . . . they smashed up things . . . and then retreated back into . . . their vast carelessness . . . and let other people clean up the mess that they made."[65]

It wasn't just Sturgis attendees who caused these problems. Others who demanded an end to mass-gathering limits, resumption of in-person dining, and the opening of large entertainment venues created the same effects. Risky met risky in these locations as well. They created externalities, just like the Sturgis attendees did.

What do we do about externalities in other circumstances? In the case of polluting firms, we stop them from polluting with laws and regulations. We don't allow them the personal choice to dump toxins into a river. If they persist in the behavior, we fine them or charge them to clean up the downstream contamination that they create, or we make them pay those they harm. When charged for their pollution and harm to others, firms have an incentive to pollute less because they must consider the full costs of their actions in their profit calculations. This helps to put costs and benefits back in balance. Economists refer to this as *internalizing* the externality of the firm.

Profit-maximizing firms prefer that others pay these costs. Britain preferred to avoid taking responsibility for keeping the Hajj safer. Restrictions such as more stringent quarantines were needed to prevent the nineteenth-century cholera epidemics from spreading throughout the world. For Britain, these restrictions would have been expensive financially and also would have cost Britain political capital among its colonial subjects in India. Because Britain was not forced to deal with this cost directly, it was able to *free ride*. Rather than pay these financial and political costs, Britain forced others to pay with their health and their lives. The same thing happened in 1918 and in 2020. Arguments in favor of free choice emboldened some to attend large gatherings, ignore mask mandates, and behave recklessly. These choices led to more infections, more hospitalizations, more chronic conditions, and more deaths. These were the costs imposed on others and on society as a whole. These were the costs of free choice and individual liberty. These were the costs forced onto others that led to less liberty for society.

Because we cannot observe the event of an infection in the same way that we can observe an act of water pollution, internalizing infectious disease externalities proves difficult. After all, the British were not even willing to admit that the cholera epidemics at the Hajj had originated within its colonial borders. With COVID-19, anti-mask protesters refused to admit that mask wearing was effective. However, let us imagine that we can trace the pattern of *all* infections in society. In this imaginary world, we know that Sheila infects Iman. Suppose we also know that Sheila is someone who had been unwilling to wear a mask before she became infected and that Iman becomes ill, loses wages from not working, and incurs various medical costs. Suppose we calculate the total costs incurred by Iman to be $20,000. In this hypothetical world in which we can trace Iman's infection back to Sheila, we could fine Sheila the $20,000 damage that her behavior forced Iman to incur. If Sheila is forced to internalize the cost that she has imposed on Iman, Sheila may regret her choice to shirk on mask wearing. If she had known of the fine in advance, she may have worn a mask and not infected Iman. If other mask shirkers were to know that such tracing and levying of fines were possible, they may be more careful too. They may wear a mask more frequently, and because of this many infections would be prevented.

This scenario may seem strange, but it is the same situation that drunk drivers currently face. If drunk drivers injure another person, they are held liable in civil court and charged for the costs incurred by the person whom they hurt. They are also placed in jail or prison for their recklessness. The infectious disease situation is identical, with one exception: we cannot precisely monitor the course of infections. Because of our imperfect observation of infectious disease transmission, we are left with a second-best solution: mandates and prohibition of risky behavior. If we could observe infections directly as a society, we could handle it exactly as we handle the externalities created by drinking and driving and by polluting. We could fine reckless people and place them in jail for making choices that endanger the lives and livelihoods of others.

Drunk-driving laws and penalties benefit society overall. Disallowing the individual liberty to drink and drive creates more liberty for everyone because we all become safer on the roads when we punish drunk drivers. When externalities are present, we often need to constrain individual liberty so that society is better off and so that more liberty is created for society in general. As John Stuart Mill wrote in *On Liberty*, "The only freedom which deserves the name is that of pursuing our own good in our own way, so long as we do not attempt to deprive others of theirs, or impede their efforts to obtain it."[66]

The unintended spread of COVID-19 in the name of individual liberty was not just a Sturgis Motorcycle Rally problem nor just a US problem. Sorting into like-minded groups and making individual decisions to ignore the safety of others occurs across the world. Located just outside of Manchester, England, Daisy Nook Country Park contains one hundred acres of footpaths, bridleways, a lake, woodlands, and meadows. The park is known for bird watching and as a habitat for wildlife. The 1953 painting *Fun Fair at Daisy Nook* by L. S. Lowry sold for £3.4 million in 2011. The painting depicts a festival in a field of the park.

On Saturday night, June 13, 2020, another festival took place at Daisy Nook. This one was an illegal rave attended by approximately 4,000 young people who danced under a banner reading "Quarantine Rave" until the police arrived to break it up.[67] This was not a lone event. Illegal raves occurred across the United Kingdom throughout the summer of 2020. As the weather turned colder, many of the raves moved indoors to abandoned warehouses in cities such as London, Leeds, and Bristol. The events became ubiquitous enough for people to question whether 2020 would surpass the "second summer of love," a term referring to the explosion of the British rave scene during the summer of 1988.

While these young English revelers had little in common with those attending the Sturgis Motorcycle Rally, their sentiments contained a fair amount of overlap. One attendee of the Daisy Nook rave stated to *The Guardian*, "No one is physical distancing. . . . There's a sense of nihilism now, like: whatever will be, will be."[68] Like those in Sturgis, these young people accepted what they determined to be their own risk of exposure to COVID-19. We know this because they were there; if they had been overly concerned, they would have stayed home, following the rules. Some accepted this behavior; one local senior citizen made tea for the revelers at Daisy Nook. Others were far more critical. Sacha Lord, owner of Manchester's music venue The Warehouse Project, tweeted, "You aren't clubbers, just selfish idiots."[69]

In these situations, risk meets risk and safety plummets for everyone. These events sat like a dry pile of kindling just waiting for the right match to land. One spark and the flames erupted. Then it only took one bridge to take the fire to even the most risk averse people. By this time in the pandemic, cases were so widespread that it was difficult to pinpoint the outflow from any single event. When all you can see are flames, you don't know which tree was set afire first. These groups probably didn't understand the damage that they were doing to others in their communities, or perhaps they did not care. Even if they did not face health risks themselves, the exposure risk that they created and passed to others resulted in disease, damage, and death. Their claim to individual liberty limited liberty for others, just as John Stuart Mill had warned in 1859.

Similar to those at Daisy Nook, young adults congregated at venues across the United States in the same time period. In March 2020, college students took spring break trips to the Bahamas and other warm locations. Many older adults were aghast to see photographs of masses of young people shoulder to shoulder at house, pool, and lake parties throughout the summer. Concern grew even more once colleges began welcoming students back to campuses in the fall. About one-third of the 5,000 colleges in the United States attempted to hold in-person classes in the fall of 2020. Many began the semester earlier than usual in order to finish before the US Thanksgiving holiday, attempting to avoid the bridges created by student travel between homes and campuses during that traditional school break.

Many colleges received negative publicity as photographs and stories of large gatherings emerged continuously in August and early September 2020. Jason Chang, a resident assistant at Cornell University, supervised 300 undergraduate students in a dormitory. He described his first week back on campus as "constant insanity and madness" as he tried to coerce students into abiding by social distancing and quarantine protocols.[70] Cornell was not the only college that struggled. Many campuses experienced outbreaks almost immediately when students returned. By mid-August, only days after welcoming students back to campus, several universities were forced to move in-person classes to remote-learning formats. Some did this temporarily, while others closed for the semester. These included high-profile schools such as Michigan State University, the University of North Carolina, and the University of Notre Dame.[71]

For many colleges there were continual struggles with cases, while others seemed to be lucky despite the challenges of maintaining testing, social distancing, and quarantines in an age demographic who often follows MacArthur's quip, "Rules are made to be broken." Not all students acted in this way, and many disagreed with the cavalier behavior of their peers. It was another situation in which sorting occurred related to beliefs about the pandemic. Those who associated lack of social distancing with high exposure risk abided by the rules. The others congregated together. The risky mingled with the risky, and outbreaks across the country were made all the worse.

Like at Sturgis, the outbreaks on college campuses were not confined to only those who participated in the gatherings. Many schools experienced outbreaks that spilled into communities near campus. A study by the *New York Times* documented links between the location of college campuses and COVID-19 infections and deaths in the surrounding communities. Making a demonstrable link was difficult because transmission could not be directly observed. Some college administrators used this ambiguity as an excuse for plausible deniability. Nevertheless, public health authorities near colleges were convinced of the cause of the outbreaks. Jeremy Eschliman, a public health director for Two Rivers Public Health Department, told the *New York Times* that he could "connect the dots" between students and deaths in high-risk populations, such as residents in long-term care facilities. "That is what has started the forest fire here," he argued.[72] Of course it is difficult to prove his assertion directly, and many college administrators across the country disagreed with him.[73]

Other school administrators felt a responsibility to the surrounding communities while also facing an unanticipated dilemma. Although colleges and universities did their best to control behavior on campus, there was little that they could do to control it off campus. Once some colleges stopped holding in-person classes and closed the dormitories, the students on these campuses were set free to act on their own without oversight.

Many students at Michigan State University live in off-campus housing in East Lansing, where they comprise a significant portion of the city's population when classes are in session. When students returned in early August of 2020, cases increased rapidly, and Michigan State was forced to cancel on-campus classes for the fall semester. By the time it did so, many students had already moved into apartments and houses near campus. They had signed leases for the year or semester and decided to stay with their roommates and friends while taking classes remotely.

Debra Furr-Holden, a Michigan State epidemiologist and associate dean for public health integration, told the *New York Times* that these students "swooped down on bars and restaurants and other places and caused outbreaks in the community. . . . We had an unintended negative consequence that these students were then not within our safety and protection and under our purview where we could better dictate testing, isolation, quarantine and all of that."[74] Linda Vail, health officer for Ingham County, told the *New York Times*, "The number of cases just exploded on us."[75]

Universities like Michigan State did their best to control the situation by increasing outreach to students to try to enhance testing.[76] Other colleges and universities went even further, based in part on a study by researchers at the Broad Institute of MIT and Harvard. The researchers developed a model of a mid-sized university of 10,000 students, faculty, and staff. Using data from Colorado Mesa University, they created a network-based model of the interactions within the university and between the university residents and their contacts in the surrounding community. They considered the possibility that the university share its testing resources with non-university contacts within the community. Because people on campus interacted with people in the community, bridges were created between these two populations every day. These populations shared exposure risk with each other. By sharing testing resources, the university could better monitor the shared exposure risk and keep both populations safer. They found that sharing 45 percent of its testing resources with community contacts lowered the rate of infection on campus by 25 percent. Varying the range of parameters within the model yielded the recommendation that the university should share between about one-fifth to three-fifths of its testing resources outside of its gates to minimize an on-campus outbreak.[77] Following this recommendation, Colorado Mesa University provided testing to any self-reported contacts of students and ran a testing center for the local community.[78]

The University of California, Davis followed a similar strategy by offering testing to anyone living or working within the city of Davis.[79] With this strategy, the university provided benefits to the university while also acting as a responsible neighbor to the community. Like firms that pollute rivers, students on college campuses may pollute communities by spreading infections into areas outside their borders. Offering testing to the wider community was an effort to clean up the infectious disease pollution that some UC Davis students had created.

Dr. Brad Pollock directed the UC Davis testing program and chaired the Department of Public Health Science. He told the *New York Times*, "What does it mean to keep your campus well when everyone else is getting sick around you? . . . The university is part of the community."[80] As goes an old saying in epidemiology, "Disease knows no borders."[81] Epidemics don't remain in Sturgis, Mecca, or East Lansing. They travel especially far when individuals do not consider the effects of their actions on others, and they grow especially large when risky individuals mix with other risky individuals. By such behavior, small actions aggregate to become big problems.

Many of us have walked across a college campus or in a public park and noticed a well-worn dirt path cutting through otherwise green grass. Almost certainly the path marks a shortcut between two points, such as between an academic building and a dorm. Sometimes the field is surrounded by a fence in an attempt to discourage people from taking shortcuts to prevent further erosion. We all enjoy lush grass stretched across a field. We all prefer that the visible dirt on these footpaths be replaced with grass. It is obvious where these well-trodden paths come from. Students late for class cut across a field to shave a minute from their tardiness. If only one student takes the shortcut, no damage is done. One person taking the shortcut on one day will not destroy the grass and wear the path into the ground. One student does little damage alone. However, when all students follow the time-cutting incentive to take the shortcut day after day over the years, the grass wears away, and the land becomes scarred.

In 1968 situations like these were collectively given the name "the tragedy of the commons" by ecologist Garrett Hardin, although the roots of the idea long precede him.[82] Imagine a resource available to all of us, such as a public park or fish in an ocean or lake. If we all do our part to maintain the resource, it is preserved in the future for all to use. However, tragedy occurs when our individual benefits do not align with the collective good. When we all allow ourselves the freedom to take as many fish as we want from the lake, the fish are depleted and disappear. In these situations when we follow only our own best interest, we, along with all of society, are ultimately harmed in the long run.

Situations like the tragedy of the commons are referred to as *social dilemmas* by game theorists. Game theory is a tool used by mathematicians, economists, political scientists, and others to study strategic interactions. It is even applied to epidemiology and problems like the tragedy of the commons. The most famous example of a social dilemma in game theory is the prisoner's dilemma, which is similar to a commons problem but concerns only two people. As an example, consider two burglars—call them Bonnie and Clyde—who commit a robbery. The police correctly suspect that they are guilty and arrest them. When apprehended, the duo resist arrest, and both can be charged and convicted of this offense and face one year in prison. However, the police don't have enough evidence to convict the duo of robbery unless one of them confesses to the robbery. After arrest, each criminal is placed in a separate interrogation room and offered a deal. The interrogator says to each individually, "You resisted arrest and face one year in prison. In addition, I know that you committed the robbery. If you confess to the robbery and your partner doesn't, I won't prosecute you for resisting arrest, and you can go home, but your partner will go to prison for ten years. If you confess and your partner also confesses, you will go to prison for eight years. If neither of you confesses, you will each go to prison for one year for resisting arrest." Both are told that their partner was offered the same deal. What should each burglar do?

Take the position of Bonnie in this circumstance. If Clyde confesses, then she is better off confessing: she goes to prison for eight years instead of ten. If Clyde doesn't confess, then she is also better off confessing: she goes home free versus getting one year in prison. Thus, no matter what Clyde does, Bonnie is better off confessing. Clyde has the same set of incentives. If both follow their individual best interest, they each confess, and each goes to prison for eight years. As a duo, this is clearly suboptimal. If they could coordinate and each avoid confessing, they could each leave prison in only one year. However, to achieve this outcome, they each need to pay a cost, namely give up the opportunity to go free if the other does not confess.

This situation is similar to the tragedy of the commons. When we face social dilemmas, choosing to follow our individual incentives leads to worse outcomes for society. The only way that we get to a solution that is best for society is if each of us gives up something of value. Sometimes we expect individuals to do this voluntarily, like roommates who take turns washing dishes. Other times we set laws and rules and impose fines to encourage pro-social behavior. We limit the number of fish that can be caught each day in a lake and fine those who cheat. Or if students don't voluntarily avoid cutting across the lawn, the college could erect a barrier and fine perpetrators who cross it.

Imagine now that the good to be preserved is not grass or an avoidance of prison time, but instead is the health of society. We have a prophylactic means to prevent the spread of an infectious disease. Maybe it is a vaccine against measles or the wearing of a face covering to prevent respiratory disease transmission. Both of these things have a cost. It may be a monetary cost or just a cost of inconvenience. No one that I know likes to be poked in the arm with a sharp object, nor do they enjoy taking time away from something enjoyable in order to be vaccinated. Similarly, masks are uncomfortable. The discomfort may be minimal, but all else being equal, we would rather not wear the mask.

What happens if one of us individually chooses to leave our mask home for the day in order to remain more comfortable? If all of us except for this one person follow the rules and wear a mask, then little harm occurs. The one without the mask is more comfortable and infections remain low because the rest of us all wear our masks. Similarly, if just one of us cuts across the lawn, nothing happens. We too are strictly better off because the person in question arrives to class on time while the lawn remains unharmed.

However, we can see the outcome if many of us follow our individual incentives and behave in this manner. If many of us shirk from mask wearing, more infections occur, more of us are hospitalized, and more of us die. We scar the health of society instead of just a lawn. The perpetrators among us have made everyone in society, including themselves, worse off because the epidemic grows larger and lasts longer. The individual liberty to shirk creates less collective liberty for all of society.

This is the pandemic dilemma.

Another effect harms the most careful when these dilemmas exist. It is sometimes referred to as the *double bind*. Imagine a lake that provides fish to a village. Each of us could catch thirty fish in a day. If each does so, the fish will be depleted and disappear, and all of us suffer. However, if all of us agree to catch only twenty fish per day, the fish population is sustainable, and everyone eats. Suppose that 50 percent of the population is reckless and catches thirty fish per day, regardless of the warning about overfishing. In this world, the cautious 50 percent of us will need to reduce our catch to only ten fish; otherwise, the fish will be depleted. We will need to catch even fewer than our share of twenty fish to keep the lake stocked. We lose in two ways.

When we behave less cautiously during an epidemic, similar things happen. Suppose a college asks students to be tested once per week for infection. If found positive, students must stay home and isolate for one week. Some students may ignore the request to be tested out of concern that they may test positive and miss classes or the chance to participate in an athletic or other extracurricular event. When these students don't get tested, they increase the exposure risk for everyone. When the exposure risk increases, there will be more infections on campus. The students who follow the recommendation to be tested might now test positive and need to isolate more frequently. They might miss more school, perhaps falling behind in their studies, and miss extracurricular activities. To avoid increasing the number of infections, the cautious students must be even more cautious than before and avoid even more activities that could lead to exposure.

Consider another example. A basketball player who follows the rules and tests positive must miss a week of practice. While this itself harms her performance, she loses out even more because the players who don't get tested and who compete with her for playing time are able to attend practice for the week. The basketball player who follows the rules loses practice time both directly and relative to the students who do not get tested. Later in the season, the student who gets tested may lose playing time to the students who don't get tested. The student who follows the rules is placed at a disadvantage relative to those who don't.

This situation played out for New York Mets baseball pitcher Chris Bassitt. After feeling sluggish during a game, he decided to get tested out of caution arising from his wish to protect his young daughter. When he informed the Mets of his positive test, he was forced to miss team practice and playing time. He regretted his decision, and in retrospect wished he had kept his test result private. He stated, "I probably won't [tell the team again]. . . . I should have never said anything."[83] He felt the double bind and wished he had held back the information in order to keep playing. Of course, he could have infected others had he done so.

The same thing happens when students who follow the rules miss classes, a school play, or a graduation ceremony. It happens when laborers miss work. They pay a price and are also placed at a competitive disadvantage relative to others who do not follow the rules. Those who are careful each pay twice for the recklessness of others, just like the conscientious fishers who take home only ten fish while the cheaters take home thirty. This situation increases the temptation to shirk on the rules all the more.

Whether it is vaccines, masks, shortcuts across the grass, or fish from a lake, it is so easy to shirk on the responsibility to play by the rules. Because the effect of our individual actions seems so small in the face of an epidemic, it may seem as if our actions do not matter. We don't notice the slight bending of a few blades of grass nor the extra exposure risk that one reckless person shares with society. Yet if many of us act in this way, we all lose because the individual effects compound and grow larger when many act selfishly.

When we ask or mandate that a person wears a mask, gets a vaccine, or is tested, the most important aim of these actions is not protecting the one person masked, vaccinated, or tested; the most important aim is decreasing the exposure risk for everyone in society. This is how we limit exposure risk so that others don't face health risks. When we all limit risks, we avoid the tragedy of the commons. That is how we avoid millions of deaths in the midst of a pandemic. In limiting our individual liberty, we create more liberty and more freedom for everyone in society because the pandemic is smaller and ends sooner. But we must do it together, collectively, in order to protect against the externalities that develop when individuals shirk their collective responsibility.

In public health emergencies, individual decisions impact others in society. Individual liberties are about individuals. Public health emergencies are about populations and societies. The actions of one impact many and this interdependence between us cannot be avoided during a pandemic.

In these situations, if we allow individuals to choose whether to take a risk or not, they are never choosing only for themselves. Each choice to wear a mask, to practice social distancing, or to accept a vaccine impacts multitudes in society because each choice contains externalities. Acts of noncompliance to recommendations or mandates increase exposure risk for everyone.

In most situations in our lives, we do not have to view the world through the lens of externalities. Most of our choices create benefits and costs for us as individuals. If you live alone, then you have the liberty to choose eggs or cereal for breakfast, and this choice affects no one but you. But we don't live alone in a pandemic world, and we must focus more on how our individual choices impact others. Our choices to mask, vaccinate, and remain socially distant affect others. If we look out only for ourselves and act with only our self interest in mind, like Bonnie and Clyde when they are arrested, then all of society is harmed. Individually minded and self-centered choices create more exposure risk for others in society. When many act without regard to others, exposure risk amplifies all the more for everyone in society.

Your safety depends crucially on the actions of others. And *your risk* is never just *your risk* because you are a part of society. When you decide to accept risk, you are making a choice for everyone. If you get an unlucky flip of the coin during a pandemic, it isn't just you that loses out on a $20 million prize. Everyone loses. Everyone is exposed a bit more if your choice goes awry. Even if you cannot see the damage of an invisible virus transmission that you create, you are still responsible. The transmission that you create ricochets throughout society because we are all connected. One infection becomes two, two becomes four, and so on. No one is alone, and we all face the pandemic dilemma together.

When we fail to control exposure risk, the largest amount of harm falls to those who are most vulnerable. When someone enters a coffee shop without a mask, they face a greater risk of being infected and of infecting others. The person may claim it is their own risk, and that they alone bear it. This argument is false. It is not that person's risk alone. They put the other patrons at risk. They put the server at risk. They put every other person that they interact with in coming days at risk. The other patrons can decide to stay home; we can all survive without a morning coffee and pastry. The server, however, may have little choice but to attend work. The server must earn money to remain housed and buy food. They may have an older or immuno-compromised loved one at home. In a pandemic economy, few extra service sector jobs exist. It isn't easy for the server to simply move to a new job with less exposure risk. Someone's choice to refuse to wear a mask forces the server to choose between health and finance. Both are essential; both are necessary.

As more and more people make these same choices to accept their personal risk, the externalities grow. Sometimes they grow very large, very fast. The largest growth occurs when we allow people accepting of risk to congregate together. Like meets like and risk meets risk at motorcycle rallies, summer raves, and college parties. This happens in less extreme scenarios too. Restaurants, small dinner parties, and family gatherings increase exposure risk as well. In all of these events, the dangers to all amplify and reverberate like feedback from an electric guitar: eventually it becomes uncomfortable for everyone.

This is the danger of mass gatherings, and it is too infrequently stated. Yes, we are worried that one could infect many, when many are present. We are worried about super-spreading. When people return home, we are worried about the bridges that they form elsewhere in the community, nation, and world. However, the risk is greater than that. When only those most accepting of risk attend these events, exposure and infection is almost guaranteed. It sets a fire that escalates and puts everyone at risk—not just those who are there and accept that risk. As the fire blazes it sits just one bridge away from everyone in society, even those who are the most cautious and most vulnerable.

When someone claims to accept the risk of the pandemic, for whom does that person speak? Likely the person means they speak for themself. But that person can't do this. Their actions affect others. We are all connected. No one bears pandemic risk alone. We bear it together. This is unavoidable because of our interconnectedness. In a pandemic, your choice isn't your risk. Your choice to be reckless is a choice that creates exposure risk for everyone near you and everyone connected to you two, three, or more steps away. It involves everyone because we are all connected in the small world in which we live.

There are positive benefits of this connection, too. Because we are all connected, each choice that we make in the name of safety reduces the risk of everyone. Each time you wear a mask, take a vaccine, or avoid a crowded gathering, you protect others. It is as if one additional blade of grass is replanted on the well-trodden path and more grass begins to grow. If we all make these small choices together in the spirit of protecting others, we can un-scar the lawn. This is our responsibility, and we can do it together, proudly, with each act that we take to decrease risk just a little for everyone else. When one has the liberty to choose during a pandemic, that one chooses for all. Whether the choice we make helps or hinders is up to each and every one of us.

Chapter 8

ROGUE WAVES

"It is time to close the book on infectious diseases, and declare the war against pestilence won." This quote, attributed to William H. Stewart, the US Surgeon General from 1965 to 1969, became a ubiquitous straw man used to argue the seriousness of the resurgence of infectious disease. The quote appeared in many places, including a PBS documentary, a *Wall Street Journal* article, and even Dr. Stewart's obituary in the highly prestigious medical journal, the *Lancet*.[1] The problem with using this quote as a setup for arguments extolling the dangers of infectious disease in our times is that it appears Dr. Stewart never uttered these words. It is a false legend with a tangled history and, like most folklore, no definitive origination.[2]

The myth of this quote came about in part because of great decreases in the incidence of infectious disease in the early twentieth century. These reductions occurred because of a multitude of factors. Great improvements occurred in urban sanitation and building ventilation beginning in the middle of the nineteenth century. Improved nutrition, at least for the average member of society, brought better levels of benchmark health. Perhaps most importantly, the germ theory of disease revolutionized how we identified and fought infectious disease. It ushered forth a remarkable string of treatments and illness preventions. Sir Alexander Fleming's accidental discovery of penicillin in 1928 saved millions of soldiers during World War II.[3] Streptomycin provided effective treatment for bubonic plague beginning in

1947.[4] Other antibiotic treatments were found to treat a range of infections. Along with these advancements in treatment came the steady development of vaccines to prevent infection and illness. The Salk and Sabin vaccines eliminated polio as a major health concern in many parts of the world during the 1950s and 1960s. The measles vaccine, discovered and licensed in the 1960s by a team led by Dr. John Enders, drastically reduced the incidence of measles. Prior to this vaccine, 500,000 measles cases were diagnosed each year in the United States alone. By the mid-1970s, cases plummeted to less than 10 percent of those in the two decades prior.

Together these treatments and vaccines led to a false hope in the public consciousness that the end to infectious disease had indeed arrived. This thinking, coupled with comments made by Stewart emphasizing the need to place greater focus on chronic health crises, such as the link between smoking and cancer, likely fed the flames of the myth.[5] Nowhere was the world's public health success more evident than with smallpox.

Smallpox has existed for tens of thousands of years. It ravaged human hosts and killed billions over many centuries of human existence. In the twentieth century alone, over 300 million people died from smallpox and up to 500 million died in the last 100 years of its existence.[6] However, it was defeated by vaccines, and the World Health Organization declared smallpox eradicated in 1980. It has not been seen, outside a lab, since.

Smallpox was not the only major infectious disease during these years. In the eighteenth and nineteenth centuries, periodic epidemics and major pandemics were simply a part of life. Cholera, measles, smallpox, typhoid fever, yellow fever, and other infectious diseases were commonplace. Mortality rates rose and fell by factors of two or three in cities across the world based on which infectious diseases happened to be present during a particular time period. Epidemics rolled into communities in waves and then receded only to splash ashore once again a few years or, sometimes, just months later.

Imagine reliving the experience of the 1793 yellow fever epidemic in Philadelphia where 10 percent of the population died during a brief three-month epidemic. If replicated in today's world, a city such as London, New York, or Tokyo would lose nearly one million people in just three months. Today this magnitude of death is unthinkable in such a short time. However, while the 1793 yellow fever epidemic in Philadelphia was large, it wasn't unique for its time. Epidemics traveled through cities across the world on a regular basis. Morbidity and mortality from infectious disease checkered the global landscape throughout the recorded history of humanity.

The mortality rates from epidemics in New York City tell a typical story for the nineteenth century. In the first half

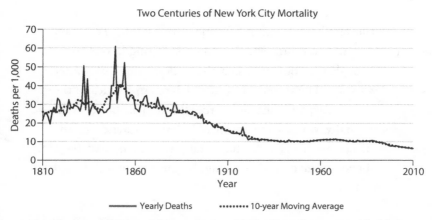

Deaths per 1,000 residents of New York City. *Data provided by Jason M. Barr*

of the century the rates of mortality swung wildly from 20 to 60 deaths per 1,000 residents.[7] These significant waves of mortality, varying from year to year, largely resulted from the arrival and disappearance of epidemics.

When cholera arrived in New York City in 1832, it found a home in the inwardly dense areas of the city that were similar to the lower city of Naples. The Lower East Side tenements and particularly the Five Points neighborhood were struck most severely. Today these neighborhoods house Chinatown and Little Italy as tourist destinations. In the 1800s these were the most inwardly dense and poor neighborhoods of the city, filled with new immigrants. Most came from western European countries like Ireland, Germany, and Italy. Jacob Riis documented these neighborhoods in words and pictures in his 1890 book *How the Other Half Lives*. In this book readers saw pictures of congestion and poverty. They saw pictures of swine roaming the streets to consume garbage in these neighborhoods where the city provided minimal sanitation efforts. They read of the conditions of families housed in tiny apartments bereft of comfort. He describes one in particular:

> The family's condition was most deplorable. The man, his wife, and three small children shivering in one room through the roof of which the pitiless winds of winter whistled. The room was almost barren of furniture; the parents slept on the floor, the children in boxes, and the baby was swung in an old shawl attached to the rafters by cords. . . . The father, a seaman, had been obliged to give up that calling because he was [infected with tuberculosis].[8]

In another apartment, "there were nine in the family: husband, wife, an aged grandmother, and six children; honest hardworking Germans, scrupulously neat, but poor. All nine lived in two rooms, one about ten feet square that served as parlor, bedroom, and eating room, the other a small hall-room made into a kitchen."[9] With the monthly rent more than a week's wages for the father, they could do no better.

In these neighborhoods, disease and death were always near in time or place. In 1832, New York City's first cholera epidemic took more than 3,500 people to the grave. Only 250,000 people lived in the city at the time. Cholera took 1.4 percent of the population in the epidemic. The worst year for infectious disease occurred in 1849. This epidemic started in a manner similar to the yellow fever epidemics in New Orleans. On a Friday night, December 1, 1848, the ship *New York* anchored with quarantine buoys off the Staten Island quarantine station. It had departed Le Havre, France, on November 9 with 352 mostly French and German passengers, along with thirty-three crewmembers. Only twenty-one passengers had the financial means to afford travel in private cabins. The remaining 331 passengers made the voyage in steerage, crowded in the chasm of the lower ship. Upon inspection Dr. Harris, the deputy health officer of the quarantine station, learned that seven steerage passengers had died of a cholera-like illness during the last week of the voyage. Others on board were ill and sent to the quarantine hospital. The remaining steerage passengers were brought ashore to quarantine, where several more became ill and died during a widespread epidemic that broke out within the hospital and quarantine station.[10]

In the communications describing these events, the quarantine station physician Dr. John Sterling also noted that "more than one hundred of the emigrants from the ship *New-York* scaled the walls and fled to the city, or adjacent villages . . ."[11] Shortly thereafter "cases of cholera began to emerge in the slums of the Five Points section of New York

City."[12] From here the epidemic spread. In 1849 more than 5,000 people died from cholera, yielding a total mortality rate of 61 people per 1,000 for the year. In both the 1832 and 1849 cholera outbreaks, mortality the year following fell to about one-half of the year prior. The cholera outbreaks had caused deaths in the city to more than double. Measles, smallpox, typhoid fever, and other infectious diseases caused large spikes in mortality in other years during the first half of the nineteenth century. As New York City moved into the second half of the nineteenth century, the mortality rate began to drop in a slow decline from an average of about 40 people per 1,000 to about 20 people per 1,000. However, the decline was not consistent. There were still periodic outbreaks of infectious disease that greatly changed mortality rates year by year.

The overall mortality rate and large spikes in mortality continued to decline into the twentieth century with one exception. The 1918 influenza pandemic caused another large spike. In this year 12,500 people died from influenza in New York City. This resulted in a total mortality rate of 18 deaths per 1,000 people. While smaller overall than the epidemics of the nineteenth century on a per capita basis, it was large for its time when typical mortality in the years surrounding 1918 were 13 per 1,000. Deaths increased by nearly 50 percent beyond the previous year from the influenza pandemic.

Following the 1918 pandemic, instances of wide-scale infectious disease mortality noticeably diminished in New York City and the rate of mortality became less volatile. With this in mind, one can better understand why people were apt to misquote Dr. Stewart in the 1960s. The dangers of infectious disease, at least of the magnitude of the nineteenth century, simply no longer existed—or so they thought. Despite this trend polio arrived in the first half of the century. Smaller influenza pandemics occurred in 1957 and 1968. The HIV/AIDS epidemic broke out in the 1980s. Clearly, the book on infectious disease was still open and the war against pestilence had not been won.

After 1850 mortality rates steadily declined due to advancements in medical technology and scientific and epidemiological knowledge, along with general improvements in sanitation, ventilation, and nutrition. Because of these advancements, it is difficult to compare the magnitude of particular epidemics that occurred in different time periods during these two hundred years. To make these comparisons across time and locations, epidemiologists frequently compare deaths in a given time period to deaths that are typical for the time period. This is called excess death analysis. We often state excess deaths in percentage terms, relative to expected deaths, in order to facilitate comparison across time or geography. For instance, in 1832 when 51 people died per 1,000 residents, the average mortality rate in New York City for years surrounding 1832 was 30 per 1,000. Thus the 1832 cholera epidemic resulted in an increase of about 21 extra deaths per 1,000 people above what was typical of the time. If we divide 21 by 30, we see that this particular cholera outbreak increased mortality by about 70 percent in 1832. The 1849 cholera epidemic resulted in an increase in the mortality rate of about 69 percent. Moving forward, the 1918 influenza pandemic caused a 38 percent increase in the rate of mortality. By using percentage increases, it is easier to compare a cholera epidemic in 1849 to the influenza outbreak in 1918, or to a spike in deaths due to World War II, or the New York City AIDS epidemic.

When I perform this analysis for New York City, the largest one-year mortality increase, in percentage terms, occurred during the 1832 cholera epidemic. The 1918 influenza pandemic ranks fifth on the list of largest epidemics in percentage terms. While there are still four years from the nineteenth century that display larger percentage increases than 1918, 1918 is noticeable as an especially large epidemic for its place in history. It is a bit smaller but roughly on par with the largest nineteenth-century epidemics in terms of a percentage increase in mortality.

Mortality rates in the decades following 1918 are far smoother than any decade of the nineteenth century. Not a single year in the twentieth century is remotely comparable to 1918. The next closest increase was the 8 percent increase in 1943 largely caused by deaths of New York City residents fighting in World War II. By comparison, the nineteenth century provided a series of epidemic waves that did not relent. During this time, wild fluctuations were the norm due to the commonplace occurrence of infectious disease outbreaks. This was not so in the twentieth century where 1918 remains the most recent severe pandemic by a shocking margin.

When looking to the past, excess mortality calculations are especially useful. In the nineteenth century health records were not as precise as they are today. It was hard to know the true count of deaths *caused* by cholera in 1832 New York City. Not all cholera deaths were recorded as such. Some in more affluent neighborhoods purposely had the cause of death omitted from the death records. They did not want a loved one confused with someone from the poor sections of the city where disease ran rampant. A cholera death would tarnish the family's reputation. However, because data on deaths in general—meaning deaths that are not specifically attributable to a cause or event—are more consistently tabulated, one can look at the changes in mortality rates over time to examine deviations from typical trends. By doing so, we can get a more accurate picture of the number of deaths that can be attributed to a specific epidemiological event. This is true today as well. We commonly use excess mortality to measure the effect of epidemics in countries without well-developed medical infrastructure and data collection. We also used it to statistically count the number of people dying "from COVID" as opposed to "with COVID" when controversies developed about the under- or over-counting of COVID-19 deaths.[13]

At the onset of COVID-19 many health agencies focused their concern on the dangers to populations in more impoverished areas of the world, particularly those with minimal access to health care. Impoverished areas in India were one area of particular concern. On March 24, 2020, India's prime minister Narendra Modi announced that "there will be a total ban of coming out of your homes. . . . Every state, every district, every village will be under lockdown."[14] He stated these words *four hours* before the lockdown took effect. For the next twenty-one days, 1.3 billion people were ordered to stay in their homes. During a lockdown, people are mandated to remain within their home, property, apartment building, or neighborhood. In certain Chinese cities, gates were erected and people were literally locked into their neighborhoods or apartment buildings. This is distinct from the "stay-at-home" orders that were common in Europe and North America. In these countries, staying at home was merely a suggestion and people could still walk in parks, shop for groceries, or perform other tasks.

The *New York Times* described the lockdown in India: "Hours before Mr. Modi's televised address [announcing the lockdown], the long straight boulevards of New Delhi, the capital, resembled deserted racetracks. All the stores in the center of town were shut, but in the poorer neighborhoods, just outside of the city, it was a different story."[15]

The *Times* goes on to describe crowded, narrow lanes, people sleeping in bus shelters, and cramped tenements all yielding the "impossibility of maintaining social distance."[16]

In the congested quarters of the impoverished districts of the city, access to food was of grave concern. One woman told the *New York Times*, "We dare not step out even to buy vegetables whose prices have skyrocketed. . . . If coronavirus does not kill us, hunger will." A house painter who had not worked in days, had the total equivalent of $50 to his name, and was overdue on his rent, stated: "All I'm thinking right now is how to put food in my children's stomachs."[17] Millions of migrant workers across India were stranded, apart from the loved ones that depended upon them for income. Many fled the cities, walking, biking, and hitching rides on cargo trucks to try to get to their families, some of whom were hundreds of miles away. Jyoti Kumari had come to Delhi to care for her injured father. As they were running out of money to buy food, she used "her last $20 to buy a hot-pink bicycle—and cycled more than 700 miles across the country in a week with her father riding on the back."[18] To return other laborers home, the Indian government created a special train service, the Shramik (meaning "laborer" in Hindi) Specials.[19] They were intended to ease the burden on this population and get them to their families in safer and more financially secure environments where housing and food were less expensive.

However, the trains were packed. So were the stations. The trips sometimes took days. The travel itself created the inward density on train cars that was bound to spread the virus. The routes into rural areas provided a multitude of bridges that spread the virus to more geographically diverse areas. Two brothers recounted a May 2020 conversation between them to the *New York Times*: "You really think we should be doing this?" The response: "What else are we going to do? We have nothing to eat and our money's out."[20]

The trains were dangerous. Although screening prior to boarding was required, the reality was different and social distancing "was nonexistent."[21] In total over 4,600 Shramik Specials ran carrying 6.3 million tightly packed passengers.[22]

However well-intentioned, the trains created health burdens. Over forty thousand railway employees tested positive and nearly seven hundred died, according to the *Indian Express*.[23] But this was just the start. Areas where the trains deposited travelers outside the cities soon became pandemic hotbeds.[24] The trains had provided bridges across which the pandemic spread outward from cities and into the surrounding areas. Other methods used by migrants to return home hastened the spread as well.

Similar patterns repeated when the country imposed new, although less strict, lockdowns during another pandemic wave in 2021. The pandemic in India would grow to be the third largest in terms of officially counted COVID-19 deaths, with over 485,000 by the end of 2021. It trailed only the United States, which had 850,000 deaths and Brazil, which had 620,000. With the huge population of India, this was viewed by some as a success. In terms of per capita deaths, India fared better than average and better than many of the more affluent countries in Europe and the United States. Had disaster been averted? Unfortunately not.

Some things did not add up. In a country as large as India, with a massive rural population and an urban slum population that lacked access to health care, it was likely that not all COVID-19 deaths had been accurately counted. This is exactly what the World Health Organization found by examining excess deaths. In 2020 and 2021, India should have suffered about 18.5 million deaths under normal circumstances. Instead, 23.3 million deaths actually occurred.

There were about 4.7 million *extra* deaths in India during these two years of the pandemic—nearly ten times the number of officially reported COVID-19 deaths. Of these extra deaths, 800,000 occurred in 2020 and 3.9 million extra deaths occurred in 2021. Measured as a percentage increase, the total deaths in India were 9 percent above normal in 2020 and 42 percent above normal in 2021.[25] For comparison, the same study found rates of death in the United States to be 15 percent above normal in both years. For the United Kingdom, rates of death were 14 and 10 percent above normal in 2020 and 2021. The increase in deaths in India in 2021 was near the levels of the large outbreaks of nineteenth-century New York City in terms of percentage increase in mortality. India did not escape the pandemic as the official numbers indicated. In fact, many of the worst fears were realized.

Rogue waves, long the subject of seafarer tales, are large, unexpected, sudden swells of water that have been known to create damage to ships at sea and, in extreme cases, the sinking of even large modern ships.[26] While their formation is not fully understood, a convergence of forces (winds, currents, and others) creates moving ridges of water that are unusually large for the sea conditions of the moment. On January 1, 1995, a single monster wave was recorded at the Draupner E drilling platform in the North Sea. This wave reached a height of 84 feet, more than twice as high as the other waves during that day.

Looking back on the pandemic of 2020, New York City will be remembered for the rogue wave that crashed upon it in March and April. The epidemic waters were choppy, and cases had popped up in cities on the West Coast in California, Oregon, and Washington. There was concern in

New York, with a scattering of infections here and there, in and around the city. Then suddenly the rogue wave washed across the metro area and into the neighboring states and regions. The catastrophic impact arrived, metaphorically speaking, in the middle of the night. By the time we awoke with a start, it was upon us, and the only thing left was to mitigate the damage that was out of control. Like a flood, there was no way to instantly remove the water. It inundated us until it seeped away slowly.

The United States Centers for Disease Control and Prevention (CDC) has published continual updates to excess deaths for the nation and individual states throughout the pandemic.[27] Most states saw epidemic peaks with a weekly excess death total 50 to 100 percent above normal. For each two people who normally died, an extra one to two were dying at the pandemic peaks. These values were not sustained throughout the year. For instance, South Dakota had weekly rates of excess mortality below 5 percent for almost the entire pandemic. The only exceptions were peaks that followed the outbreaks in meat packing plants in the summer of 2020 and a large wave in the fall of 2020 that continued into winter. This wave started in early fall not long after the Sturgis Motorcycle Rally. It would crest at a weekly percentage of excess deaths of just over 100 percent above normal in late 2020. This means that for every one person expected to die, one additional person died.

New York City, in late March and early April 2020, was very different from any other large city at the time. Deaths were so great that one school carpenter, who normally works repairing doors, floors, and other school infrastructure, was tasked with building makeshift caskets inside of a high school gymnasium.[28] Freezer trucks lined streets outside hospitals when burials could not keep up with deaths.

As late as November of 2020 there were still about 650 unclaimed bodies in freezer trucks at Sunset Park in Brooklyn, which was the site of one improvised pandemic morgue.[29] The number of deaths in New York City during this time period peaked at rates 600 percent greater than normal. For every death expected in normal times within New York City there were six additional deaths at the height of the spring 2020 COVID-19 pandemic. It is hard to fathom this. There isn't a good comparison in modern history. In World War II, over 400,000 US soldiers died fighting in a little over three and a half years. The war was gruesome and horrible. On D-Day alone, 2,501 US soldiers died.[30] In New York City, at the height of the 2020 pandemic, nearly five thousand people were dying from COVID-19 each week. Over twenty-four thousand people died in a seven-week period when the pandemic wave first hit New York City. This was the tsunami of rogue waves.[31]

The city fared far better in the other periods of the COVID-19 pandemic, yet the rogue wave of spring 2020 left the city with deaths 43 percent higher than expected for the year. This places it fourth on the list of largest epidemics in the city over the past 200 years. When measured as a percentage above normal, excess deaths in 2020 were 9 percent higher than those that occurred during the 1918 influenza pandemic. The only years that eclipse 2020 by a large margin are the historic cholera epidemics of 1832 and 1849.

The difference between the year 2020 and the decades immediately prior stand out more than anything. One can pinpoint excess deaths from polio, World War II, the 1968 influenza pandemic, and the HIV/AIDS epidemic. These were all huge and tragic events; many books have been written about each. However, no single year of these events compare to what transpired within New York City in 2020. (However, cumulative AIDS deaths in New York City ex-

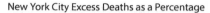

New York City Excess Deaths as a Percentage

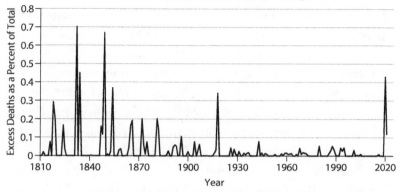

Excess deaths as a percentage of expected deaths in New York City. *Underlying rate of death data provided by Jason M. Barr. Excess death calculations by the author*

ceed 100,000 lives lost, a total far greater than cumulative COVID-19 deaths in the city to date.)

Philadelphia in 1793 experienced a rogue wave in the midst of a metaphorical hurricane. New York City's rogue wave in 2020 appeared out of calm seas. Will the next one hundred years return us to the frequent storms of the eighteenth and nineteenth centuries or the calm waters that existed for the last eighty years of the twentieth century? There are arguments in both directions. Medical technology, health care, and sanitation all far exceed that of the 1800s. At the same time, population expansion, deforestation, and global warming has put humanity in contact with different and novel microbes each and every day. The world has also experienced another revolution of global travel. The invention of the steamship hastened global travel and the spread of infectious disease in the early nineteenth century. This travel can be faulted for the epidemic peaks of the nineteenth century as much as microbes. Yet that advance is nothing like the explosion of international air travel during the past fifty years. In 1970 there were 310 million air passengers per year. In 2019 there were 4.6 *billion*. In fifty years, air travel has increased by a factor of fifteen. In the last decade alone air travel has doubled. An epidemic in one corner of the globe spreads across the world in days or weeks in today's hyper-conencted and hyper-mobile world. It isn't yet clear whether hurricane season has returned or if calm seas will prevail after the rogue wave of COVID-19.

Even though the pandemic washed over all parts of New York City, the pandemic did not threaten all equally. Some neighborhoods, particularly those that had greater levels of inward density, suffered more. These neighborhoods contained higher proportions of people of color. The peak of the epidemic across New York City created deaths 6 times greater than normal. For white residents of the city mortality increased 3.9 times normal rates at the peak of the pandemic. While this is shocking and large, people of color fared far worse. The Black population died at rates 7.2 times greater than normal. Deaths in the Asian population were 7.7 times greater than normal. Members of the Latinx population died at an astounding 9.6 times the normal rate.

These were the differences in outcomes at the peak of the epidemic. The differences between people of color and the white population continued over the entire year. Overall, in 2020 the increase in the rate of mortality was about 25 percent for the white population of the city. As a historical comparison there are only a handful of nineteenth-century epidemics that exceed this rate of excess mortality. Yet it is not unlike the multitude of spikes we see throughout the nineteenth century that were around 20 percent or higher. People of color, however, had much worse outcomes. During the year 2020, people of color had an increase in rate of mortality of over 50 percent. The pandemic tsunami for people of color was twice as large as that of white individuals. The Latinx population in particular suffered a mortality rate increase of 63 percent. These rates are close to those of the cholera epidemics of 1832 and 1849.

However, we need to be careful in making this comparison. The data presented earlier concerning these nineteenth-century epidemics is for the city as a whole. It is an averaging of the experiences of all of the neighborhoods and all populations of the city taken together. Just like the year 2020, it is certain that the poorer neighborhoods, like Five Points, had outcomes much worse than other areas of the city in the 1800s. Jacob Riis noted that residents of the Gotham Court block of Fourth Ward had mortality rates during the "last great cholera epidemic" at the unprecedented rate of "195 in 1,000 inhabitants."[32] He noted elsewhere this epidemic "scarcely touched the clean wards."[33] It wasn't just cholera that menaced these neighborhoods. "A sanitary official counted 146 cases of sickness in [Gotham Court], including 'all kinds of infectious disease' from small-pox down, and reported that of 138 children born [on the block] in less than three years 61 had died, mostly before they were one year old."[34] Going back to the nineteenth century and exploring the origins of this neighborhood will help us to understand why it stood out as unique.

Collect Pond was a forty-eight-acre body of fresh water near the site of present-day Chinatown in Manhattan. Sixty feet at its deepest point, it was fed by an underground spring. As depicted in Archibald Robertson's 1798 painting, the area around it provided a bucolic setting.[35] Bayard Hill rose 110 feet above its banks. It was surrounded by a diverse ecosystem of trees, berries, and wildlife. The pond was used for picnicking in summer and ice skating in winter.[36] Until the beginning of the 1800s it was a primary source of drinking water for Manhattan's growing population.

The area around Collect Pond changed rapidly as population and industry grew. Land near this water source provided prime real estate for slaughterhouses, tanneries, and breweries that needed water to operate or discard waste. These industries came to surround the pond. The commercial activities all liberally dumped discarded animal remains, refuse, and other pollutants into the pond. Pollution and the accompanying stench grew to a point that intervention was needed. The city decided to build a series of canals to drain the pond through the marshy land nearby. Bayard Hill was leveled into the pond and the remaining area was backfilled with construction debris, trash, and any other materials the builders could find.[37] With an open-top canal continually draining water from the underground spring and passing through polluted land, the odor of the area was putrid. In order to remedy the stench, the city began converting the canal into the equivalent of an underground sewer, which was completed in 1821. When it was fully covered and lined with trees it became known as Canal Street, which still exists in the city today.[38]

With the new land available atop the former pond, and the tanneries and slaughterhouses having left, developers entered. They constructed new high-end apartments and named the area Paradise Square.[39] Unfortunately, it would not live up to this name. Built atop marshy land with new water continually entering underneath from the natural spring, Paradise Square began to sink. Buildings tilted and settled unevenly like the Tower of Pisa. Further, the odors from the polluted land began to manifest again. Rain and snow produced flooding and muddied the stench-filled streets. Those who could afford better environments left the newly built but sinking apartments and homes; they were replaced by poorer residents who sought inexpensive housing. Landlords began subdividing their structures into smaller dwellings. While describing other tenements created from larger dwellings in nearby Gotham Court, Riis wrote, "Their large rooms were partitioned into several smaller ones, without regard to light or ventilation."[40] The developers capitalized on the influx of low-income residents seeking nothing other than minimal quarters. Soon, the buildings "became filled from cellar to garret with a class of tenantry living from hand to mouth."[41] The new residents were frequently immigrants seeking a fresh start in the New World. A spiral began and continued unabated as those with more wealth fled and the less well-to-do arrived in wave after wave of immigration. At the bottom of the spiral, the Five Points neighborhood of Manhattan was born.

Named for the oddly shaped intersection of Anthony, Cross, and Orange Streets, Five Points was easily the most notorious nineteenth-century slum in America. Charles Dickens described scenes from the neighborhood in his *American Notes for General Circulation.* "This is the place, these narrow ways, diverging to the right and left, and reeking everywhere with dirt and filth. . . . Debauchery has made the very houses prematurely old. See how the rotten beams are tumbling down, and how the patched and broken windows seem to scowl dimly, like the eyes that have been hurt in drunken frays."[42] He continued, further in the passage:

> What place is this, to which the squalid street conducts us? A kind of square of leprous houses, some of which are attainable only by crazy wooden stairs without. What lies beyond this tottering flight of steps? . . . A miserable room lighted by one dim candle and destitute of all comfort, save that which may be hidden in a wretched bed.

Beside it sits a man: his elbows on his knees: his forehead hidden in his hands. "What ails that man?".... "Fever" he sullenly replies without looking up.[43]

Not only was Five Points infamous for debauchery, crime, and poverty, it was known equally so for its connection to infectious disease. The subdivided rooms that created more apartments lacked sanitation and fresh air. This problem grew worse as the already dense population of the sixth ward that included Five Points increased by over 80 percent from 1830 to 1855. Most of this increase occurred as immigrant populations, many fleeing abject poverty in their home countries, flooded the neighborhood. By 1855, 89 percent of adults in Five Points were foreign born.[44]

Much of the original housing in Five Points consisted of two- to three-story houses. Measuring approximately 25 × 25 feet, these buildings were originally designed to hold a place of business, a proprietor and family, and sometimes a few employees or an apprentice. As the neighborhood grew and slowly changed, these buildings were converted into sets of two to five apartments along with space on the ground floor for a storefront or pub. Many of the converted apartments consisted of a single room that housed an entire family. Most lacked windows and the ability for air to circulate.[45] In terms of creating the ideal breeding ground for an infectious disease such as tuberculosis, measles, or smallpox, this was particularly hazardous. Equally harmful in terms of spreading a disease like cholera, most tenements of the district were not connected to sewers. Heavy rains and accompanying floods washed excrement carrying cholera bacterium from outhouses into basements and streets, where it eventually reached the water supply.[46] Then it was nearly impossible to stop the contagion. Even worse, at the time of the great cholera epidemics of the mid-nineteenth century, the source of the infection was unknown.

No building in New York City was more notorious as a representation of the living conditions in Five Points than the Old Brewery, which sat on Cross Street one block to the west of the Five Points intersection and adjacent to Paradise Square. This location is approximately where the New York County Supreme Court sits today. Formally, the building had been constructed by Coulthard's Brewery at the height of commercial activity on the banks of Collect Pond in 1792.[47] The brewery used the pond as its water source for brewing. As the neighborhood fell into disrepair so did the brewery. By 1837 the building had become "so dilapidated that it could no longer be used for its original purpose."[48] That, however, did not stop it from being converted into tenement housing with minimal updating.

By all accounts the conditions of the Old Brewery were nearly beyond description. With such infamous squalor, separating fact from myth can be a challenge. As the story goes, one cavernous dwelling room, nicknamed the Den of Thieves, was rumored to house seventy-five men, women, and children. The Old Brewery was also home to a passageway dubbed Murderers' Alley. The storage cellar was converted into twenty rooms. The upper part of the brewery contained seventy-five more rooms. At one point, a murdered young girl allegedly lay in a corner for five days before being buried. Twenty-six people who lived together in one basement room had not been outside for more than a week in their entire time living there. Children born here in windowless apartments lived until their teens without seeing the sun or breathing fresh air.[49] Of course, much of this is hyperbole, folklore, and in some cases, outright fiction. Separating fact from fantasy in the lore of the building is a challenge even for serious historians. Even contemporaneous accounts are filled with exaggerations.

Historian Tyler Anbinder provides a fact-check and a more serious investigation of the living conditions of the Old Brewery. The building was large. It covered both the addresses of 59 and 61 Cross Street and was at least 100 feet deep. Because of this immense size, it did indeed contain a maze of windowless apartments in its most interior hallways. However, it is unlikely that anyone spent their entire childhood within an apartment and excluded entirely from sunlight. An 1850 census found 221 people living across thirty-five apartments, including one containing sixteen people.[50] Anbinder recounts first-hand descriptions of outright squalor. Of course, even these first-hand descriptions of Five Points likely come with a bit of exaggeration. However, there is little doubt that the Old Brewery lived up to its labelling in the *Police Gazette*, as quoted by Anbinder, of "the wickedest house on the wickedest street that ever existed in New York."[51]

Density, poverty, and lack of sanitation led to epidemic outbreaks throughout nineteenth-century New York City. Neighborhoods like Five Points and the Old Brewery were ground zero for pestilence. Neighborhoods that had better sanitation, less congested living conditions, and less inward density in general fared better than their more impoverished counterparts, even in nineteenth-century conditions. We can see this in quotes about how the cholera victims were viewed by other residents. In 2008 historian Kenneth Jackson discussed an exhibition titled *Plague in Gotham! Cholera in Nineteenth-Century New York* at the New York Historical Society. He stated, "Other New Yorkers looked down on the victims. If you got cholera it was your own fault."[52] In the view of many nineteenth-century New Yorkers, infestation of infectious disease was in part due to living conditions and poverty, but also in part due to vice that brought

God's judgement. In this view it was the inhabitants' choice to live this way. Many from the upper classes felt the poor were solely at fault for disease in the city and did not deserve sympathy. As Tyler Anbinder quotes from the *Mercury News* during the 1832 epidemic, "The broken down constitutions of these miserable creatures, perish almost instantly on the attack [of cholera]."[53]

The exhibit also contained contemporaneous letters from John Pintard, who founded the New York Historical Society. In one letter to a daughter concerning the 1832 epidemic, he wrote that the epidemic "is almost exclusively confined to the lower classes of intemperate dissolute and filthy people huddled together like swine. . . ." In another, he wrote "Those sickened must be cured or die off, and being chiefly of the very scum of the city, the quicker [their] dispatch the sooner the malady will cease."[54] People like Pintard blamed the cholera victims for their plight—if they would just move to a better location and choose not to live in squalor they wouldn't suffer. To Pintard it was the poor's own fault that they died and the sooner the city was cleared of these leeches the better.

Even people working for reform viewed the residents of these neighborhoods with an air of contempt. In the introduction to *How the Other Half Lives*, Jacob Riis wrote, "In the tenements all the influences make for evil; because they are the hot-beds of the epidemics that carry death to the rich and poor alike." Similar to the pauper pilgrims of India in this same period of time, the most concern for this population came because of their ability to carry infectious disease to the wealthier population. It wasn't care for the poor that troubled the wealthy, who worried exclusively about their own survival and the effect that the poor had on them. Riis continued his description of evil in the tenement neighborhoods: "The nurseries of pauperism and crime that fill our jails and police courts; that throw off a scum of forty thousand human wrecks to the island asylums and workhouses year by year; that turned out in the last eight [years] . . . half [a] million beggars to prey upon our charities; that maintain a standing army of ten thousand tramps with all that implies; because, above all, they touch the family life with deadly moral contagion."[55] As long as moral contagion, cholera, and other infectious disease stayed in the tenements and didn't expand to more affluent people, most in nineteenth-century New York City didn't care about those in the tenements. When infectious disease did expand more widely, the poor were blamed for both their own plight and the effect that infectious disease had on the affluent.

Additionally, those in the tenements were not seen as true Americans by many who lived in New York at the time. The perspective told in history books of America as a great melting pot where all were equal contains a fair amount of fiction. Recent immigrants from western Europe and everywhere else were seen by many as outsiders. Riis wrote, "One may find for the asking an Italian, a German, a French, African, Spanish, Bohemian, Russian, Scandinavian, Jewish, and Chinese colony. Even the Arab. . . . The one thing you shall vainly ask for in the chief city of America is a distinctly American community."[56] Riis worked for reform to lift those in the tenements out of poverty and squalor, yet even he saw all of these groups in the tenements as un-American. This *othering* of the immigrant groups in the tenements made it all the easier to blame them for their destitution and, when infectious disease arrived, their death.[57] According to this view, it was their own fault.

Misplaced blame occurred in more distant periods of history, too. In one contemporaneous account of the plague in 1349, Franciscan Friar Herman Gigas wrote, "Some say that [the plague] was brought about by the corruption of air; others that the Jews planned to wipe out all the Christians with poison and had poisoned wells and springs everywhere."[58] During this time the penalty for spreading contagion was often death. From another account during the same time period: "All the Jews between Cologne and Austria were burnt—and in Austria they await the same fate."[59] During the 1630 round of plague in Milan, a group of four Spaniards were tortured until they confessed to spreading plague. After continued abuse, including the severing of their hands and being broken on the wheel, they were burned at the stake.[60] Jews throughout Europe were also tortured. To the British, the pauper pilgrims were to blame for cholera outbreaks in the 1800s, as well as the poor who suffered the "beggar's disease" in Vienna in the 1600s.[61] In each of these instances, outsiders were blamed for infectious disease.

Some people blamed Chinese and other Asian populations for COVID-19, too. Racist comments were made about Chinese culture, such as when Luca Zaia, president of the Italian region of Veneto, claimed on February 28, 2020, that Italy would handle the COVID-19 pandemic better than China because of differences in their hygiene. He stated in a television interview, "The hygiene that our people, the Venetians and the Italian citizens, have, the cultural training we have, is that of taking a shower, of washing, of washing one's hands often. It is a cultural fact that China has paid a big price for this epidemic because we have seen them all eat mice live or things like that."[62] Zaia later apologized, sort of: "My words came out badly, I agree. If anyone was offended, I am sorry."[63] How could anyone, Chinese or not, be anything other than offended by his comment? It had the same cultural sensitivity as those made in the nineteenth century and earlier.

In the United States, early in the pandemic, President Trump continually made statements referencing the "China virus" and Secretary of State Mike Pompeo spoke of the "Wuhan virus."[64] This othering rhetoric by these political leaders and many additional people led to increases of anti-Asian racism and violence. On February 3, 2020, a sixty-one-year-old Filipino American named Noel Quintana was slashed across the face from ear to ear with a box cutter when a masked man attacked him.[65] On July 14, 2020, an eighty-nine-year-old Chinese woman was slapped in the face by two men who then set her clothes on fire as she walked outside her apartment in Brooklyn.[66] According to the FBI, anti-Asian hate crimes increased by 73 percent in the United States during 2020.[67]

Anti-Asian violence also increased across the world. In Birmingham, England, a Chinese student's jaw was dislocated as he was "punched, kicked, and subjected to racial taunts" on February 3, 2020. On April 15, 2020, in Melbourne, Australia, two Chinese students at the University of Melbourne were attacked and one was punched in the face after being accosted with "go back to China," "get out of our country," and "you fucking immigrants."[68]

Along with violence and hostility to Asian people, some in the United States came to blame the groups of hospitalized and dying people for their plight. In June, Ohio Senator Stephen A. Huffman extended blame to the Black population. "Could it be that African Americans—the colored population—do not wash their hands as well as other groups? Or wear a mask? Or do not socially distance themselves? Could that just be the explanation of why there's a higher incidence?"[69] Senator Huffman wanted to wash his hands of the responsibility of the social circumstances that led to disproportionate Black deaths in his state by blaming the victims. He was not the only one.

During a May 17, 2020, interview on CNN's *State of the Nation*, US Secretary of Health and Human Services

Alex Azar was interviewed by Jake Tapper about the high rates of COVID-19 deaths in the United States. Azar gave this explanation: "Unfortunately, the American population is very diverse and . . . it is a population with significant unhealthy morbidities that do make many individuals in our communities, in particular African American, minority communities, particularly at risk here because of significant underlying disease health disparities and disease comorbidities." Tapper then responded, "I want to give you an opportunity to clear it up, because it sounded like you were saying that the reason that there are so many dead Americans is because we're unhealthier than the rest of the world." Azar then clarified, "We have a significantly disproportionate burden of comorbidities in the United States, obesity, hypertension, diabetes. These are demonstrated facts . . . that do make us at risk for any type of disease burden."[70] While Azar did continue by saying it would be absurd to blame someone for their health conditions, his previous statement did just that. He blamed the high rates of COVID-19 mortality in the overall US population specifically on "African American" and "minority community" disease comorbidities. What he didn't say made his feelings clear. He didn't follow up and discuss how the comorbidities arise within these populations due to a lack of access to health care and nutritious food. He didn't discuss how these issues related to racism and poverty. Nor did he mention that comorbidities disproportionately affect low-income and uninsured individuals regardless of race and ethnicity.[71] Azar singled out people of color only. He didn't mention the added exposure that people of color faced as a result of their jobs, living conditions, and financial constraints. All of these factors were leading to people of color dying at higher rates than white people. Like Huffman, he wanted no responsibility for their circumstances.

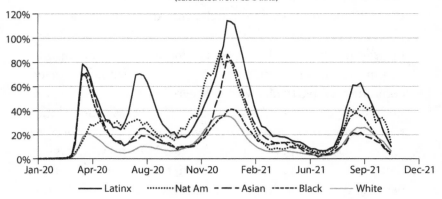

United States excess deaths measured as a percentage above normal through the Delta wave of the COVID-19 pandemic. *Underlying data gathered from the United States Centers for Disease Control and Prevention's web page (www.cdc.gov). Calculations by the author*

The virus that caused COVID-19 didn't seek out populations of color directly. Viruses do not see color. Yet social circumstance, economic inequality, lack of access to health care both before the pandemic and in the midst of it, along with other factors led people of color to stand directly in the path of the coming rogue wave.

Throughout the pandemic, the white population had much lower rates of excess mortality. At various times over the course of the pandemic, Asian, Black, and Latinx populations all reached a weekly peak percentage of excess deaths of at least 65 percent. At this peak, three extra people died for every five that normally die. Through the fall of 2021, the white population experienced none of the exorbitant peaks like the other ethnic and racial groups in the United States. This group hovered in a band of excess mortality typically below 25 percent. It only exceeded this value for a two-month period in the winter of 2020 into 2021 with a peak of just over 35 percent. The Latinx population was above 35 percent excess mortality for almost the entire first year of the pandemic. During nearly the entire first year of the pandemic, the Latinx population had a rate of excess mortality that was greater than the most dire one-week period for white Americans. All groups other than the white population were rarely below 20 percent excess mortality until the effect of vaccines took hold during spring of 2021.

This isn't to say that white Americans were not affected by the pandemic. They were. A 20 or 30 percent increase in rates of mortality is huge. In my lifetime the United States has never experienced such an event. Neither have baby boomers or the generation before them. Even World War II did not cause this level of excess mortality in the United States. COVID-19 was a historic pandemic not rivaled unless we go back more than a century in history to 1918. Nonetheless, the COVID-19 pandemic was woefully unequal.

The waves have rolled in and out throughout the pandemic, but each time their effect has been larger on the least fortunate groups. Urban economist Jason Barr and I performed a demographic analysis of these different waves of the pandemic.[72] The 2020 summer wave was a dramatic shift. It was a movement away from an urban inward density-based epidemic to an epidemic of rural poverty.

Each year for eight years, Marco Antonio Galvan Gomez left his wife and daughter behind in Mexico and traveled 1,200 miles north to the small, 8,000-person town of Dalhart, Texas.[73] Dalhart sits on the border of Dallam and Hartley counties in the northern panhandle of Texas, a short distance from New Mexico and Oklahoma. Together, the two counties have a population of 12,500 people spread across a little less than 3,000 square miles. Population density is a little more than four people per square mile, which is a world far different than New York City in the 1800s or present day.

In early July 2020, forty-eight-year-old Mr. Galvan arrived in Dalhart on an H-2A visa as a temporary contract employee. He worked at the 45,000-acre Larsen Farms, one of the largest potato producers in the country. With production facilities in four states, Larsen provides products to customers as diverse as Whole Foods and Wendy's. At Larsen Farms, Mr. Galvan was one of four hundred other employees and about one hundred other H-2A contract employees. The contract workers lived in a group of sixteen trailers and bunkhouses where up to eleven people crowded together in an inwardly dense environment. Originally hired as a truck driver, Mr. Galvan's duties shifted to work in a warehouse, where he toiled from sunrise to sundown without bathroom or lunch breaks for six days a week.

Ten days after arriving, on July 12, 2020, Mr. Galvan began to feel ill. He developed a fever, sore throat, and body aches before collapsing on his work shift. After telling his wife that he "couldn't possibly go to work,"[74] he arrived the next day for his normal shift but was transferred to the potato fields, where he hoed in 101-degree heat. Speaking by phone that night, he told his wife that he feared he might lose his job if he could not work. She begged him to return home. A coworker accompanied Mr. Galvan to the Larsen Farms office the next day. They were told "no one had permission to leave."[75]

Mr. Galvan tested positive for coronavirus at a local clinic the next day and was placed in an isolation trailer with two other employees. He relied upon the generosity of coworkers for food. No one followed up with him from the local health office after his positive test. He received no medical treatment and relied upon only over-the-counter medications to treat his symptoms while housed in the isolation trailer. On July 19, he spoke to his wife. She told the *Texas Observer* that he "could hardly breathe or speak."[76] He said, "Talk to me. Talk to me. I need to be listening to you because it gives me the strength to continue fighting." This was their last conversation. The next morning, on July 20, 2020, he died.

After Mr. Galvan died, Larsen Farms attempted to charge his family $2,500 to have his ashes returned home. The farm argued that he had not died of COVID-19 but instead had died of a heart attack. A heart attack was listed as the immediate cause of death on his death certificate, with underlying causes of "respiratory distress, possible blood clot, and COVID-19."[77] His family received no worker's compensation benefits. The company's insurance would pay for an accident at work but it would not pay for a COVID-19 death. Eventually the family was informed that Larsen Farms would cover the cost of shipping Mr. Galvan's ashes home.

One would think that the circumstances of Mr. Galvan's death would bring about national outrage. He was neglected despite his work being essential. Yet no one has written extensively of his passing other than Dana Ullman of the *Texas Observer*, from which I based my description of his passing.[78] The ease with which his demise went unnoticed by most was reminiscent of the deaths of immigrants in nineteenth-century New Orleans and New York City. Like many who perished during large epidemics in those times, Mr. Galvan was an immigrant who died in harsh living and working conditions. The country depended upon people like him for essential services during COVID-19, just like they depended upon Irish immigrants to dig canals in New Orleans. His living situation at the farm was crowded and congested, just like it was for immigrants living in New York City tenements. In terms of people per square mile, Mr. Galvan was not in a traditionally dense area. Yet the trailer in which he lived was inwardly dense with up to eleven people living together in a small space. The country depended upon people like him to remain functioning. We needed people like him in order to be able to feed our families. Once he was infected, he was left to die in a quarantine trailer without medical attention. Each year, he left his family to earn the wages that supported them. He didn't want to leave Larsen Farms that summer because he needed the job. He and his family needed the money. Yet if he didn't work, Larsen would find someone else. To them and their bottom line, he was as easily replaceable as a hoe to use in the fields. Their view was little different than that of employers in nineteenth-century New Orleans. However, to his family he was indispensable for more than the wages that he earned. He was a loving father and husband and now he is gone. For them, he can never be replaced.

Even if Larsen Farms had sought medical treatment for Mr. Galvan, it may not have mattered. The local hospital in Dalhart, Coon Memorial, had no cardiac or surgical ICU services. The small rural hospital contained a total of twenty-one in-patient beds. When the hospital became flooded with COVID-19 cases later in the fall, they grew over-whelmed like other rural hospitals. They had no room for patients. They became short-staffed as doctors and nurses tested positive and isolated, and others needed to quarantine from exposures. Many hospitals nearby confronted the same shortages of space and staff. They had no room to take over-flow patients from area hospitals. They lacked beds and ICU care just like Coon Memorial did. This shortage forced Coon Memorial to transfer some critical patients as far as San Antonio, nearly 600 miles away.[79] For a rural area in

America's heartland, this was not unusual. Many small towns throughout middle America faced the same circumstances.

After the summer of 2020, the COVID-19 waves continued to climb and spread further across society. The pandemic crested in the largest wave in the early winter of 2021. In this wave again, the white population continued to fare better than all other groups. At the same time, the Latinx population crested at its worst period of the pandemic with increases in mortality of over 110 percent. This peak for the Latinx population was over three times higher than the peak for the white population. The peak for the Native American population also occurred in the winter of 2020 and 2021 wave. It resulted in nearly a 90 percent increase in deaths. This exorbitant peak was also caused in part by a lack of health care resources and poverty.

The Navajo Nation was established by treaty in 1868, with land covering 27,000 square miles of the states of Arizona, New Mexico, and Utah. This area is slightly larger than the state of West Virginia. About 180,000 people (approximately half of the tribal members) live within this land. Like the panhandle of Texas where Mr. Galvan worked, the Navajo Nation is sparsely populated, with about seven people per square mile. Yet at least one-quarter of the population lives in an overcrowded home, according to the department of Housing and Urban Development. This level is ten times higher than the percentage of people living in overcrowded housing across the United States.[80] While Navajo Nation is not dense by traditional measures, it is inwardly dense. Multigenerational homes are common. The Navajo Nation is poor overall. The median household income is about $27,000 per year. This is less than half of the median household income in the United States. About 40 percent of all people and 50 percent of children within the

Navajo Nation live in poverty.[81] More than one-third of the population lacks running water or electricity in their homes.[82]

During the 1918 influenza epidemic, the Navajo Nation and its communities of Diné people had rates of mortality far greater than the general population in the United States. One recent study places their rate of mortality at 12 percent of the population.[83] When the COVID-19 pandemic moved to the rural United States in the late spring and early summer of 2020, Navajo Nation was one of the first areas to be struck. By early May it had passed New York State in cases per capita.[84]

Melvina Musket spoke to *USA Today* in October 2020.[85] She lived in Gallup, New Mexico, which abuts Navajo Nation, on a sheep ranch in a four-generation household. Her father was a former Marine, a retired mechanic, and a church board member. The family respected the danger of the pandemic. They wore masks and were careful to shop in stores they felt were safe, sometimes driving up to five hours round-trip for groceries when they felt customers in their local store weren't being cautious enough. In early May, Melvina's father began coughing. "Twelve hours later, he was gasping," she said.[86] Despite their best precautions, Dikos Ntsaaígíí-19, which translates from Navajo to mean "cough that kills" or the "big cough," had found the Musket family. Benjamin Musket was taken to the Gallup Indian Medical Center run by the United States Government's Indian Health Service (IHS). When concern grew over the condition of his heart, he was flown to a larger hospital over 100 miles away in Albuquerque. Most of the family in the Musket home subsequently tested positive for COVID. Melvina's mother was hospitalized and transported to Albuquerque too. Her parents died only five days apart in early June.

As winter approached in November and December, the Navajo Nation was overcome with cases, hospitalizations, and deaths. In announcing an extension of the "Stay-At-Home Lockdown," Navajo Nation President Jonathan Nez wrote, "Navajo area IHS has reported that nearly all ICU's [sic] beds are at full capacity . . . we are at a point where our health care providers are going to have to make very difficult decisions in terms of providing medical treatment to COVID-19 patients with very limited resources such as hospital beds, oxygen resources, medical personnel, and little to no options to transport patients to other regional hospitals because they are also near full capacity."[87] Limited resources at Indian Health Service in Navajo Nation, which was already short of medical resources before the pandemic began, were disappearing by the day.

The Indian Health Service was created in 1955 as a division of the United States Department of Health and Human Services. Its primary mission is to provide direct medical care and public health assistance to Native American tribes and Alaskan Native people. In 2020 the national budget included $6 billion for the division. This amounted to a per capita expenditure of about $4,000 per person, an amount less than half of per capita health care spending in the United States.[88] For the Navajo, IHS medical facilities provide about two hundred hospital beds—one for every nine hundred residents of Navajo Nation. This is about one-third of the national per capita rate in the United States.[89] When pandemic relief efforts were allocated, the Navajo once again received fewer per capita resources than the country at large. A total of $714 million was allocated to the Navajo, which was about $4,500 per person on the reservation.[90] The allocation for the entire package across the country was about $6,700 per person. Health care resources were already underfunded for the Navajo before the pandemic. This resulted in worse health outcomes during normal times. The Navajo were a community that was exceptionally vulnerable and needed more assistance to escape the pandemic onslaught. Instead of receiving extra resources because of their vulnerability, they received fewer resources per capita on the reservation than the rest of the country. As a result, 1,808 Diné residents of Navajo Nation died of COVID-19 as of mid-year 2022.[91] This was over 1 percent of the population of Navajo Nation at a rate of 10.5 deaths per 1,000 residents. The rate of death for the US population overall at this time was 3.1 per 1,000.

Taking the year of 2020 in total, the pandemic created an increase in mortality of about 13 percent across the country according to CDC estimates.[92] Being the majority, the white population tracked this total relatively closely, with a 10 percent increase in mortality. People of color, however, had an increase of 23 percent—over twice that experienced by the white population. Latinx people were hit the hardest, with an increase in mortality of 33 percent, more than three times what the white population experienced. The year 2021 was not significantly different in magnitude. Rates of excess mortality were 15 percent for the country as a whole. This was made up of a 13 percent increase for the white population and 25 percent increase for people of color. The effect on the Latinx population was again the most pronounced, with a 37 percent increase in mortality. These were rates of excess mortality similar to those that existed in the middle of the nineteenth century.

There are a few things that stand out when considering the overrepresentation of people of color in the US pandemic mortality statistics. We know people of color more commonly live in inwardly dense and multigenerational homes. They also more commonly work front-facing essential jobs and live closer to the poverty line on average. These types of occupations and neighborhoods face more exposure risk in a pandemic

Finances play a role too. The quintile of most impoverished counties had 43 percent more deaths per capita than the quintile of the least impoverished counties. The difference was even greater during the pandemic peaks in the summer months of 2020 and in early fall of 2021 (the Delta wave). Here, the most impoverished counties had rates of death that were 300 percent and 275 percent greater than the least impoverished counties.[93] It truly was a pandemic of poverty and a pandemic of inequality across race, ethnicity, and income.

Viruses don't choose the people they infect. They don't target specific groups of the population. Instead, they are opportunistic and invade those who happen to cross their path. People of color faced circumstances that placed them in the path of this oncoming tsunami. Their living conditions caused them to experience more exposure risk, and financial constraints didn't allow them the mobility to flee.

Once a person is infected, it becomes important to have experience with the health care system. Like many infectious diseases, COVID-19 was an opportunistic killer. Discussion of the role of comorbidities and general health factors on morbidity and mortality is better left to medical professionals. However, from the social science perspective, one issue stands out: access to health insurance, which leads to preventative care and familiarity with the health care system.

Prior to the passage of the Affordable Care Act (ACA) in March 2010, a consistent 17 percent of non-elderly Americans lacked health insurance. By the time President Barack Obama left office, this value had fallen to 10 percent, largely due to the ACA.[94] A decrease in the number of non-elderly uninsured occurred across all racial and ethnic groups.

Yet percentages of uninsured were still vastly unequal. As of 2019, 20 percent of the Latinx population and 11 percent of the Black population were uninsured in the United States, compared to 8 and 7 percent for the white and Asian populations of the country.[95]

Why does the lack of health insurance matter? First, according to the Kaiser Family Foundation (KFF), people who lack insurance tend to have less access to preventative medical care, such as regular checkups and physicals, than those who are insured. These services provide protection against chronic disease like diabetes and heart ailments, which led to increased health risks from COVID-19.[96] Further, the uninsured population less frequently seeks medical care when health issues occur. KFF claims that "three in ten uninsured adults in 2019 went without needed medical care due to cost."[97] When we search for areas most disrupted by the pandemic, we find exactly those areas that have high rates of uninsured individuals.

Over the course of the first year of the pandemic, the counties in the quintile with the most uninsured individuals had 48 percent more deaths per capita than the quintile of counties with the fewest uninsured individuals. The summer 2020 wave and the 2021 Delta wave stand out even more strongly. During the summer 2020 wave, the least insured quintile of counties had over 360 percent more deaths than the quintile of counties with the highest insurance rates. The summer 2020 wave, which had such a discrepancy in deaths for the counties with the most uninsured individuals, was also the wave in which deaths among Latinx individuals far outpaced all other groups.[98]

There are misconceptions in the general public about who lacks health insurance. First, 73 percent of non-elderly uninsured individuals have at least one full-time worker within their household and another 11 percent have at least one part-time worker.[99] A lack of insurance isn't due to a lack of employment. Uninsured people are far more likely to work than not. Finances do play a large role, however. Approximately 18 percent of families who live below the poverty line are uninsured.[100] And about 25 percent of families in poverty with two or more full-time workers are uninsured.[101] This is 8 percent *higher* than the uninsured rate for people without labor market jobs. Low-income families with two full-time workers but with income less than double the poverty threshold also have high rates of being uninsured, at 22 percent. Those facing the harshest uninsured rates are working families who have low-income jobs. They are the working poor. This underscores the largest reason given for lack of coverage. It is not affordable for many low-income working families.

Where does this come from? We have a tradition in the United States of tying health insurance to employment. It is a perk of the job. This perk goes along with jobs that pay well, and low-income jobs frequently lack this benefit. Because the working poor do not earn a large sum of money, they cannot afford private health insurance. Of uninsured individuals, 74 percent state that lack of affordability is the reason for not being insured.[102] These are large swaths of the population who work hard jobs and cannot afford health insurance. A family with a full-time worker earning $20 an hour makes about $40,000 per year. Non-subsidized health insurance for a family of four costs between $1,000 and $1,500 per month, or $12,000 and $18,000 per year.[103] For a family making $40,000 per year, this is 39 to 45 percent of before-tax income! This family would be well above the federal poverty line of $26,200 and would not qualify for Medicaid in most states.[104] Because this family cannot afford health insurance, they receive worse health care and develop more chronic conditions. Then they die in a pandemic tsunami when they face both more exposure risk and more health risk.

Bloomberg News described the situation of the Bobbie family, which includes parents Joe and Corinne, and two children, Sophia and Joey. Sophia was born with a heart defect along with other ailments. By the time she was three years old, her medical bills had already totaled over $1 million. Luckily, they were covered by Medicaid. However, when Sophia turned two, the family was told that they no longer qualified for Medicaid. With Sophia's pre-existing conditions, in a pre-ACA world, no insurer was willing to cover Sophia. In the *Bloomberg* article, Corinne is quoted as saying, "Every door, every option, everything was just slammed in our face."[105] Their solution was to take a pay cut in order to continue receiving Medicaid. They had to give up wages in order to maintain Sophia's care and to keep her alive. It is absurd that a country as wealthy as the United States puts people in this position. They never could have paid for her care on their own. Once the ACA was enacted in 2014, the Bobbies were able to find a policy for Sophia. However, with a $55,000 per year income, they could not afford a policy that covered the rest of the family.[106] This family earned nearly median income and could not afford health insurance for their family. While Sophia and the Bobbie family's medical situation is unique, there are many working-class families like them across the country who also cannot afford health insurance.

What jobs have the largest percentage of uninsured individuals? Workers in agriculture (31 percent), construction (30 percent), and the general service sector (22 percent) lead the list. These are demanding professions that are physically taxing, and some have high rates of on-the-job injuries.[107]

It isn't that these populations couldn't receive health care if needed. They can seek care at urgent care centers for emergency situations. However, their unfamiliarity with the health care system puts them at a natural disadvantage. An insured person who receives regular checkups has experience with the health care system. They have regular doctors who know them. They know the typical questions to ask of their health care provider and have experience seeking specialists for treatment when needed. Fifty percent of non-elderly uninsured people report that they have "no usual source of care." Only 11 percent of non-elderly insured people with employer-provided insurance and 12 percent of Medicaid recipients lack a usual source of care.[108] Insured people likely had a primary care physician to contact if they began to experience COVID-19 or other symptoms. They knew where to get care if needed. They had doctors they trusted who knew their health history and who provided advice on preventative measures. One-half of the uninsured population lacked this important resource when the pandemic began.

In addition to relying upon overcrowded urgent care systems where doctors did not know their health history, the poverty status of uninsured individuals may have made it more difficult for them to access online appointments for COVID-19–related ailments or other health problems. The waiting list of patients for non-essential medical procedures and appointments likely made it even more difficult for the uninsured to receive health care services.

The populations listed above of ethnic and racial minorities who were in or on the brink of poverty, worked in front-facing industries, and lacked health insurance had to deal with the more difficult challenges presented by the pandemic of anyone in the United States. These populations faced heightened exposure risk, and at the same time their status of near poverty and lack of insurance placed them at the greatest health risk if infected. This double risk likely cost many of these individuals their lives. For many of these populations, it was a return to the dangers of a time we once thought was long gone, to a time when the book on infectious disease sat wide open. It was as though these people were reliving the pandemic waves of the nineteenth century.

In the future, it is certain that another pandemic will arrive. It may be soon if we relive the nineteenth century, or it may be another hundred years if we relive the twentieth. We don't know the date of arrival. We do know that when it arrives, nothing will be different if we continue the patterns of the past. If our "return to normal" is a return to the patterns of a 2019 health care system, the same tragedies of the COVID-19 pandemic will be repeated. Will we still leave low-income people in the path of the tsunami? Will we improve access to health care for the working poor? Will people of color still live with existing levels of inequality in income and wealth? All of these issues create exposure and health risk. Will these same groups be blamed for their plight like the pauper pilgrims of the 1800s? Will we care about their plight if the next pandemic doesn't affect the more-wealthy? We were not significantly better at protecting the vulnerable and marginalized in the twenty-first century than we were in the two prior. We could have asked these exact questions in 1832, 1849, and 1918 and we could have acted to provide better health care and less risk for our vulnerable populations. We have choices as a society. If we maintain the status quo, the next pandemic, which will surely arrive someday, will leave us asking these same questions yet again.

Chapter 9

A CURIOUS PRACTICE

Born in England in 1689, Lady Mary Pierrepont was raised by a governess who filled her education with superstitious tales and false notions. Overcoming this barrier, Lady Mary used her family library to learn Latin and read literature. In 1712 she married Edward Wortley Montagu. Shortly after marriage, the couple had a son, Edward. After this joy, Lady Mary met tragedy. Her brother died from smallpox the next year and Mary contracted smallpox herself in 1715. Although she recovered, the common scars from smallpox marked her face for life.

At the time of Lady Mary's infection, smallpox was a common affliction in Europe. The eighteenth century saw around 400,000 deaths annually from a population of 200 million. While there were peaks and valleys in infections and deaths from year to year, two-tenths of a percent of the population died from smallpox each year on average. A death toll like this, with today's population in Europe or North America, would result in 134,000 deaths in the United Kingdom and 600,000 deaths in the United States each year for a century. Those are shocking totals, but this was the year-by-year existence of eighteenth-century life. Of those infected with smallpox, 20 to 60 percent died, and most who survived were left with severe scars.[1] Earlier epidemics of smallpox were even more devastating. Smallpox was likely the agent of the Plague of Antoine, which caused 7 million deaths—10 percent of the Roman Empire.[2]

Shortly after this series of infections in her family, Mary's husband was appointed ambassador to Constantinople and was tasked with negotiating an end to the Austro-Turkish War. Mary traveled with him to the distant land. She recorded her experience with the customs and hospitality while abroad in voluminous letters and journals.[3] In particular, the writings detailed her introduction to a curious practice that she witnessed and wrote about to Sarah Chiswell in April of 1718:

> The smallpox, so fatal . . . amongst us, is here entirely harmless by the invention of engrafting. . . . They make parties for this purpose . . . the old woman comes with the best sort of smallpox, and asks which veins you please to have opened. She immediately . . . puts into the vein as much venom as can lie upon the head of a needle. The children or young patients play together all the rest of the day, and are in perfect health until the eighth [day]. Then the fever begins to seize them and they keep to their beds for two days, very seldom three . . . in eight days time they are as well as before their illness. . . . Every year thousands undergo this operation. . . . I intend to try it on my dear little son.[4]

The practice she described came to be known as variolation. A doctor extracted a small amount of pus from a smallpox blister and introduced it into a non-infected person through a small piercing of the skin on an arm or leg. The recipient typically developed a mild case of smallpox and recovered to live free of future infection. The procedure was an early means of inoculation.

Eager to avoid infection for her children, particularly given her and her brother's experience with the disease, Lady Mary instructed the embassy surgeon to inoculate Edward in 1718. Later, after the family returned to England, she had her daughter inoculated when a smallpox epidemic overtook London in 1721. This is believed to be the first recorded inoculation in England.

The Ottoman Empire established inoculation well before Lady Mary's arrival. The practice originated in China or India with the first known written recording of the procedure published in 1549. Who exactly invented the procedure was not documented. References were made to a Taoist or Buddhist monk or nun, or it may have developed independently in multiple locations across time. Stories exist that indicate prisoners were the first experimental subjects.[5]

The procedure was not without critics. Occasionally the effects, intended to be mild, grew severe, and extreme cases resulted in death. Sometimes the infection was passed to others before the mild symptoms abated and immunity was granted. While not one of these early critics, Ben Franklin failed to inoculate his young son, Francis, because he was ill. When he later died from smallpox, Franklin was filled with regret. He wrote in his autobiography: "In 1736, I lost one of my sons, a fine boy of four years old, by the small-pox, taken in the common way. I long regretted bitterly, and still regret that I had not given it to him by inoculation."[6]

Despite the risks, the tenfold decrease in the case-fatality rate led to the widespread adoption of the procedure in Europe across the aristocracy and to a lesser extent, among the common people.[7] King Frederick II of Prussia inoculated all of his soldiers, as did other European armies, including many of the British forces in North America.[8] This proved important in the coming Revolutionary War.

For the British forces in North America, few inoculations were needed due to previous exposure and infection of their soldiers in Europe. Furthermore, because of this natural exposure, the risk that an inoculation could result in a more widespread outbreak within their ranks was slight. Because the Continental Army lacked this exposure, General George Washington feared that inoculations could trigger an epidemic within his army. This concern prevented him from implementing the tactic. His opinion changed after Quebec.

In September of 1775, two legions of the Continental Army moved north toward Canada with the hope of securing the city of Quebec. Troops led by General Richard Montgomery moved north past Lake Champlain and captured Montreal on November 13, 1775. Colonel Benedict Arnold led a second legion through the forests of Maine and arrived outside Quebec in mid-November. After the British rejected his demand for surrender, Arnold waited for Montgomery to arrive with additional troops and supplies. On December 31, 1775, the Continental Army attacked. General Montgomery was killed in the initial battle, and Arnold was wounded in the leg. After being rebuffed in the initial attack, the Continental troops continued the siege through the winter and into the spring.[9] At some point the British sent people infected with smallpox outside the city gates in an attempt to seed an epidemic among the Continental troops. The ploy succeeded. In the last two weeks of May 1776, 1,800 of the 7,000 Continental troops in Quebec died of smallpox.[10] When British reinforcements arrived, the Americans abandoned the siege of Quebec. It was the first defeat in the Revolutionary War for the Americans.[11] Of the ordeal, John Adams wrote, "Our misfortunes in Canada are enough to melt the heart of stone. . . . The smallpox is ten times more terrible than the British, Canadians, and Indians together. This was the cause of our precipitate retreat from

Quebec. And, it has been claimed, the main cause of the preservation of Canada to the British Empire."[12]

Washington eventually switched course and had the entire army inoculated in 1777. In a letter to Dr. William Shippen Jr., Washington ordered the mass inoculation. He wrote, "Necessity not only authorizes but seems to require the measure, for should the disorder infect the Army . . . we should have more to dread from it, than from the Sword of the Enemy."[13]

While the benefits of traditional inoculation continued to be proven, some looked for a safer alternative. Dairy maids in England were rumored to be immune to smallpox due to a common infection from a similar but less dangerous disease, cowpox. Medical doctor Edward Jenner documented this relationship and then devised an experiment.[14]

In May 1796, Jenner drew pus from the cowpox lesions of a dairy maid named Sarah Nelms. He then inoculated eight-year-old James Phipps, the son of his gardener. The boy developed a mild fever and loss of appetite but no other significant symptoms. Jenner then inoculated the boy a second time in July—this time with smallpox. No symptoms resulted, not even the traditional mild case that accompanied traditional variolation. Jenner concluded from this that the cowpox inoculation was sufficient to provide protection from smallpox.[15] Jenner called his procedure *vaccination*, derived from the Latin words for cow (*vacca*) and cowpox (*vaccinia*).[16]

This advance in the safety of variolation led to Jenner being known as the father of vaccinations in England, alongside its mother, Lady Mary.

The cowpox vaccine worked because of cross-immunity. The body's reaction to cowpox primed the immune system for invasion from smallpox. This was not understood during Jenner's time. The germ theory of disease did not come into acceptance until the mid- to late eighteenth century largely due to the scientific discoveries of Robert Koch and Louis Pasteur.[17]

Pasteur was next in line to take the process of vaccination forward. His work came at the forefront of a movement that understood diseases as distinct entities that could be classified by the symptoms present in those infected. This revolution occurred within the Paris School of Medicine.[18] Pasteur applied the newly developed power of the microscope to disease. An early discovery centered on the spoilage of wine and milk. Pasteur identified that the spoilage was due to the presence of bacteria as opposed to a chemical process, which was the standard theory before his identification. By examining and cultivating the bacteria in his laboratory, Pasteur discovered that heat was able to destroy the bacteria without harming the wine or milk. This new process was called "pasteurization."[19]

Pasteur's discovery of the effects of heat on bacteria led to the development of a host of vaccines using a similar methodology. He believed in "nonrecurrence," a form of acquired immunity from disease that could be used to develop universal vaccines. Scientists faced the problem of learning how to create this immunity without harming the subject through infection and the dangers that it entailed.[20]

In 1878 Pasteur worked on culturing the bacterium that caused fowl cholera. Using these cultures, it was easy to induce the disease by inoculating chickens with the bacterium.[21] By chance he observed that an older culture that had been left in the summer heat would not induce the disease in a set of chickens as the other cultures had done. His prior discovery of pasteurization gave him the idea for an experiment. He took a fresh batch of live and healthy bacteria and inoculated these same chickens again, along with a new set of chickens. The chickens that were initially inoculated with the old bacteria did not develop disease, while the new chickens did. Pasteur found that the procedure was repeatable. Heating the bacteria weakened it to a form that would not harm those inoculated with it, and this procedure allowed the recipient to acquire immunity from future infection. This led to the development of the first attenuated, or weakened, vaccine.[22] Pasteur developed other attenuated vaccines for infectious diseases such as anthrax and rabies.

Shortly after Pasteur developed the first attenuated vaccine, Theobald Smith made a related discovery. He developed a vaccine for fowl cholera by killing the bacteria with heat, which also conferred immunity for the chickens.[23] These two discoveries of live-attenuated and killed-bacteria (and subsequently virus) vaccines led to the proliferation of vaccine development.

As new diseases emerged, scientists raced to find new vaccines to protect society. One of the most famous searches resulted in the discovery of a vaccine for polio. Poliovirus, which causes poliomyelitis or more commonly polio, existed for centuries but was not formally documented until the late eighteenth century by Michael Underwood.[24] At the time of identification it was not a common disease; but its incidence grew over the course of the nineteenth and twentieth centuries. Three different strains of poliovirus cause polio. Poliovirus 1 caused 85 percent of cases that resulted in paralysis and death.[25]

Polio infection had two features in common with COVID-19. First, a large majority of infections are asymptomatic. Only about 25 percent of polio infections resulted in symptoms and illness. Second, many symptomatic infections resulted in minor ailments of fever, headache, and fatigue. It was only one out of every two hundred of the symptomatic infections that resulted in severe disease and paralysis.[26]

Many severe cases of polio appeared without a known contact with another infected person because of the large prevalence of asymptomatic and unidentified carriers. Similarly, many contacts of infective people seemed to pass exposure unharmed with no symptoms.

It wasn't until 1916, when a large epidemic occurred in the northeastern United States, that polio attracted widespread attention. The epidemic started in Brooklyn and spread across the northeast, resulting in over twenty-seven thousand cases of paralysis and six thousand deaths.[27] Following this outbreak, epidemics of polio became more common in the United States and Europe. About three-fourths of the cases occurred in children, which made the disease all the more tragic in the public eye and the focus became more acute. Over the twentieth century, it resulted in one million deaths and twenty million people were disabled.[28] The visible nature of paralysis after infection, especially in children, made concern for the disease even more palpable. One wonders if more concern would be given to long COVID if its debilitating effects were as visible to the world as those of polio.

Within these polio epidemics lived a significant difference in class and racial perception that repeated history. Professor of the History of Medicine Naomi Rogers wrote, "Epidemiologists initially saw wealthy white polio patients as anomalies, best explained by an unlucky association with infected members of the urban poor."[29] Once it was recognized that polio transcended class among the white population, it was not recognized as a medical concern for the Black population. In the first major study of racial differences in polio, Paul Harmon argued in 1936 that statistics from the 1916 polio epidemic in New York City, which displayed a "Black morbidity rate of 241 per 100,000 of population compared with 383 for whites, suggested 'that the disease is relatively infrequent in the colored race.'"[30] While the Black population had a lower rate than the white population in this particular epidemic, it was certainly not infrequent as Harmon stated.

Other examples where Black morbidity and mortality occurred at higher rates than white rates were seen as anomalies that defied explanation. There came to be a mistaken belief that polio was a "white disease." Rogers argued that this belief led to incorrect training for medical professionals, segregated "second-hand" hospitals for the treatment of Black patients, and ultimately "medical racism and neglect."[31] Even as the perception shifted to accept Black susceptibility, inequality and segregation remained. The Roosevelt Warm Springs Institute for Rehabilitation, founded by Franklin Roosevelt in 1927 to treat polio patients, remained a white-only facility. With the politics of this segregation troubling to his re-election, Roosevelt pushed for the opening of a new Black-only facility in Tuskegee, Alabama. The uniqueness of the facility was remarkable enough that its opening ceremony was broadcast on national radio. Yet it contained only thirty-six beds and, as Rogers wrote, "could help only a fraction of the patients who sought its care."[32] At a minimum, recognition grew that polio was not an only white disease, but the myth of Black immunity was not resolved nor corrected. In 1951, "a white physician speaking for the March of Dimes" referenced an unusual Black polio outbreak as odd because "usually polio strikes blonde, blue-eyed persons at a far greater rate."[33] This misperception would lead to further problems as the race to find a vaccine continued.

The first significant polio vaccine trials were performed in 1935 using a virus from infected monkeys. None proved effective.[34] Even worse, the attenuated vaccine resulted in paralysis in 1 in 1,000 of those vaccinated and, in some cases, death.[35] It wasn't until 1953 that Jonas Salk developed an inactivated (killed) vaccine using a virus grown on the kidney cells of monkeys. It was tested on 1.6 million children in North America and Finland and found to be highly effective. The trial results were announced to the world from the Poliomyelitis Vaccine Evaluation Center at the University of Michigan. Salk's vaccine was 80 to 90 percent effective. The vaccine was adopted, and cases dropped precipitously from 13.9 cases per 100,000 in 1954 to 0.8 per 100,000 by 1961.[36]

The vaccine drew criticism, however. There was a tragic incident at one of the vaccine production centers shortly after distribution began. Two pools of vaccine from the Cutter Laboratories in Berkeley, California, were produced incorrectly and resulted in the distribution of 120,000 doses of vaccine that contained the live virus. Weak symptoms resulted in forty thousand recipients, but fifty-one were permanently paralyzed and five died.[37] This incident did not stop widespread adoption in the United States. However, there were further, though less obvious, difficulties.

The drop in cases unexpectedly stalled. Even worse, it reemerged, particularly in impoverished urban neighborhoods.[38] Epidemic historian Frank Snowden reports the *New York Times* found "the incidence of polio among African Americans in inner cities and among Native Americans on reservations was four to six times the national average."[39]

Two particular outbreaks in 1959—one in Des Moines, Iowa, and the other in Kansas City, Missouri—made the problem clear. Tom Chin and William Marine tracked the outbreaks of polio in these two cities during outbreaks in 1952, 1954, and 1959.[40] In doing so, they found a distinct change in the pattern of the outbreaks. In the earlier two epidemics, the cases were evenly spread across the neighborhoods of each city, but the 1959 outbreak was different. The cases in each city were concentrated in the urban center and more importantly in the most impoverished neighborhoods of the cities. They write, "The attack rate for [Blacks] in Des Moines was 20 times higher than for the upper [class] whites, and in Kansas City, it was 32 times higher."[41]

The reason for the difference was clear: the underlying rates of vaccination. In Des Moines, 65 percent of the upper-class white children between zero to four years had received three or more doses of vaccine; in the Black population, it was 30 percent. For older children, the discrepancy was 90 percent to 43 percent. The vaccination rates were two times higher in the affluent white population than in the Black population. Kansas City had similar discrepancies.[42] Similar concentrations of infections in lower socioeconomic groups occurred in Chicago,[43] Washington, D.C.,[44] and Detroit.[45]

Snowden quotes the CDC's chief of epidemiology, Alexander Langmuir, from 1960: "An overestimate of potential vaccine acceptance was made. Large islands of poorly vaccinated population groups existed in our city slums, in isolated and ethnically distinct communities, and in many rural areas."[46] The difficulties appeared to be centered around access to the vaccine. In a white world that believed in separate but equal treatment, Black children were disadvantaged. In Mobile, Alabama, Black children traveled to white schools to receive the vaccine. They waited on the lawn to be vaccinated and were not allowed to use the bathrooms inside the building.[47] This occurred in the same month, May 1954, that the Supreme Court ruled in *Brown v. Board of Education* that separate but equal treatment violated the Fourteenth Amendment.

Despite the ruling, change was slow. Historically and into the present day, impoverished and rural populations have had less access to medical care. There were fewer hospitals and other medical facilities in rural areas. Rural residents faced constraints of time and forgone wages as they traveled to distant health care providers. Race-based housing segregation led to fewer medical options and less access to care for residents of Black neighborhoods in urban and rural areas. Further, because the Salk polio vaccine required three doses, all of these barriers had to be overcome three times. This made the unequal access to care even more prominent in the fight against polio.

However, another vaccine arrived on the heels of Salk: the Sabin oral vaccine. Unlike the Salk vaccine, the Sabin vaccine contained attenuated live virus. The Sabin vaccine had a number of practical advantages over the Salk vaccine. First, it could be taken orally and in one dose. Second, it did not require extensive training to administer. The Salk injection required medical training to inject and was usually provided at a physician's office. This was a particular challenge if it were to be administered worldwide in the global fight against polio. By contrast the Sabin vaccine was placed in a droplet on top of a sugar cube. Literally in Mary Poppins fashion, a cube of sugar "helped the medicine go down." Third, it was inexpensive in comparison to the Salk vaccine. The price of the Salk vaccine was $25 to $30 for each dose and required three doses. This was a significant amount of money. In 1960, the median household income in the United States was $5,600 per year. Three doses of the Salk vaccine amounted to 1.5 percent of yearly income for the median family in the United States. The Sabin vaccine was significantly cheaper at $3 to $5 per dose and required only one dose.[48] The cost was paid by the government, but the financial advantage of the Sabin vaccine was important. All of these factors made the Sabin vaccine easier to distribute widely across the population.

With the new vaccine available, the United States set out to eliminate polio within its borders. The country did so with a new model for vaccine distribution. Instead of requiring recipients to visit physicians, they attempted to take the vaccine to the people. Epidemiological historian Frank Snowden gives credit to Cuba for pioneering this idea. Cuba created a door-to-door census to locate every child within the country. Once a child was identified, a vaccinator would return to their home to administer the vaccine. The program was immensely successful and allowed Cuba to become the first country to eliminate polio.[49]

With the model of Cuba in mind, similar programs within the United States began. Pediatricians in Arizona's two most populated counties, Maricopa and Pima, created a festival atmosphere with games and attractions where children received a vaccine at a local school for a cost of only $0.25. If a recipient could not afford the fee, the vaccine was given at no charge. No one was turned away. The program was labeled "Sabin Oral Sundays." More than 700,000 people, 75 percent of the state's population, were vaccinated in the first two months of 1962.[50] Programs like these became the model across the United States. By the end of the 1960s the number of cases of paralytic polio had dropped into the double digits and the United States has been polio free since 1979.[51] Further efforts have been made to eradicate polio worldwide. In 1988 there were still an estimated 350,000 cases. Today, while not fully eradicated worldwide, there are only a handful of cases each year.

Present-day vaccines are a highly effective and safe method to combat many infectious diseases. Yet the existence of a vaccine is not a foolproof tool to end a pandemic. Vaccines work through averages to reduce the reproduction number of an infectious disease. The reproduction number needs to be below one for an epidemic to recede. From a public health perspective, each effective vaccination leaves one fewer person to be infected and one fewer person to infect others. It lowers the reproduction number by reducing the number of susceptible people in a population, the S in DOTS. Vaccines get us to herd immunity more quickly and safely than by naturally occurring and more dangerous infection. However, the match of the vaccine to the virus and the *average* response in the population is only one part of the story.

Vaccines vary in effectiveness. The influenza vaccine is 40 to 50 percent effective in the average person but it varies from year to year depending on the match of the vaccine to the most commonly circulating influenza strains in a particular year. Some years the vaccine is more effective, and some years it is less effective.[52] The effectiveness also varies individually. On average, effectiveness is much lower in the elderly population that holds the most health risk from infection. This makes it all the more important for middle aged and younger people to be vaccinated in order to lower the exposure risk for the elderly. When people are vaccinated for influenza it lowers the exposure risk for others around them because they are less likely to be infected and therefore less likely to pass the infection to others. Even if these vaccines are not perfect, they create a barrier against infection in the most vulnerable populations. Like influenza vaccines, the COVID-19 vaccines also are less effective in older and immunocompromised populations.[53] As with influenza, the immunity granted by the COVID-19 vaccine wanes over time, resulting in the need for booster shots to re-energize the immune response.

No vaccines are perfect at preventing infection and transmission. The measles, mumps, and rubella (MMR) vaccine is considered the gold standard because it provides about 97 percent effectiveness at preventing severe illness after two doses. Still, this highly effective vaccine does not work 100 percent of the time.

Even when we have effective vaccines, lack of use can be problematic. Because the externalities created by vaccines limit exposure risk in a population, it is sometimes necessary to encourage their use even for people who do not hold health risk from infection. For over a century, national and state governments have made some vaccines compulsory in order to increase usage. In 1853 England passed its first law requiring that all children be vaccinated for smallpox. The law was modified multiple times later in the nineteenth and early twentieth centuries including the levying of a fine of twenty shillings for noncompliance in 1867. This was a hefty fine as laborers in London earned payment of about three to six shillings per ten-hour workday.[54] The fine was equal to a few days' wages.

The first law in the United States requiring smallpox vaccination was passed by the state of Massachusetts in 1809. Several other states followed soon after. Strong opposition occurred in some areas and many states repealed the mandatory vaccination laws until the Supreme Court ruled in 1905 that states had the authority to enact vaccine mandates.[55] Mandates followed for polio, measles, and other infectious diseases. Shortly thereafter came exemptions for medical, religious, and personal beliefs. The passage of these bills and their specific language became a political battle in many locations. A bill was held up in Michigan for over a year until language was added allowing freedom from the mandate for "religious or other objection." Democrats held up a similar law in Ohio over the right of "freedom of choice."[56] A 1961 polio vaccination mandate in California originally contained language allowing for exemptions for "religious beliefs." When a movement arose to broaden the exemption, the word *religious* was removed, allowing for a very broad interpretation of personal beliefs that lasted for over half a century.[57]

The most recent wave of US vaccine mandates occurred in the 1970s and concerned measles. Like polio, the new mandates were a response to the persistence of measles in impoverished urban areas. In the new laws, many of the previous exemptions were carried forward. California was one of the states where this occurred.[58]

Because of concern about the overuse of what came to be known as personal belief exemptions, as opposed to religious belief exemptions, California changed its law in 2015. It eliminated the personal belief exemption and only allowed exemptions for religious or medical reasons. As of the last year of personal belief exemptions being available, about 95 percent of kindergarteners received the MMR vaccine in the state of California. This was only a slight decrease from the 96 percent vaccination coverage in 2000. The use of personal belief exemptions increased from 0.7 percent of kindergarteners to 1.9 percent between 2000 and 2015.[59] However, the rate was not the most important part of the change in behavior. More important, the use of personal belief exemptions became increasingly concentrated in specific pockets of the population and increasingly used by those who were financially well-off.

Using the reproduction number for measles and the level of vaccine efficacy, one can calculate that the level of vaccinations required to reach herd immunity is a little under 95 percent. In 2000, 25 percent of schools in California were below this level of vaccine coverage for entering kindergarteners, and only 12 percent of schools had fewer than 90 percent of kindergarteners vaccinated for measles. By 2015, these numbers had grown to 32 percent and 15 percent.[60] Even though there was a slight uptick in the use of personal belief exemptions and the overall vaccination rate was relatively consistent, nearly one-third of schools were under the vaccination levels needed for herd immunity. Unvaccinated children were becoming increasingly concentrated in specific schools.

The change in vaccination rates in private schools, frequently attended by children of wealthy individuals, was even worse. Here personal belief exemption usage increased from 1.3 percent in 2000 to 4 percent in 2015. In 2015, 45 percent of private schools had vaccination rates of less than 95 percent and 28 percent of private schools had rates less than 90 percent.[61] Nearly half of private schools in California lacked herd immunity against measles. Non-vaccinated children were more frequently being sorted into the same schools. Risk met risk again. The at-risk students were mixing with each other every day in the same buildings, the same classrooms, and at the same lunch tables.

Schools that fall below herd immunity put themselves at risk. More importantly, they put neighboring school districts at risk along with children in the vicinity of the schools with low vaccination rates. The decisions of parents made these schools hubs of exposure risk. One infection in the school meets one bridge to another community, and a widespread outbreak occurs. Because the least vaccinated schools were private schools the students at risk were from a wider geographic area and thus created more bridges to a wider set of geographic communities. These bridges created connections to immunocompromised children and to children too young for the vaccine.

In an ironic sense, the success of the measles vaccine fueled this behavior. While measles is not eradicated, the vaccine saved millions of lives since the 1960s. In 2014 the World Health Organization estimated that over seventeen million lives had been saved by the measles vaccine in the twenty-first century alone.[62] The decreased incidence of measles caused many to deem the exposure risk it poses to be negligible. When there were only a few hundred cases of measles each year in the United States, it was psychologically easy for parents to forgo the vaccine. When most other children were vaccinated, a parent could calculate that their child was already safe. They could free ride on the choices of others. Thus, measles vaccines, and other vaccines, tend to stall out right at the edge of herd immunity as the exposure risk of infection drops to near zero. Similar to young adults who forgo influenza or COVID-19 vaccines because of their lower health risk, parents could choose to forgo measles vaccines because their children faced limited exposure risk. In addition, many of the parents forgoing a vaccine for their child in a private school expect to receive high-quality medical care if their child is infected. Their health risk is lower than others whose exposure risk they increase with their vaccine refusal.

The number of measles cases grew in part as a result of this behavior. In the decade from 2000 to 2009, the maximum number of measles cases in a single year within the United States was 140 in 2008.[63] In the years 2010 to 2019, there were six years with more than 140 infections, including a high of 1,282 in 2019. The largest local outbreak occurred in New York City, which experienced a fall 2018 to spring 2019 epidemic. During this time period, 535 cases were reported to the New York City Department of Health. Most of the cases occurred in the neighborhoods of Williamsburg and Borough Park, which contain large Orthodox Jewish communities with low rates of MMR vaccination.[64] This one single outbreak in New York City was almost four times larger than the largest yearly total across the entire nation in the decade from 2000 to 2009. All it will take is one spark for a similar-sized epidemic to occur in one of the affluent private schools in California or another area with low vaccination rates.

Europe had an even larger problem with measles vaccination. There a series of measles outbreaks resulted in over eighty-two thousand cases and seventy-two deaths in 2018.[65] In the United Kingdom, measles infections grew from below one hundred per year at the beginning of the twenty-first century to a peak of almost two thousand in 2012.[66] In 2018, the United Kingdom lost its "measles-free" status from the World Health Organization. At this time, 95 percent of children under five had received a first dose of vaccine, but only 87 percent had received the required second dose that nearly guarantees immunity.[67] In France, fewer than 85 percent of children were vaccinated, and in 2011 they had nearly four thousand measles infections.[68]

Of most concern, the rate of measles infections per 100,000 was greatest among those under one year of age.[69] The vaccine wasn't recommended by physicians to be given until late in the first year of life or early in the second. Children too young for the vaccine were most frequently infected. Those who could be vaccinated but refused were responsible for these infections. They ignored their social responsibility and others paid the price. This was a part of the externality created by vaccine hesitancy. The effects of the externality in Ukraine were even worse.

In 2008, Ukraine had a measles vaccination rate of 94 percent.[70] Then a seventeen-year-old boy died shortly after being vaccinated.[71] Although a medical report documented that his death was not caused by the vaccine, a false internet rumor blamed vaccination for his death. Vaccine skeptics fueled the lie. Following the rumor, vaccination rates began to wane. Growing vaccine hesitancy, coupled with a vaccine shortage due in part to a military conflict with Russia, led to Ukraine vaccinating only 42 percent of infants under two years old in 2015. Further, only 31 percent of six-year-old children received the recommended booster in 2015.[72] By 2016 Ukraine had the second lowest measles vaccination rate across the world for children under twenty-three months. Only the country of Chad was worse.[73]

With rates plummeting, a measles epidemic emerged within the country that pushed its way throughout Europe. In 2016 Ukraine had 102 measles infections. The next year it had over 4,700. Then it exploded to over 50,000 in both 2018 and 2019.[74] These were the largest outbreaks in Europe in over two decades.

In addition to the low rates among children, there also appeared to be a problem with a batch of vaccine that Ukraine received from Russia in 2001. Of those infected in 2018, twenty thousand were adults who were vaccinated in 2001. One such adult was Serhiy Butenko. Serhiy was an eighteen-year-old medical student living in Vinnytsia, Ukraine. He had recently fallen ill with mononucleosis, a contagious viral infection caused by the Epstein-Barr virus that is common among teens and young adults. Shortly thereafter, Serhiy contracted measles despite having been vaccinated and boosted at the recommended ages. His physician told the BBC, "This mononucleosis weakened his immune system, so it could not fight properly against the measles virus." Serhiy died in early 2019, eighteen months into his medical studies.[75]

No one will ever know if the measles vaccines of Serhiy's youth were faulty. Nor will we know if avoiding mononucleosis would have spared his life. We do know, however, that if vaccination rates had not plummeted in Ukraine the epidemic that took his life would not have happened. There were only 102 cases of measles in Ukraine just three years earlier. Had they stayed at this low level, it is almost certain that Serhiy never would have been exposed. Anti-vaccine behavior and false rumors created the exposure risk that killed Serhiy.

As noted above, when measles exploded in Ukraine the epidemic did not remain within its borders. Cases spilled outward to other areas of Europe. There were only five thousand measles infections in all of Europe in 2016. In 2018 there were over eighty thousand.[76] Serbia and Georgia, neighbors of Ukraine, had significant outbreaks despite vaccination rates in the mid-nineties. Vaccination coverage was near all-time highs across the European continent.[77] Yet measles still broke out of Ukraine into other areas of Europe.

Ukraine's epidemic spilling outside its borders into areas with high rates of vaccinations demonstrated a misunderstanding that many have about herd immunity. Herd immunity from vaccines develops when a population has too few susceptible people for the reproduction number to be above one. If an infection occurs, there are not enough susceptible people to fuel an epidemic fire. The common understanding of herd immunity represented in mass media misses some of the subtleties of the concept, particularly how herd immunity depends on space.

Imagine a forest of trees spread out across a geographic area. Now suppose that a fire starts somewhere in the forest. If the trees are densely packed together, the fire spreads from tree to tree and grows larger. This is what happens when the reproduction number is above one. One tree on fire becomes two, two becomes four, and so on. Now imagine that we could reach down and pluck a bunch of trees from the forest so that when the fire starts, the remaining trees are too far apart for the fire to spread.[78] The lone tree that catches fire is not close enough to other trees to spread the blaze from one to another. This is herd immunity.

Imagine further that this spacing of trees in the forest is accomplished by removing 50 percent of the trees. Notice, however, that when we select these trees to remove they need to be evenly spread about the forest. For instance, we could remove every other tree across the entire forest and reach herd immunity. In comparison, suppose that we remove 50 percent of the trees but do so in a different manner: we start in the north and remove every single tree as we move south. We stop when we hit the 50 percent mark. This process entirely clears trees in the northern half of the forest but leaves the southern forest untouched. This does not create herd immunity. If a fire were to start in the southern half of the forest, it will burn in this area just as it would have done before removing the northern trees.

The ability to reach herd immunity depends on how many vaccines are given in combination with where the vaccines are allocated. One cannot be separated from the other. In most cases, an uneven geographic distribution of vaccines causes the level of vaccines needed to reach herd immunity to be higher than if the vaccines are spread evenly.[79] If you vaccinate all the people in Georgia but no one in Florida, then Florida is no more protected than it was before. Further, because people in Georgia and Florida interact with each other, Georgia is also less safe because Florida will share its exposure risk with Georgia. While this example and the forest example are more stark than reality, the uneven distribution of vaccines occurs often.

Urban centers in Des Moines and Kansas City had low rates of polio vaccinations in the late 1950s. Limited measles vaccinations in Ukraine caused outbreaks in Ukraine and in other parts of Europe. California private schools sit in danger with student populations at risk of measles. In the United States, COVID-19 vaccination rates were much lower in certain counties and states than others. The problem was particularly pronounced early in vaccine rollout in urban centers and in southern rural states and counties that had limited access to the vaccine.

Many media reports that discussed herd immunity during the summer of 2021 were misguided. Numerous statements were made about whether or not a certain city, state, country, or geographic area had reached the requisite level of vaccinations for herd immunity. The statements implicitly assumed that a certain state, such as New York or Utah, could reach herd immunity on their own if roughly 70 percent of the state's population were vaccinated. Many journalists seemed to think that these vaccinations were evenly spread. These reports ignored the fact that each of these states had populations interacting with populations of other states, just as the country of Ukraine interacted with Serbia, Georgia, and the rest of Europe. They ignored that people traveled to neighboring countries and states for business and tourism or for events like bike rallies. The level of vaccinations needed for herd immunity depended upon the interactions of their citizens with each other and their interactions with citizens in other areas, along with the level of vaccinations in these other areas. Even this is a simplification. There is no reason to consider only state or national borders. We could think about this same example at the county level, or even at the neighborhood or block level within a city or town.

In this sense herd immunity can't be stated in terms independent of geography and the interlinkages between geographic units. We can't say a given state, Michigan for example, has reached herd immunity without considering how the vaccine is distributed within Michigan. We also need to consider the interactions of residents of Michigan with those of Indiana, Ohio, and Wisconsin and the vaccine distribution in these states. We also need to consider Ontario, the rest of Canada, and the rest of the world.

Uneven vaccine distribution often occurs as a function of wealth. It is morally responsible to distribute vaccines across the globe regardless of wealth. However, providing vaccines to other parts of the world doesn't have to be entirely altruistic. To quote Dr. Saad Omer, director of the Yale Institute of Global Health: "Vaccine equity is not a zero-sum game."[80] Protecting populations outside of the arbitrarily drawn borders of a map increases protection for everyone on the map. Just as testing for coronavirus outside of a university campus helped the community as well as the campus, providing vaccines outside of a geographic area of interest has benefits for all geographic areas. Yet economic and political incentives drive populations to protect their own first. This is another form of the pandemic dilemma. We cannot be shortsighted, however. If we allow diseases like COVID-19 to grow anywhere in the world, we will continually be visited by new virus variants in our communities and homes. Vaccine advocates such as Dr. Peter Hotez constantly make this point. We need to vaccinate the world in order to create the safety we desire.[81] Failing to do so helped to form the Delta and Omicron variants of coronavirus.

The effects of uneven vaccine distributions keep repeating. Rolling out vaccines and not taking account of these distributional issues is irresponsible. We saw with polio that we cannot expect vaccines to reach vulnerable populations without specific efforts to get the vaccine to them. Sabin Sundays were a solution that took the polio vaccines to the people and allowed a broader range of society access to the vaccine. Across the world, unequal COVID-19 vaccine distribution was still a problem. Like polio, simply having the vaccine available was not allowing access to everyone across the world.

As of the first week in December 2021, much of western Europe was highly vaccinated against COVID-19. The European Centre for Disease Prevention and Control reported that countries such as Denmark, Ireland, and Portugal had over 90 percent of their adult populations fully vaccinated. Many other western European countries had rates well into the 80 percent range. Moving east in Europe revealed a different reality. Romania had less than half of its adult population fully vaccinated. Bulgaria had less than a third. Most other countries of Eastern Europe sat in the 60 to 70 percent range.[82]

However, even the areas with lower vaccination rates in Europe outpaced other areas of the world. Asia had rates of full vaccination for its entire population of about 50 percent. Some countries such as India, at 35 percent, trailed this average by a significant margin. South America had rates similar to Europe and North America, yet it too had outliers far below continental averages. Bolivia, Paraguay, and Venezuela only had about three in eight people fully vaccinated.[83]

The worst coverage by far occurred in Africa. As a continent, the percentage of the population that was fully vaccinated was below *10 percent*. Many countries in central Africa had vaccination rates of 2 percent or less, including Chad, Ethiopia, and Nigeria. Countries in the southern portion of the continent had rates around one in four to one in five.[84]

When the vaccines for COVID-19 were first developed, the ability to provide coverage in lower income countries was of paramount concern. COVAX, or COVID-19 Vaccines Global Access, was created to provide low-income countries access to the newly developed vaccines. It was run by Gavi, the Vaccine Alliance, the Coalition for Epidemic Preparedness Innovations (CEPI), and the World Health Organization (WHO).[85] Unfortunately, it was plagued by missteps. Initial goals for vaccine acquisition were not met. Even as vaccines were acquired, difficulties with distribution mounted. The *New York Times* reported hundreds of thousands of doses going unused and spoiling.[86] As of early December 2021, Chad and Nigeria had used about half of the vaccine doses delivered to their country. Ethiopia had used about 70 percent. Other countries such as Ghana, Uganda, and Zambia, as well as several others, had used less than 40 percent of the vaccines delivered.[87] At the same time, the number of doses received was small. Ghana received only thirty-six doses per one hundred people. Uganda received thirty-five. Ethiopia and Nigeria received twelve and ten doses per one hundred people. Chad received only three.[88]

There were multiple reasons for the failure to distribute vaccines in Africa. Many countries in Africa, particularly those with the lowest income, received minimal amounts of vaccines. If distribution had been perfect, with no spoilage, the low-income countries in Africa still would have been severely under-vaccinated. Imperfect distribution compounded the problem. Funding for distribution lagged behind the arrival of doses. There were shortages of freezers to store the vaccine.[89] Perhaps most importantly, vaccine hesitancy arose in a population distrustful of both their governments and Western medicine based on a history of being used as guinea pigs in the past.[90] Many failures conspired to ruin the vaccination distribution process: lack of vaccine, lack of distribution, and vaccine hesitancy all cascaded together, leaving the African people little better off than had the vaccines not been developed at all.

Much of this was predictable to public health experts. Dr. Omer told the *New York Times*, "Almost no investment in vaccine education or promotion has gone into low-income countries. Why do we expect that all we have to do is drop vaccines at an airport, do the photo op, and people will come running to the airport and grab the vaccine?"[91]

Despite the difficulties, the fight to more equitably distribute COVID-19 vaccines continues. For instance, a group led by Dr. Elena Bottazzi and Dr. Peter Hotez developed a COVID-19 vaccine at the Baylor College of Medicine using donated money. The vaccine is patent-free and can be produced by any low- or middle-income nation.

It wasn't just low-income countries that ran aground in the first months of vaccine distribution and vaccine equity. Similar though less severe problems struck the United States and other high-income western countries. "I have no idea where I would go," seventy-three-year-old Nancy Spencer told Boston 25 News in February 2021, concerning where she could find a COVID-19 vaccine.[92] In South Carolina, a retired military veteran in his seventies, Joe Pepper, knew where to find a shot in a pharmacy nearby. However, without a car, getting to an appointment would be a challenge. In March 2021, he told *New York Magazine*, "It's not really walking distance, but it's reasonable. I know it would take me a long time now because my back bothers me a lot. By the time I've walked about a mile, I have to sit down."[93]

On the other end of the economic spectrum, affluent populations had time and resources to seek out vaccines. In early 2021, ninety-year-old Seattle resident Frances H. Goldman searched for a vaccine appointment for a month. She enlisted her daughter and a friend to help her. Finally, persistence and luck provided her an appointment at Seattle Children's Hospital. On the morning of her appointment, a storm arrived and deposited ten inches of snow. Undaunted, she donned her hiking boots and walked three miles in each direction to receive her vaccine.[94] Ms. Goldman was in good health and had been the recipient of a hip replacement the year prior. She also had the ability to search countless times for a vaccine appointment. Had she lacked either of these things, she would not have gotten the vaccine as early as she did.

Once COVID-19 vaccines became available, acquiring the shot to begin the return to normalcy was a challenge for more people than Ms. Spencer, Mr. Pepper, and Ms. Goldman. Vaccine deserts are areas with a lack of nearby vaccination sites and/or too few vaccination sites to serve the population size. They tend to occur in a bimodal relationship with population density. Rural areas often have few services because of the distance to medical facilities and pharmacies; 177 counties in the United States have no pharmacies located within their borders.[95] Urban areas often have too many people relative to the number of medical facilities in the area; it isn't possible to serve all of them.

As of June 2021, over forty-five million people in the United States (14 percent of the population) lived in a vaccine desert. This included nearly one-third of census tracts in the mountain region of the United States and slightly over one-third of those in the eastern south-central region of the United States.[96] Of most concern is that vaccine deserts impacted populations who were older, poorer, and more likely to be uninsured. These areas also had larger rates of COVID-19 health risks and greater exposure risk.[97] The deserts were frequently in areas of the rural poor and composed of census "tracts with a higher proportion of Black residents, Hispanic residents, and older residents."[98]

In addition to challenges of spatial access, vaccine deserts also occur because of a lack of access to information. Nearly one in five residents in census tracts categorized as vaccine deserts lack internet access.[99] This was a problem for locating vaccination sites and scheduling appointments once a site was found.

Even when internet access was available, the technological challenges of the internet were problematic for older adults who faced the most health risk. As eighty-four-year-old Annette Carlin told the *New York Times*, "It's very frustrating. I feel like everybody else got the vaccine, and I didn't."[100] Ms. Carlin can't afford a computer. She is not alone, as twenty-two million older Americans lack access to broadband internet.[101]

Even when access is available, the technological struggles are real and frustrating for many older adults. Seventy-four-year-old Cheryl Lathrop told the *New York Times*, "I don't know where to go. I get frustrated with the computer and then I just give up."[102] Eventually her daughter found an appointment for her. Many other older adults relied on their children to find vaccines. Yet it remained a challenge. Children of the elderly struggled to book appointments that disappeared in front of their eyes. As one daughter of a seventy-three-year-old woman described, "It became a secondary job. I was doing all these searches at all times of the day and evening."[103] The time to conduct these searches was a luxury that many in lower socio-economic circumstances did not possess.

Together the lack of access to vaccines along with challenges of finding information and scheduling appointments led to disproportionate rates of vaccination across the country in the early months of vaccine rollouts. By the end of June 2021, 47 percent of white Americans had been fully vaccinated compared to only 39 percent of Latinx Americans and 34 percent of Black Americans in the states reporting racial and ethnic breakdowns.[104]

Florida, Iowa, and South Dakota had rates of white vaccinations that were over twice as large as Black vaccinations. Colorado had a vaccination rate for white residents that was over twice the rate for Latinx residents. South Dakota had a shocking vaccination rate of only 3 percent among Latinx residents.[105] Other rural southern and south-central states had low vaccination rates across the board for all racial and ethnic groups. These were states such as Alabama,

Louisiana, Mississippi, South Carolina, Tennessee, and Virginia. They all had rates of vaccination below or just above one out of three individuals.[106]

The vaccination desert problem extended beyond rural areas, as cities experienced overcrowding of vaccination sites. One study reported that vaccination sites in high-poverty districts of Brooklyn served areas containing 65 percent more residents per square mile than low-poverty districts. The authors of this study concluded, "Vaccination efforts in NYC have been focused primarily in white, middle-to-upper class neighborhoods."[107] We were repeating the ineffective distribution of the Salk polio vaccine.

This unequal distribution became more important when the COVID-19 pandemic surged with a vengeance in July 2021 after an early summer respite. This resurgence occurred after significant portions of the US population had been vaccinated and rules on mask wearing and social distancing were relaxed. Large swaths of the population lived in areas with low vaccination rates. This was where the *Delta wave* wreaked the most havoc.

While vaccines were in short supply when first released, access improved greatly by July 1, 2021, just prior to the beginning of the Delta wave.[108] At this point in time, counties in the top quintile of vaccination coverage had average vaccination rates over 60 percent, while those in the bottom quintile had average rates below 30 percent. Many of the least vaccinated counties were in the southern and southeastern part of the United States. Twenty percent of all counties in the bottom quintile were in just two states: West Virginia and Missouri. Three-quarters of the counties in the bottom quintile of vaccination rates were located in just a dozen of the fifty states: Alabama, Arkansas, Florida, Kentucky, Louisiana, Mississippi, Missouri, Nebraska,

Ohio, Oklahoma, Tennessee, and West Virginia. These states were mostly located in the same region of the country. Each of these twelve states borders at least one of the others. All but Nebraska and Florida border at least two. Arkansas borders five of the states listed.

Uneven vaccine distribution would have been a much smaller problem if the under-vaccinated counties were evenly dispersed around the country. If each of the fifty states had a small number of counties with low levels of vaccinations, then it would have created a situation like the forest with only a handful of trees evenly spaced about. If this were the case, the high vaccination status of the counties near the under-vaccinated counties would have offered some protection. The under-vaccinated counties would have received a bit of insulation from their neighbors. This is what an approach to herd immunity does. It allows the decision of one to protect others. However, when the under-vaccinated counties are all clustered together, we get the opposite effect. It is an effect similar to when risky individuals congregate in bars, in restaurants, and at bike rallies. The pandemic grows in the areas with low vaccination rates and spills into neighboring regions. When those neighboring regions also have low vaccination rates, the pandemic grows there as well. The pandemic then spills into even farther geographic regions.

When externalities spill from an under-vaccinated region into other under-vaccinated regions, the damage is compounded rather than dampened. Danger is increased for everyone. When like interacts with like, and both are high risk, the danger and risk to each grows larger. The lack of vaccine usage in the southern United States was like a bike rally many times larger than Sturgis. It fed the Delta wave, which grew to be one of the largest and deadliest waves of the pandemic. But it didn't need to be that large. It would have been dampened with more even vaccine distribution.

Instead, like other waves, it was notoriously unequal. Deaths per capita in the counties in the lowest quintile of vaccine coverage were more than 2.8 times higher than deaths in the counties in the highest quintile of vaccine coverage. What were the characteristics of these counties with such exorbitant deaths? They were poor and uninsured. Compared to the most vaccinated quintile, the counties in the least vaccinated quintile had rates of poverty over 40 percent higher and contained nearly 50 percent more uninsured individuals.

Of course, the elephant in the room was politics. The under-vaccinated counties were overwhelmingly Republican and supported President Trump in the 2020 election. In the least vaccinated quintile of counties, the average vote share for Trump was over 75 percent. However, the Trump factor didn't apply to everyone. It applied mostly to low-income Trump supporters. According to the United States Census Bureau's Household Pulse Survey COVID-19 Vaccination Tracker, 91 percent of individuals with a bachelor's degree or higher had received at least one vaccine dose.[109] The profile of these under-vaccinated locations was clear. They were poor, uninsured, and rural.

It wasn't just the lack of vaccinations that harmed this population, however. Lower rates of health insurance led to less experience with the health care system and less knowledge about where to go and what to do when serious illness struck. Even further, the options for care in many of these counties was severely limited. Rural areas were underserved by critical care resources. In the lowest quintile of counties for vaccine coverage, there were about eight intensive care unit (ICU) beds per 100,000 residents. This was less than half of the seventeen ICU beds available in the highest quintile of counties. This is a huge discrepancy—yet it understates the issue. Of the counties in the lowest quintile of vaccine coverage, 68 percent had no ICU beds within the entire county. Not one single ICU bed.

Many residents in these unvaccinated counties had to cross county lines just to receive ICU care if needed. Beyond vaccine deserts, these unvaccinated individuals lived in barren critical care deserts. Medical care wasn't available just down the street when COVID-19 symptoms progressed. Care was many miles and minutes (or even hours) away. They were small towns like Dalhart, Texas, that had to send patients 600 miles to San Antonio for treatment. Many of the least vaccinated areas of the country were in the worst possible place for handling a pandemic surge.

In normal times, the lack of ICU care isn't as damaging. If a particular county or hospital is overrun, patients can be transferred to another hospital in a nearby town or county. This happens when there are massive traffic accidents on highways. Patients are dispersed to a range of hospitals so that all can receive care. This wasn't possible at a pandemic peak. All the hospitals were overrun. There was nowhere to go nearby, as every hospital in the area was at or reaching capacity. Nearby hospitals were in the same position as Coon Memorial in Dalhart, Texas. When these small hospitals were overrun, care could only be received hundreds of miles away.

A study by the US Department of Agriculture investigated the patterns of rural and urban mortality in the first years of the COVID-19 pandemic. Differences in rates of infection over the course of the pandemic were relatively small. Rates of mortality had much greater disparities and evolved over time. In the initial wave of the pandemic, both cases and deaths per capita were much higher in cities than in rural areas. By the end of 2020, per capita cases were marginally higher in rural areas, but deaths per capita were three times higher in rural areas than urban areas.[110] These rural areas had over seven times higher rates of dangerous underlying health conditions; residents of rural areas had to travel on average thirty times as far to get to an intensive care hospital; and the percentage of people without health insurance in rural areas was double that in urban areas.[111]

All of these issues worked together. Rural areas of poverty are underserved by health care. They tend to have lower rates of vaccination, even when vaccines are not a hot-button political issue. The counties least vaccinated for COVID-19 had lower rates of influenza vaccination prior to the pandemic. Residents of these counties were more frequently uninsured. These people had less experience with the health care system partly because of low incomes, high poverty, and no insurance, but also because access to health care was not nearby. It was not nearby because a for-profit health care system does not make large profits in sparsely populated low-income areas. All of these issues, even without Trump-based politics, were interconnected, harmful, and dangerous. Then–President Trump's rhetoric of COVID denial made things much worse. However, the residents of these areas wore pandemic targets even without Trump needing to pin them on their chests. These areas were already the nexus of all types of potential risk.

If these people hadn't been poor and uninsured, or if they would have had access to ICU centers nearby, or if they would have had more experience with the health care system, then far fewer people in these areas would have died. The problem was that these things are not independent in the United States. They go together. The United States did not and does not provide uniform access to high-quality health care across society. As during the polio epidemic with its "second-hand hospitals" and "whites only" care facilities, this inequality when paired with COVID-19 cost people their lives. These same problems occur even in normal times, but we don't often notice. When the pandemic arrived, it exposed and magnified the failure to provide quality health care access to all. The cost of this failure was many lives needlessly lost.

Chapter 10

COMPASSION, NOT TOOLS

"The most terrible outbreak of cholera which ever occurred in this kingdom, is probably that which took place in Broad Street, Golden Square, and the adjoining streets, a few weeks ago. Within two hundred and fifty yards of the spot where Cambridge Street joins Broad Street, there were upwards of five hundred fatal attacks of cholera in ten days."[1] So began Dr. John Snow's description of the London cholera outbreak of 1854. Snow had long been suspicious of the prevailing miasma theory of infectious disease, in which noxious bad air emanated from the ground and caused disease. He believed cholera and many other infections of the time to be communicable in a more direct manner. For cholera specifically, he believed that the disease was transferred through contaminated water. His theory was unorthodox for the time, and few believed him.

In this particular outbreak, Snow focused on a water pump that sat at the intersection of Cambridge and Broad Streets in the Soho section of London. In an initial examination of eighty-nine deaths, Snow found that seventy-nine of these deaths occurred in homes where the Broad Street pump was the nearest water source. Of the ten outliers, five used the Broad Street pump instead of the pump nearer to them because of a preference for the taste of the Broad Street water. Three others had children in schools near the pump.

This left only two of the eighty-nine deaths that did not have a known connection to the Broad Street water pump. With this evidence, Snow continued to dig deeper.

Some locations near the pump were puzzling for a lack of infections and death. A nearby workhouse had no deaths out of 535 inmates, other than a few who arrived to the workhouse already ill. The workhouse was surrounded by buildings that contained infections. Why were they exempt from the epidemic? Snow found that the workhouse had its own water well and received additional water from an independent water works. A brewery in the vicinity of the pump had only two cases with minor illness out of seventy workmen. During interviews with the proprietor, Mr. Huggins, Snow learned the men were allowed to drink malt liquor during work and, in addition to the brewery having its own well, Mr. Huggins believed the men "do not drink water at all," only liquor.[2]

There were other cases of cholera in the outbreak not clearly connected to the pump. However, one by one, Snow began documenting a heretofore unknown connection. A nearby coffee shop that used water from the pump had nine customers dead from cholera. A group of seven men who lived outside the area of the pump all died. Each was employed at the same factory making dental equipment. These factory workers used the Broad Street pump for refreshment during the workday. A man from Brighton died from cholera. Snow discovered that he had visited Soho to tend to his brother's death, ate lunch, and died the next evening after drinking water at his deceased brother's home. A fifty-nine-year-old woman in West End died without ever having been in the neighborhood of the pump. The death was puzzling until her son revealed that she received water delivered from Broad Street each day. Her niece, from a "high and healthy part of Islington," had also perished after visiting her aunt and being refreshed with Broad Street water.[3] Snow continued documenting: A cabinetmaker who had recently worked in the area, schoolchildren who regularly passed near the pump, a tailor who worked on Broad Street. Case after case connected to the Broad Street pump. Snow carefully plotted their location and connection to the water pump on a street map. He had no doubt as to the source of the epidemic, and he spoke to the Board of Guardians of St James's parish on the evening of September 7. He convinced them to remove the handle from the pump. By the end of the month, the cholera epidemic was over. The Broad Street pump had indeed been the source.

Yet to prove his theory of waterborne contagion more forcefully, Snow needed to convince others. He needed to identify how the pump came to be contaminated. Snow had a staunch critic in twenty-nine-year-old Reverend Henry Whitehead, who published his own account of the epidemic prior to Snow's 1855 book. Whitehead disputed Snow's conclusion. He believed in the standard miasma theory of bad air and set out to interview as many people in the area of the pump as possible in the hope of finding evidence to prove Snow wrong. He was not able to do so. In his June 1855 report, "Special Investigation of Broad Street," he wrote, "I find it necessary to state my conviction, slowly and I may add reluctantly adopted, that the use of this water [at Broad Street] was connected with the commencement and continuance of the outburst in a very remarkable way."[4] What had changed his mind? In part, the identification of a probable cause in the case of an early victim located at 40 Broad Street.

A young girl, Frances Lewis, aged five months, died of cholera on September 2, a few days into the outbreak. Frances's father, police constable Thomas Lewis, died five days after his young daughter.[5] At first Whitehead had thought this case not significant until he conducted additional interviews with the girl's mother, Sarah. Then he realized that the young girl had not perished quickly as most cholera victims did. Instead, she had been ill for days with diarrhea prior to her death. "The child was attacked [with illness] on Monday, 28th August . . . the [excrement] were collected in napkins, which . . . were immediately steeped in pails, the water from which was poured partly into a sink in the backyard, and partly into a cesspool in the front area."[6] Whitehead notes this cesspool sat in "dangerous proximity . . . to the pump well."[7] A subsequent excavation revealed that the cesspool leaked into the well. Snow's harshest critic had identified the initial source of the outbreak in Soho and proved Snow correct. Although Snow died in 1858 before his contributions were fully appreciated by the world, he would become known in the twentieth century as a father of epidemiology and public health largely due to his work identifying cholera transmission.

Parallel to Snow, a new movement developed at the Paris School of Medicine which would be transported to England via a controversial figure. Edwin Chadwick, a barrister from Manchester, was a social reformer. An acolyte of Jeremy Bentham, Chadwick laid the foundation for England's New Poor Laws. Chadwick was a harsh critic of relief for the indigent, and he felt that too much public assistance created dependence and slovenliness. In the New Poor Laws, he advocated for workhouses where the poor would be required to work for their assistance. The conditions of the poorhouses were designed to be so foul and labor-intensive that they would be avoided by all means possible. Thus, only the most deserving poor, those who had no other choice, would seek to remedy their poverty through the wretched conditions of the workhouse.[8] As Charles Dickens wrote in *Oliver Twist*, "So they established the rule that all poor people should have the alternative (for they would compel nobody, not they) of being starved by a gradual process in the house, or by a quick one out of it."[9] The poor laws were seen as sinister by many other than Dickens. Yet with the poor laws in place, Chadwick turned to the issue of health and sanitation.

The prevailing theory of the time indicated that miasma created illness. As such, Chadwick believed that the dirt, filth, and squalor of the living conditions of the poor brought about their near constant affliction with disease. The noxious odors of trash, dirt, and human waste brought morbidity and mortality to the poor. In turn, this ill health created destitution. With this framework in mind, Chadwick set about improving the sanitary conditions of England through a vast public works program. In his vision, water would circulate through a city much as blood circulated through the body.[10] Cesspools were removed and replaced with more modern sewers that would carry waste away from homes and remove the necessity of discarding waste into them or onto alleys and streets. Streets were swept and cleaned daily to separate humans from the miasma that would theoretically contaminate them. While Chadwick was wrong in his theory of infection, his methods brought about vast improvements in hygiene that would pay dividends through to modern day. Frank Snowden has argued that these improvements in cleanliness in the streets ushered in an era of cleanliness inside the home that also proved beneficial to overall health: "Ordinary people armed themselves against disease through multiple daily rituals of washing their bodies, food, utensils, clothing, and homes. Cleansing and vigilance became integral parts of daily routines."[11] This view of cleanliness inside and outside the home, plus Snow's discovery of cholera transmission and the coming revolution of the germ theory of disease, ushered in a new discipline of public health.

Perhaps no one better understood and advocated for a more nuanced and all-encompassing view of public health than Rudolf Virchow. As a first calling, Virchow was a German physician and the founder of cellular pathology. He was credited with identifying, describing, and naming leukemia. In the founding of public health, Snow sought to prove a cause-and-effect relationship between contaminated water and cholera. Chadwick saw disease and poverty interlinked with disease acting as the causal force that drove people into poverty. Virchow saw connections between health, poverty, sanitation, employment, living conditions, and politics. In the view of Virchow, all these forces acted together in a tangled web of interdependence.

This worldview emerged for Virchow when he was assigned to a commission investigating a typhus epidemic in the Upper Silesia region of Prussia in 1847 and 1848. The outbreak followed a series of crop failures and a famine. He reported that "in a single year 10% of the population died in the Pless district, 6.48% of starvation combined with the epidemic, and, according to official figures, 1.3% solely of starvation. In 8 months, in the district of Rybnik, 14.3% of the population were affected by typhus, of whom 20.46% died."[12] Virchow's report noted further that "at the beginning of the year, 3% of the population of both districts were orphans."[13] Virchow was shocked to see Prussia, "which took so much pride in the excellence of its institutions,"[14] in such a miserable state of affairs.

Virchow's report of the outbreak emphasized the social circumstances of peasants and their poverty along with the failures of government that combined and led to disease. Prussian laws were intended to provide food, excellent

schools, sanitary policies, and a litany of civil servants to assist in each of these endeavors. Yet all of these did little
good in practice during the Upper Silesia outbreak. "The law
existed, the civil servants were there—and the people died in
their thousands from starvation and disease. The law did
not help, as it was only paper with writing. . . . The whole
country had gradually become a structure of paper, a huge
house of cards, to be toppled in a confused heap."[15] Out of
indifference or incompetence, the government was failing
to protect its people.

Virchow saw a government and an aristocracy using impoverished miners, farmers, and laborers as tools for their
own gain: "The feudal aristocracy used its money to in-
dulge in the luxury. . . . The plutocracy, which [drew] very
large amounts from the Upper Silesian mines, did not recognize the Upper Silesians as human beings, but only as
tools."[16] Virchow tied these circumstances to the epidemic,
"for there can now no longer be any doubt that such an epidemic dissemination of typhus had only been possible under
the wretched conditions of life that poverty and lack of
culture had created in Upper Silesia. If these conditions
were removed, I am sure that epidemic typhus would not
recur."[17]

In the view of Virchow, the causal link between disease
and poverty ran contrary to the views of Chadwick. To
Virchow the solution to curing this epidemic and others like
it, along with the prevention of similar epidemics in the
future, was greater financial prosperity, education, and
culture, along with a reduction in economic inequality.[18]
Virchow's view was more nuanced than poverty leading to
disease, however. As Klaus Lang wrote, "According to Virchow, inadequate social conditions rendered a population
more susceptible to other causal factors, none of which

would suffice in isolation to produce an epidemic."[19] A combination of factors led to the poor suffering more than the wealthy from epidemic disease. Virchow deemed social science as essential in combatting disease. He wrote later in life, "Medicine is a social science and politics is nothing else but medicine on a large scale. Medicine as a social science, as the science of human beings, has the obligation to point out problems and to attempt their theoretical solution; the politician, the practical anthropologist, must find the means for their actual solution." One can see within this quote several strands of Virchow's worldview. While he was a well-known pathologist, he recognized a social component to disease that could not be separated from biology. An essential part of curing disease needed to include social circumstances, social science, and politics. As such, medical practitioners had a responsibility to work for social change in order to fully care for their patients. He called upon medical practitioners to become political activists. Virchow's recognition led to his dedication toward increasing access to medical care for the poor and vaccines for children, as well as to projects to increase sanitation in impoverished areas.[20]

In the figures of Chadwick, Snow, and Virchow we see the birth of the field of public health in the nineteenth century. In many ways, this view of public health was short-lived. Robert Koch and Louis Pasteur arrived to bring forth the germ theory of disease. Initially there were complementarities between this new paradigm of science and the social medicine of Virchow. Laws requiring indoor plumbing, open windows, and ventilation in housing served dual purposes in line with both social medicine and germ reduction.[21] These advances in sanitation all limited exposure risk. Similar complementarities continued into the early twentieth century.[22]

Historians note that medicine and public health then separated. Medicine increasingly moved into the laboratories. Hospital construction, new medical technology, vaccines, antibiotics, and other pharmaceuticals all became paramount in medicine and in the treatment of illness.[23] As the medical profession rose in stature, health services provided by public health agencies were seen by physicians as threatening. In the late nineteenth and early twentieth centuries, physicians did not hold the stature or earnings potential of today. They needed to protect their limited market. Public health, which often provided duplicate services at a limited or non-existent fee, threatened the marketplace of physicians.[24] Further, physicians saw public health data collection as infringing on the patient-physician relationship and privacy.[25] These conflicts developed into a professional rivalry.

At the same time, public health changed. Following medicine, public health also moved closer to the laboratory. In *The Atlantic*, Ed Yong wrote that "Public-health practitioners thought that by cleaving to the same paradigm [as physicians], 'they could solidify and extend their authority and bring public health up to the same level of esteem and power that medicine was beginning to enjoy.'"[26] Public health didn't entirely remove itself from social circumstance. However, it increasingly moved away from advocacy for social reform and toward scientific and statistical identification of individual and environmental risk factors. As it did so, it moved further away from the politically volatile issues of social reform. As public health "prioritized objective science over social reform and alliances with relatively powerful progressive constituencies such as labor, charity, social welfare organizations, and housing reformers, the field was marginalized and left with no political base."[27] Because of all of these factors combined, "medicine generally triumphed [over public health] in direct political conflicts."[28]

Over time, the distinction between medicine and public health deepened and medicine rose in prominence relative to public health. Medicine came to be associated with "care and treatment of the individual," curing illness, and "objective and reductionist . . . science."[29] Public health concerned itself with prevention of illness and "on ameliorating the social and environmental conditions producing disease."[30] Medicine focused on the individual, while public health focused on the population. The disciplines separated into an "I" and a "we" approach to health. In H. Holden Thorp's editorial in *Science*, epidemiologist Gregg Gonsalves was quoted as saying that medicine today is "about private risk and private choices."[31] Public health is about the health of populations. In making this distinction, Professor Gonsalves struck a point of emphasis, not an all-encompassing difference; it was not that physicians did not care about populations nor that public health professionals did not care about individuals. However, they had different organizing principles and structures of thought in their training and methods. Both approaches were valuable and necessary.

In recent decades, public health has returned toward its roots. In the 1960s Thomas McKeown laid out a controversial theory: the large decreases in mortality during the industrial revolution were not due to medicine but to improvements in the overall standard of living, diet, nutrition, and overall better economic circumstances.[32] Although much of McKeown's work has been supplanted by subsequent research, his legacy lives in the influential question at the heart of his research: is public health most improved by targeted interventions of medicine or by broad efforts to better the economic circumstances, living conditions, and equality across society?[33] This question, along with an increased emphasis on preventative health in medicine and a renewed emphasis on the social and political determinants of health, led to a re-emergence of understanding social factors as instruments of health in recent decades.[34]

Even with the increased emphasis on social and political causes of ill health and a rise in preventative medicine, twenty-first-century society still was overreliant on medicine and medical technology to find a cure for afflictions. When too much focus goes to individual health risk and private adjudication of this health risk, we lose sight of the population and the dangers of exposure risk. When we do so, we put ourselves into the pandemic dilemma where individual choices can lead to collective failure for the population.

We saw this result in 2021 and 2022 when countries, particularly the United States, gave up the fight to mandate social precautions and non-pharmaceutical interventions while the COVID-19 pandemic still raged. Vaccine mandates, social distancing requirements, and mask mandates largely disappeared even in locations where they were not widely opposed. It wasn't that the pandemic was over. School mask mandates in New York ended in late February 2022 when the country was still losing an average of 1,000 lives per day to the pandemic. Only one month prior, we had been losing over 3,000 lives per day. The primary argument for lifting the school mask mandate: a coronavirus infection was "just a cold" for most children and there was no need to protect them unless their parents felt they were at risk. By risk, of course, they meant health risk. They were ignoring exposure risk and the additional infections that children would introduce into society. National and state leaders ceded authority to individuals. Adjudication of personal (health) risk and personal choice became the new pandemic policy, perhaps because it was too costly in political terms to do otherwise.

With this political decision we entered the pandemic dilemma where individuals now not only made choices for themselves, but more importantly they also made choices for the public. Many did not consider this second factor. Individuals were allowed to choose their exposure risk that they shared with society. If individuals chose to pollute society by enhancing exposure risk, they were given the liberty to do so despite the consequences and infringements on liberty that they created for others. People more accepting of risk would meet in public spaces, maskless, with little precaution. As of early 2023, when this manuscript was still being completed, we did not yet know the cost of these decisions. As a society, we hoped that new vaccines and treatments would arise quickly enough to combat any new strains. We trusted in technology once again. We also trusted that we could distribute any new resources widely and equitably. This was a leap of faith, as it was a task that we have never done well in the past. We were set on a course to allow individual decisions to trump collective protection and hoped that this would not create a dangerous precedent in a future infectious disease crisis.

In the early twenty-first century, people lived in a world filled with technology. When new problems developed, science and technology were expected to find the solution. In late 2020, the first COVID-19 vaccines arrived. Many expected them to quickly end the pandemic and bring normalcy back to the world. Most of these same people never gave thought to how the vaccines would be distributed. We had forgotten the misfortune of the past barely a half century earlier when the arrival of Salk's polio vaccine was similarly lauded but didn't end the polio epidemic overnight. In the 1950s there were holes in our social fabric, in our distribution of medical care, and in our public health system that didn't deliver the vaccine to all. It would take the Sabin vaccine and its more efficient distribution to fully end polio in most areas of the world. In many ways, this process repeated with COVID-19. Unequal access to the vaccine led to some being protected and not others during early periods of vaccine availability. The inequity became readily apparent during the Delta wave in the fall of 2021.

This wave, along with waning immunity and the evolution of new subvariants, led public health officials to call for a "vaccine plus" strategy of pandemic mitigation. Vaccines were to be used in combination with a range of measures to limit exposure risk, such as continued indoor mask use, social distancing when possible, and frequent testing, especially in situations that created interactions with vulnerable individuals or where large groups of people were congregated. This vaccine plus strategy was based upon the "Swiss cheese model" of public health that originated with psychologist James Reason.

In 1990 Reason published a book titled *Human Error*.[35] Out of this book and subsequent publications, Reason developed linkages between the concepts of human error and system design to prevent an individual error from cascading into a catastrophe. The world didn't want one ill-designed O-ring to lead to the destruction of the space shuttle nor one inattentive safety inspector to lead to a nuclear power plant meltdown. Reason recognized that humans are prone to mistakes. We make errors and take missteps. We don't have the skills to perform a task that we think we can or we don't follow a rule that we know we should. We lack timely knowledge to make an informed decision in a critical situation. We are tired and we don't recognize something unusual that would cause alarm if we were more attentive at a crucial moment. Reason argued that errors such as these are an unavoidable part of human decision making.

Reason delineated two views of mistakes—the person approach and the systems approach.[36] The person approach blames the individual. If we could just keep the person more attentive or give him more training and knowledge then the failure would not occur. The person approach tries to avoid human error by improving the human. Conversely, the systems approach recognizes that humans are fallible no matter how well trained, knowledgeable, or rested. It argues that rules, procedures, and organizations are only reliable and robust if their system of defense is built to expect and overcome these inevitable failures of people. As opposed to fixing the human, the systems approach builds our institutions, organizations, and procedures with redundancies in order to be robust to our inevitable shortcomings.

Automobiles are dangerous. Some accidents will happen. To prevent harm from these accidents we implement laws about speeding and safe driving and add stop signs and traffic lights to our roads. Each of these safeguards limit the probability of an accident—they limit exposure risk. If an accident does occur, we have other protections. Seat belts, air bags, and crumple zones in high-impact areas of our cars all limit our health risk when an accident occurs. The hope is that when one piece of this system fails, other safeguards protect you to avoid a catastrophe such as serious injury or death. We build checks and redundancies like these into the way we live our lives and the institutions we create. In public health, this thinking led to what became known as the "Swiss cheese model."[37]

In mid-2020, Ian M. Mackay, a virologist at the University of Queensland, set about promoting the Swiss cheese model in hopes of slowing the COVID-19 pandemic.[38] Imagine that for any infectious disease there are a series of protections that one can take. Individually, each of these protections lowers risk, but none are foolproof. They all have holes like a piece of Swiss cheese. Now imagine that we take many of these protections and apply them all at one time. It is unlikely that they will all fail simultaneously. Like a series of randomly chosen slices of Swiss cheese all stacked on top of each other, it is unlikely that a series of holes will line up to provide a path through the entire stack of cheese slices. At least one of the randomly placed slices will cover any hole. Mask-wearing, hand-washing, avoiding congested spaces, and limiting large gatherings all combine to greatly limit our chance of being infected and spreading the infection to others. If we are infected, other protections limit our risk of a severe health outcome. Even if none of these protections are perfect, any failure in one of these protections is covered by at least one of the other protections to keep us safe.

Some people in the population are able to accomplish these multiple layers of protection with relative ease. When a pandemic arrives, a family moves to their second home in rural Vermont. The parents work their white-collar jobs remotely. The children attend high-quality suburban schools with resources available to provide high-quality remote learning. It isn't as good as in-person learning but they make do the best they can. At the height of the pandemic, the family orders groceries to be delivered to the front steps of their cabin, or they shop in the small grocery of their temporary hometown at non-busy hours when it is never crowded. Still, even with these protections, they wear a mask, use hand sanitizer, and avoid large social gatherings. Even though they are separated from friends and family they do their best to maintain mental health and connections to those they love. They schedule group Zoom meetings on high-speed broadband internet to keep in touch with family.

Friday night remains family game or movie night, perhaps with grandparents or another family visiting with them over Zoom. Children still socialize at lunch over group FaceTime calls with the same friends that sit at the cafeteria lunch table in normal times. When a vaccine becomes available, they have the resources and time to search a multitude of state facilities, pharmacies, and hospitals to find an appointment to receive the vaccine.

If a family member somehow becomes infected, the infected person remains isolated in his bedroom, and one of the multiple bathrooms in their house is used exclusively by him. His isolation makes it unlikely that other family members will be infected. The family schedules a telehealth appointment for the infected person with the family physician who has known him for years. The physician knows the infected person's health history and any dangers that this history may hold for his infection. However, complications are less likely because his white-collar job provides high-quality health insurance, and this physician has consulted with him for years on preventative medicine and addressed issues of high blood pressure and high cholesterol in the past. He has avoided dangerous comorbidities through these methods and lives in good health. If there is still concern, an anti-viral drug such as Paxlovid is prescribed and gathered quickly from the local pharmacy. He and everyone else in this family are more likely than others to pass through the pandemic lightly scathed. Everyone in the family has lower exposure risk because of the layered protections in place. If someone is infected, health risk is low because their health care resources are easily mobilized and provide additional layers of protection. At every step in the pandemic there is a level of protection that helps to prevent catastrophe. The holes in the Swiss cheese slices never line up. The members of this family are never 100 percent safe. Long COVID remains a possibility, as does death. However, each of these are un-likely occurrences because of the layers of protection that each family member holds. Not everyone matches this ide-alized description of safety.

Isidoro Flores Contreras stands on a sidewalk in Sand City, California, a small town near the southern shore of Monterey Bay.[39] Passengers in the cars that pass by see the Costco store and a set of McDonald's arches behind Mr. Contreras. The cars have just driven past the Porsche dealership that sits a short distance to the south on Del Monte Boulevard. Soon they will reach the local shopping mall, one of the local beaches, or the local high school. Each of these are common destinations a short distance from where Mr. Contreras paces as he waves bouquets of flowers at passing cars. The sun beats down on Mr. Contreras. He wears a hat and seeks shade from a large tree that stands alongside the road. A sign reads $15. A set of three white plastic buckets sit farther back from the street containing ad-ditional bouquets. Mr. Contreras has sold flowers on this street for ten years, rarely missing a day until the pandemic arrived and his business was shut down for fifteen days due to a stay-at-home order. While the job is not glamorous, he makes a steady income of about $300 most weeks. With this he must make do financially. He pays about one week's earnings for rent each month. This leaves him about $1,000 per month for food, utilities, transportation, health care, and other living expenses. The fifteen days he misses work because of the pandemic make his normal budget untenable.

After work, he goes home to Alisal, a neighborhood within the small city of Salinas, California. Here he shares a two-bedroom house with four other people. Most days it takes between sixty and ninety minutes to commute from Alisal to Sand City by public transit. Mr. Contreras sleeps in the living room of his home while the four other people share the bedrooms. If any household member were to become infected, it would be impossible to isolate. Where would the others go? Where would they sleep and eat? The likelihood that someone in the home becomes infected is high because of the neighborhood in which they live and the jobs that they hold. Alisal's population is primarily Mexican and Mexican-American, and their culture leads there to be many multigenerational homes in the area. Many residents work at nearby farms in essential jobs that do not stop when the pandemic arrives. Few here work remotely. Alisal is inwardly dense. It measures as the most overcrowded zip code in Monterey County. Overcrowded housing and essential work strongly overlap in this area and throughout California. There is at least one essential worker in 65 percent of these overcrowded homes. These dual risks of exposure amplify each other during an epidemic. Essential workers are more likely to be infected and overcrowded housing allows each of these infections to spread more widely. Alisal is poor too, with 22 percent of its residents living in poverty. Once infections reach this neighborhood they spread quickly and easily in these conditions. In 2020 Alisal contained just 14 percent of the Monterey County population, but it had about 33 percent of COVID-19 infections in the early months of the pandemic.

We cannot ascertain the health insurance situation of Mr. Contreras from viewing him on the street. Given his income and profession, it is certain he does not have high-quality employer-provided health insurance. Given his limited budget, he likely cannot afford private health insurance, but he may qualify for Medicaid. As he paces on the sidewalk selling his flowers, we can notice a persistent limp in his gait. He is a bit overweight. We can imagine that he does not see a physician on a regular basis. When he does, he likely visits a crowded urgent care center, an emergency room, or a public health clinic that does not allow for lengthy patient consultations. He sees whoever is on duty. This physician will not know his health history well, nor his personal history. In the short time allotted for the visit there will not be time to fully reveal this information. The physician will only know what is written on his chart. We can also imagine that Mr. Contreras does not have regular physicals or screenings for chronic illnesses like cancer. He makes do with what he has in health, health care, and money. This leaves him with high levels of exposure risk and high levels of health risk. He lacks almost every protection that a more affluent family holds.

The dichotomy between Mr. Contreras and the fictional family in Vermont helps to illustrate the differences in pandemic outcomes. The family in Vermont has done nothing wrong. They have protected themselves, as they should, with the benefits that affluent families have built into their everyday lives. They have methods to limit exposure risk. In the event that one of the family members is infected, existing levels of good health and access to health care add other layers of protection that lower their health risk. Any exposure or health risk they hold is covered by another layer of protection in another dimension of their lives. The other half lives as if the holes in the block of Swiss cheese are purposefully aligned. A pandemic tunnel leads them directly to exposure and health risk. Their circumstances leave them targeted in a pandemic, and everything in their lives leads them to have greater exposure and health risk.

The wisdom of the Swiss cheese model lies in the fact that deficiencies in protections are uncorrelated. An askew mask is not the result of a faulty handwashing; these things are independent. However, when we think about the big things that create exposure and health risk, they are all correlated. Poverty, lack of education, overcrowded housing, essential front-facing work, lack of health insurance, and lack of access to health care and vaccines all go together. They all lead to increased exposure risk and increased health risk. If you have one of these features in your life, you likely have many. It is nearly impossible to separate one from the other because they are so tightly connected. These overlapping exposure and health risks and incidents of infections and deaths led people like Chadwick, Snow, and Virchow to sometimes get the causality wrong in the nineteenth century. It was impossible to know which element was a cause and which was an effect. They were all entangled and intertwined. That is true even today. Hong Kong, Naples, and NYC tenements of the nineteenth century, although more extreme, had the same essential features of the neighborhoods that were inwardly dense and contained multigenerational homes with many essential workers commuting by public transit who died from COVID-19. The people in these neighborhoods faced a simultaneous host of exposure and health risks. All of these things worked together to bring about the great disparities in pandemic outcomes.

Many of the people in the pandemic tunnel today are people of color. There is no getting around this fact and its link to US history. Although they have long preceded other groups, Native Americans are seen as outsiders on the fringe of society. The Asian, Black, and Latinx populations have lived here for centuries. Despite their long histories, many within our population do not see these racially and ethnically diverse groups of people as "true Americans," in *their* image of the founding fathers.

To this day people of color face an empathy gap. Psychological research shows that white Americans do not sense pain in people of color as strongly as they sense pain in people of their own ethnic backgrounds.[40] It is an example of what W. E. B. Du Bois called *peculiar indifference* in the nineteenth century when speaking on the condition of the Black population. "The most difficult social problem in the matter of Negro health is the peculiar attitude of the nation toward the well-being of the race. There have . . . been few other cases in the history of civilized peoples where human suffering has been viewed with such peculiar indifference."[41] This indifference to health disparities is not a relic of the past and has continued into modern times.[42] It is little different than in the 1800s when people such as Chadwick saw the plight of impoverished laborers as a result of their choices, as if a simple decision not to be poor was enough to change their circumstances. Many of those indifferent to the plight of the poor in the twenty-first century hold similar views. These people feel that if the poor would just work harder they could avoid today's equivalent of the nineteenth-century poorhouse that leads to their ill health. These feelings were implicitly revealed in the privileged claims of the need to return to normal commerce and normal education without recognizing the effects of these actions on those less fortunate. The fictional family in Vermont likely intends no harm. They do no wrong until they return to Boston or Manhattan and argue for the reopening of in-person restaurants and maskless schools without concern or a plan for how to protect the most vulnerable while doing so.[43]

Outsider status remains for people of color. Violence against Asian people increased across the world from misplaced blame for the COVID-19 outbreak. In the United States, agricultural workers were left to essential tasks on farms throughout the pandemic. Many of those farms were staffed with temporary workers brought to the country on H-2A visas that have increased nearly 350 percent in the past decade. When these workers arrive to the country, their visa status requires that their employers house them, but these employers are not required to house them well. Most of these workers are stuffed into overcrowded bunkhouses. When a pandemic arrives these bunkhouses and farms contain high levels of exposure risk. Some die in these conditions like Mr. Galvan in Dalhart, Texas. Why do we use these temporary visa programs instead of more permanent programs? In part because it makes the workers expendable like a broken tool that can be discarded when it doesn't perform.

The situation parallels how Irish and German immigrants were used in nineteenth-century New Orleans. If those workers died or were injured digging canals, the firms simply hired another worker from the lot of the Irish Channel. Virchow's observations of Upper Silesian miners being used as tools were little different. We did the same with the workers brought to the country on H-2A visas. If they were infected or died, they were simply sent home to be replaced by another worker. They were neither protected nor valued. The United States needed these people for essential work but had no interest in investing in them long term. The country only valued them as long as they were able to harvest fruit and vegetables. If they were unable to do the task because of illness or injury, their employers replaced them with another worker just as they might replace a broken tool.[44] There was no respect for their humanity.

The workers on H-2A visas faced extreme circumstances, and other essential workers lived on the same gradient. They were tasked with dangerous work that exposed them to the pandemic. Many of these same workers faced increased exposure risk at home. Their exposure may not have been as extreme as the workers on H-2A visas, but it was close. Multi generational and overcrowded homes within inwardly dense neighborhoods created bridges and multiple levels of heightened exposure risk throughout communities. Lack of high-quality and consistent health care created heightened health risk once someone was infected.

As we move down the financial gradient all of the same exposure and health risks increase.

In early 2021, Corina Knoll of the *New York Times* wrote a story about Magalie Salomon and her family. Ms. Salomon was born in the Bahamas before immigrating to the United States. In the spring of 2020, she lived in an apartment in Brooklyn, New York, with her two children, sixteen-year-old Adriana and eighteen-year-old Xavier. She worked overnight shifts as a home attendant. Described as a woman with a "scathing sense of humor," she was "generous and gregarious."[45] She provided lavish gifts to her children on their birthdays such as brand name clothes and special restaurant dinners. In late March 2020, Ms. Salomon began to feel unwell. Adriana too began to feel unusually fatigued. COVID-19 tests were not widely available in their neighborhood at this time. Ms. Salomon's condition worsened and she called an ambulance on March 31, 2020. Before she left in the ambulance, she hugged both of her children. She was a breast cancer survivor. She was tough and her children assumed she'd be okay. She continuously texted and chatted on FaceTime with her children upon arriving at the hospital, but her condition continued to deteriorate. Just before midnight three days later, Xavier received an urgent telephone call from the hospital. His mother had gone into cardiac arrest—should they resuscitate her if it happened again? "Do whatever it takes," he told them.[46] Xavier and Adriana had lost their father to lymphoma nine years earlier when he was just thirty years old. Their mother was all they had—the lifeblood of their home. They must save her—they must. Another call, another plea to resuscitate her. Finally, a third call. Ms. Salomon had passed away, and Adriana and Xavier were alone.

Where to now?

Being barely an adult, Xavier felt he couldn't care for his sister. Adriana moved in with family friends in Queens and then an aunt in Brooklyn. She spent two weeks on vacation visiting her half-brother in North Carolina. Xavier started classes at City College of New York. He focused on studies to become a civil engineer. He wanted to stay in his family's apartment, but his limited earnings at Burger King made that difficult. He sold his prized sneaker collection to pay for water, electricity, and phone bills. He discontinued cable and landline telephone services. He ate inexpensive ramen noodles and fast food to minimize his spending. Adriana struggled in school despite being a top student in previous years. Their struggles brought the siblings closer. Conversations with his girlfriend and her family helped to ease the pressure that Xavier felt mounting in his life. His sister moved back in with him, although they stayed in the family apartment only briefly. It was time to move on.

Xavier took care of his sister as best he could, and Adriana likewise helped at home. They were forced to be adults before their time and did their best to live up to their mother's image. Xavier is now engaged, committed to doing well in school, and thinking about the future with a post-college career and a home and children of his own. On Adriana's birthday Xavier took her to the mall, just as his mother would have done, and showered her with gifts. "On Xavier's own birthday, when he turned 19, he worked an eight-hour shift" at Burger King.[47] He was becoming the image of his mother and doing the best that he could for his family, as many of his classmates were studying, making friends, and enjoying their youth.

As the world began to emerge from the pandemic, we continually heard about a return to normal. What is a return to normal for Adriana and Xavier? A pre-pandemic "normal" can never exist for them, nor for others in similar circumstances. As of June 2021, 167,000 children in the United States had lost a caregiver to the COVID-19 pandemic.[48] The children most likely to lose a caregiver were those belonging to American Indian or Alaskan Native populations. They were 4.5 times more likely to lose a caregiver than a white child. Black and Latinx children were 2.4 and 1.8 times more likely to lose a caregiver than a white child.[49] Five million children around the world lost a caregiver to COVID-19.[50] When we consider the trauma that these children face, normal no longer exists for them. The loss of a parent will carry forward for the rest of their lives. It will affect their future education, their jobs, and their mental health. In turn, it will affect that of their children and their grandchildren. Their grandchildren will carry the residual effects of the history of the pandemic with them. Trauma and inequality pass from generation to generation. It doesn't disappear overnight.

We are a product of our history. For some this history provided advantages and for others it did not. When some of these orphaned children rise up in their lives to do great things, it doesn't mean that they had equal opportunity. When Xavier Salomon becomes a civil engineer and starts his own firm in a decade or two, he will have earned it in the most difficult manner possible. His Horatio Alger story will not mean that everyone can do what he has done. There are many who will struggle even more greatly and will not overcome their circumstances. For Adriana, Xavier, and all these other children like them, normal has forever been changed.

For many, the normal that we longed to return to was not a dream to seek. After all, as Ed Yong wrote in the *Atlantic*, "Normal led to this."[51] If the next pandemic arrives tomorrow, the circumstances that Adriana and Xavier will face will be the same ones that they and their mother faced in 2020. In the short run, what choices would change their lives? Xavier was doing all that he could. He had a job and supported his sister. He was going to college and had dreams of a family and a career. If the next pandemic came tomorrow, he and his sister couldn't flee. They would be trapped as they were in 2020. The circumstances that they faced would be the twenty-first-century equivalent of the Athens war refugees congregated and trapped inside the Long Walls with body lying upon body. Neither had anywhere to go to gain safety.

Many parallels exist between the pandemic conditions then and now. Families in the inwardly dense apartments of Jackson Heights resembled all too closely nineteenth-century immigrants and laborers of the Irish Channel and Pinchguts. Working-class children watched the exodus of New York and Philadelphia in the eighteenth and nineteenth centuries as yellow fever and cholera invaded their homes. In the twenty-first century, essential workers saw affluent areas of cities empty again, leaving behind those too poor to flee. Children were orphaned and watched their mothers depart in a box in the past and present. Grandparents had no room to isolate when illness arrived in crowded multigenerational homes then and today. Women of the working poor remained trapped in an economic nether land scrounging for food to feed their children as if they lived in an 1800s tenement. Pauper pilgrims journeyed in the cavernous underbelly of a ship, while the British were unwilling to recognize the danger and offer precautions because it was too costly. "Un-American" immigrants of Five Points were looked upon with disdain for their brazenness of choosing to live next to disease, as if they had a choice. Alongside them workers congregated together in meat packing plants and congested restaurant kitchens during the twenty-first century. Immigrant workers were left to isolate and die in a trailer with no medical attention. Native Americans were stuck on barren land with less access to health care for decades and then expected to rise above a pandemic with fewer resources than the rest of the country. Residents of eldercare homes were connected across the country by countless bridges created by health aides whose wages were so low that they had to work multiple jobs to survive. The working poor in Los Angeles rode the bus with eyes averted, hoping no one would sit next to them as they commuted daily to their jobs that we deemed essential.

All the while, the wealthy sit above these people in nineteenth-century Naples and Hong Kong and in twenty-first-century condominiums with views of Central Park. Others work from basements, dens, and extra bedrooms, finding safety in isolation like the patrons of steamships and lazarettos who could afford to purchase private rooms. Centuries ago, politicians and royalty fled to the spacious countryside. Today politicians arrive at Walter Reed National Military Medical Center, where state-of-the-art therapeutics save their lives.

When the next pandemic arrives, the current normal will lead us down the same path once again. We cannot, with a clear conscience, allow this to happen. The pandemic created a new awareness of these issues and how they are interlinked. Melinda Gates recently stated, "This pandemic has magnified every existing inequality in our society—like systemic racism, gender inequality, and poverty. And it's impossible to pick one issue as more serious because so many people live at the intersection of all of those challenges."[52] Yet we knew this before. Rudolf Virchow saw this in the 1800s when he recognized that the epidemic in Upper Silesia would not occur without the dire economic circumstances of those who suffered and the indifference of those with money and power. The same issues were present and visible in Mumbai, Naples, New Orleans, and New York City throughout the nineteenth century. The next century brought pandemic inequality in the 1918 influenza pandemic and in the polio epidemics. The HIV/AIDS epidemic in the United States was an epidemic of stigmatization and discrimination, as well as an epidemic of health. Inequality still prevails each and every year in the deaths of *millions* from AIDS, malaria, and tuberculosis in some of the most impoverished areas of the world. Yet many sit with peculiar indifference unable or unwilling to relate to the plight of these populations. In 2010 public health experts called attention to the large socioeconomic, racial, and ethnic disparities that would result from a major influenza pandemic.[53] In response, we did nothing. A decade later we faced a different virus, but their predictions hit the mark of rising inequity and disadvantage for people of color.

The world has recognized these problems for nearly two centuries. Yet we chose to ignore the issues. We cannot allow the pattern to continue. So what do we do now?

We can start by guaranteeing better access to high-quality health care for everyone. A 2022 study by a group of epidemiologists, public health experts, and economists estimated that over 300,000 lives would have been saved in the first two years of the pandemic in the United States alone if it had universal health care. It would have saved $105 billion in costs of hospitalization during the height of the pandemic. In a non-pandemic year, the move to universal health care would save over $400 billion.[54]

We have a unique system in the United States with high-quality health insurance tied to employment. This relationship is the result of an unusual history that encompasses the rise of the medical profession and the health insurance industry.[55] It is archaic. Imagine if a child lost access to education because their mother or father lost a job. It would make no sense and we wouldn't stand for it. Why should we continue to accept this absurdity for health care? We need high-quality health care for all so that everyone has access to preventative medicine with regular visits to health care providers who will know them and know their health histories. When baseline health care is high, health risk is low.

A change from the current health care and insurance system is not easily attained in the current political climate of the United States. However, lives are on the line not just during a pandemic, but each and every day. We cannot accept the status quo of unequal access to health care.

Unfortunately, we were regressing not progressing with respect to COVID-19. As I finished writing this book in January 2023, President Biden announced his intention to end the official pandemic national emergency. In May 2023, the government would begin phasing out payment for COVID-19 tests, vaccines, and treatments such as Paxlovid. For the wealthy or those with high-quality health insurance, this would matter little because their health insurance would cover these items and they could afford any co-pays or direct payments. Many others described in this book, those with low-quality or high co-pay health insurance, or no health insurance at all, would need to pay out-of-pocket. These were exactly the people who faced the most exposure and health risk. They now would need to pay $10 for each at-home test, $130 for each vaccine, and $530 for each course of Paxlovid. A family may need to pay these amounts multiple times. The government was set to shift a financial burden onto the people who could least afford these items but needed them the most. In January 2023, when President Biden announced his intention to end the national emergency, around four hundred people were still dying from COVID-19 every day. If left to persist, these totals would accumulate to 140,000 deaths in one year. This was four times the typical number of yearly influenza deaths. In May 2023, many would be left behind and further exposed to the ongoing pandemic.

In the workplace, workers need to be seen as more than tools used to meet profit goals. Small business owners often see the humanity in their workers. They have direct relationships with those who work for them. They know them as people. They understand when the child of a worker is sick and they can't attend work. They know when a worker's parent or grandparent is suffering. They know when the family of a worker faces some crisis. Many times they understand and they lend assistance in some way. At a minimum they are compassionate because they know the person apart from the worker. They do not see the worker as just another tool. This compassion needs to pervade our relationships of employment throughout society. We need to consider employee happiness and well-being as an integral part of corporate performance. Our society has come to expect that market forces will drive out bad policies at a firm. We expect that if a firm treats its workers poorly, then good workers will move to other firms and the bad firms will suffer. We can't trust compassion to markets, especially when there is vast inequality. This leaves some with a choice between physical and mental health and wealth. We saw the result of workers being forced to make this choice in 2020. It was the modern equivalent of the choice between starving slowly or quickly.

We need workers to earn living wages. When Xavier Salomon needs to eat cheap fast food and inexpensive non-nutritious ramen noodles to pay his rent, we can't have health equity. Lack of nutrition creates health risk. Food deserts that don't allow for consumption of nutritious foods need to be remedied. Living wages that allow room in a consumer's budget for high-nutrient foods will bring more groceries with higher quality products to these areas. We need paid sick, family, and eldercare leave for all workers so that workers aren't forced to choose between family and finances, or between exposure and economics.

Domination of for-profit health care leaves vast critical care deserts and preventative care deserts across our society. Areas with fewer people are underserved by health care that is run by corporations looking to maximize profits. We shouldn't demand a Mercedes dealership in every community of rural Kansas. It isn't profitable. However, we should demand high-quality health care in each of these communities. Health care should not be left to decisions of profit maximization. We need a stronger re-integration of public health services and clinics into areas that will never be high-profit centers for corporate medicine. If we continue to let corporate medicine dictate the location of health services, rural areas and areas of urban poverty will continue to be underserved. We manage to put public schools in every community. We need high-quality public health care in every community as well.

We need to recognize the fault lines in exposure and health risk and take direct action to mitigate each. We cannot forget that epidemics and pandemics will never be a great equalizer. Instead they capitalize on, create, and maintain inequality. When outbreaks arise, we need to pay special attention to the most physically and financially vulnerable. It isn't up to each individual to mind his own risk. It is up to each of us to look out for the other. This was a broad miscalculation at the onset of the pandemic. We touted *individual* protection when discussing masks, hand-washing, and wiping down groceries. Yet we never acknowledged or lived up to the responsibility that fighting pandemics must be a collective effort. We were too familiar with looking out for our own individual health risks with medicine and technology. We didn't recognize that those were not available or easily accessible to all and that many were going to face greater risks than others.

How do we protect people? We limit their exposure risk through public health interventions. That is our responsibility because exposure risk is a collective risk. Limiting pandemic devastation is never about protecting ourselves, it is about protecting our neighbor and our neighbor's mother in the nursing home across town. That is how pandemics are defeated. This isn't done with medicine and technology alone. This isn't done with individual decisions about personal risk. This isn't done with peculiar indifference to those less fortunate. It is done by recognizing the less fortunate and seeing them as human beings and not as tools. It is done by demonstrating care and compassion for everyone in society, regardless of social or economic status.

Speaking at Riverside Church in New York City, Reverend Martin Luther King Jr. once said, "True compassion is more than flinging a coin to a beggar. It comes to see that an edifice which produces beggars needs restructuring."[56] Our society and institutions need restructuring, or we are doomed to once again repeat our sins of the past when the next pandemic arrives.

ACKNOWLEDGMENTS

My mother and father were always supportive of my formal education in the classroom. But more importantly, Mom and Dad, thank you for the lessons of hard work and dedication to craft and family that will be with me forever. These lessons are essential in everything that I do, personally and professionally. Stephanie, thank you for being a great sister and friend throughout our lives and for providing a sounding board on pandemic life and education in the heartland.

A long series of academic homes all played a direct or indirect role in producing this book. At the University of Iowa Department of Economics, one important person kept us all on path while also being a joy to be around every day. Thank you, Rena Jay, for your dedication to students throughout the college. The University of Michigan Center for the Study of Complex Systems provided an intellectual haven where my interests at the intersection of economics and epidemiology were born. I never felt more at home in an academic community than during my time there. Similarly, the New York City Computational Economics and Complexity Workshop provided a great intellectual community, from our first dinner in that small diner two decades ago (with Jason, Leanne, and Nobi) and still today. I thank the economics department and administration at Fordham University for giving me the intellectual space to find research areas of passion inside and outside of economics. I appreciate the Fordham IPED program for supporting my economics and epidemiology courses. This book was completed in part with funding from a Fordham University Faculty Fellowship, and I am grateful for the financial support.

Fil Menczer and Scotte Page are each a great source of inspiration to me because of their intellectual breadth and courage to follow nontraditional paths of research. In addition, they are both incredibly kind and generous people. Thank you for your mentoring, advice, and friendship. Thank you to Myong-Hun Chang and Phil Polgreen for being great colleagues and friends during our joint projects combining economics and epidemiology. It has been a joy to work with you both.

I appreciate the many friends and colleagues who read portions of the book as it was being written and provided comments or discussed its core issues at length with me. In particular, Duncan James and Pam Papish both read the book from cover to cover and provided detailed feedback on every chapter. I am forever in your debt! Thank you to Kristen Alten, De Combs, Danielle Kaley, and Tom Kaley for comments and conversations. You each made this a better book.

In 2016, I attended a reading of Jason Barr's fabulous book, *Building the Skyline: The Birth and Growth of Manhattan's Skyscrapers*. Afterward, Jason signed my copy with the inscription "no Troy=no book." I laughed because it certainly wasn't true. But now the shoe is on the other foot. Jason advised me on proposal preparation, finding an agent, and choosing a publisher. He read everything I wrote, from my early drafts of a book proposal to the entire manuscript. He provided insightful and practical comments at every step. He gave me confidence when I had doubt. Without hesitation, I can state today, "no Jason=no book!" You've been a great friend for two decades! Thank you.

Kristina Perez jumped aboard this project immediately. I am incredibly lucky to have you represent me. You've been a champion of my work and an essential guide throughout the process. Every time that I talk to my editor, Robin Coleman, I'm energized to get words on the page and to write better and more clearly. Robin, your advice and guidance about how to step outside of writing for academic journals and toward this new venue and audience has been invaluable. Thank you to both Kristina and Robin for believing in me and the book!

I am grateful to a number of people at Johns Hopkins University Press for their help editing, designing, and publicizing this book. Jane Medrano helped me get image rights and manuscript materials organized. Kris Lykke and Kait Howard got the book in front of people and made them take notice. Julie McCarthy, Sarah Cline Mabus, and the editors at Inksplash made the book sing better than I could ever do on my own. I thank Chris Tobias for designing a perfect cover that represents the book so well. Hilary Jacqmin did a great job keeping everything together as production manager. I thank Sergey Lobachev for his work producing the index. I know that there are many anonymous people behind the scenes that worked on the book; I appreciate all that you did!

My at-home editorial team is second to none. I began writing this book in the midst of the pandemic during winter 2021. At that time, my children were part-time in-person and part-time online students. During his at-home school lunch break on the first day that I put words to the page, my son Nick, then in fifth grade, read my morning's work. He marked numerous typos and grammar errors while eating a bowl of soup. When he finished writing the corrections, I asked him what he thought. He responded, "Hmm, I would probably find it interesting if I was older." I took that as a compliment, made the corrections that he had marked, and marched forward. Katherine, then in eighth grade, also provided insightful editorial advice when I started writing. She was rarely direct with criticism, but I could always tell when she liked something or didn't like it.

It was only after the fact that she let her true feelings be known with comments like, "This is a LOT better than last time!" or, my personal favorite, "This title is much better. The last one sounded like a bad middle-school essay." Thank you, Katherine and Nick, for your perfect editorial advice and your love. I am proud of you both every day. And I love each of you more than anything.

My wife, Mary Beth, is my intellectual partner. I couldn't have written this book without her encouragement, advice, and love. From start to finish, she read each of my words with the care of a poet. Every suggestion was spot-on. She always knew where I needed a little more or a lot less in the book. She immediately recognized what was clear and what was muddy, what was important and what was trivial. On the days when I couldn't get the words onto the page or the words weren't right and I couldn't find a way to fix them, she was always more patient with me than I was with myself. This book wouldn't exist without her. Mary Beth, I love you dearly and I thank you for our life together.

NOTES

Preface

1. Thomas Dekker, *A Rod for Run-awayes: Gods tokens, of his fearefull iudgements, sundry wayes pronounced vpon this city, and on seuerall persons, both flying from it, and staying in it. Expressed in many dreadfull examples of sudden death* (London: G. Purslowe for Iohn Trundle, 1625). Early English Books Online Text Creation Partnership, https://quod.lib.umich.edu/e/eebo/A20080.0001.001.

2. Ryan J. Hackenbracht, "The Plague of 1625–26, Apocalyptic Anticipation, and Milton's Elegy III," *Studies in Philology* 108, no. 3 (2011), 403–38, http://www.jstor.org/stable/23055998.

Chapter 1. The Most Important Letter

1. Quotes in this paragraph are from Thucydides (trans. Richard Crawley), "Thucydides on the Plague," Livius, https://www.livius.org/sources/content/thucydides-historian/the-plague/.

2. Jona Lendering, "Athens, Long Walls," Livius, https://www.livius.org/articles/place/athens/athens-photos/athens-long-walls/.

3. Anders Frøland, "Thukydid: Pesten i Athen i 430 før vor tidsregning. Et skridt på Athens vej mod undergangen som stormagt" [Thucydides: The plague in Athens in 430 BCE. A step on Athens' path towards the downfall as a great power], *Dan Medicinhist Arbog* 38 (2010): 63–80. Danish. https://pubmed.ncbi.nlm.nih.gov/21560771/.

4. "Thucydides on the Plague."

5. Robert J. Littman, "The Plague of Athens: Epidemiology and Paleopathology," *Mount Sinai Journal of Medicine* 76, no. 5 (2009): 456–67, https://doi.org/10.1002/msj.20137, https://pubmed.ncbi.nlm.nih.gov/19787658/, and Burke A. Cunha,

"The Cause of the Plague of Athens: Plague, Typhoid, Typhus, Smallpox or Measles?," *Infectious Disease Clinics of North America* 18, no. 1 (2004): 29–43. Published online March 1, 2005, https://doi.org/10.1016/S0891-5520(03)00100-4.

6. Lucretius, *De Rerum Natura, On the Nature of Things,* William Ellery Leonard (translator) (New York: E. P. Dutton and Co., J. M. Dent and Sons, 1916), http://data.perseus.org/citations /urn:cts:latinLit:phi0550.phi001.perseus-eng1:6.1138-6.1173.

7. Frank M. Snowden, *Epidemics and Society: From the Black Death to the Present* (New Haven: Yale University Press, 2019).

8. Snowden, *Epidemics and Society.*

9. Snowden, *Epidemics and Society.*

10. Data from Frank M. Snowden, *Naples in the Time of Cholera, 1884–1911* (Cambridge University Press, 1995), 107 (table 3.2).

11. Snowden, *Epidemics and Society.*

12. Notes on the life of Ronald Ross are taken from Adam Kucharski's *The Rules of Contagion: Why Things Spread and Why They Stop* (New York: Basic Books, 2020).

13. Kucharski, *The Rules of Contagion.*

14. Alfred W. Crosby Jr., *The Columbian Exchange: Biological and Cultural Consequences of 1492* (Westport, CT: Praeger, 2003).

15. Emmanuel Le Roy Ladurie, "Motionless History," *Social Science History* 1, no. 2 (1977): 115–36, www.jstor.org/stable/1171054.

16. Jeffrey G. Williamson, "Migrant Selectivity, Urbanization, and Industrial Revolutions," *Population and Development Review* 14, no. 2 (1988): 287–314, www.jstor.org/stable/1973573.

17. Jeremy Atack, Robert A. Margo, and Paul Rhode, "Industrial-ization and Urbanization in Nineteenth Century America," National Bureau of Economic Research Working Paper 28597, March 2021, https://doi.org/10.3386/w28597.

18. United States Census Bureau, "Urban and Rural Areas," https:// www.census.gov/history/www/programs/geography/urban_and _rural_areas.html. Last accessed July 8, 2022.

19. Jason M. Barr, *Building the Skyline: The Birth and Growth of Manhattan's Skyscrapers* (New York: Oxford University Press, 2016).

20. Jason Barr and Teddy Ort, "Population Density across the City: The Case of 1900 Manhattan," unpublished manuscript available at http://www.jasonmbarr.com/wp-content/uploads/2016/12/BarrManhattanDensityApril2014.pdf.

21. Barr and Ort, "Population Density across the City."

22. Barr and Ort, "Population Density across the City."

23. Aanchal Malhorta, "When the 1897 Bubonic Plague Ravaged India," *Mint,* April 26, 2020, https://www.livemint.com/mint-lounge/features/when-the-1897-bubonic-plague-ravaged-india-11587876174403.html. Last accessed July 8, 2022.

24. K. David Patterson and Gerald F. Pyle, "The Geography and Mortality of the 1918 Influenza Pandemic," *Bulletin of the History of Medicine* 65, no. 1 (1991): 4–21, http://www.jstor.org/stable/44447656.

25. Maura Chhun, "1918 Flu Pandemic Killed 12 Million Indians, and British Overlords' Indifference Strengthened the Anti-Colonial Movement," *The Conversation,* April 17, 2020, https://theconversation.com/1918-flu-pandemic-killed-12-million-indians-and-british-overlords-indifference-strengthened-the-anti-colonial-movement-133605.

26. Going back further in history, it is often stated that bubonic plague in medieval Europe was class neutral. Economic inequality did decrease after the initial bouts of plague. However, this isn't a general result of all epidemics. See for discussion Guido Alfani, "Economic Inequality in Preindustrial Times: Europe and Beyond," *Journal of Economic Literature* 59, no. 1 (March 2021): 3–44.

In terms of mortality, however, even the plague wasn't class neutral. For instance, during the London plague outbreak in 1636–1637, 84 percent of the people quarantined in St. Martin in the Fields parish in central London couldn't afford to pay the four pence per day fee charged for quarantine housing. See Kira L. S. Newman, "Shutt Up: Bubonic Plague and Quarantine in Early Modern England," *Journal of Social History* 45, no. 3 (2012): 809–34, http://www.jstor.org/stable/41678910. Part of this destitution came from middle-class families falling into poverty during the plague, yet it appears that people in poverty were more frequently quarantined. Further, historian Paul Slack wrote that the plague "picked the narrowest alleys and poorest houses" when describing its spread in Bristol during the same time period. Paul Slack, *The Impact of Plague in Tudor and Stuart England* (UK: Clarendon Press, 1985).

27. Svenn-Erik Mamelund, "A Socially Neutral Disease? Individual Social Class, Household Wealth, and Mortality from Spanish Influenza in Two Socially Contrasting Parishes in Kristiania 1918–19," *Social Science & Medicine* 62, no. 4 (2016): 923–40, https://doi.org/10.1016/j.socscimed.2005.06.051.

28. Winston A. Reynolds, "The Burning Ships of Hernán Cortés," *Hispania* 42, no. 3 (1959), 317–24, https://doi.org/10.2307/335707.

29. Joshua S. Loomis, *Epidemics: The Impact of Germs and Their Power over Humanity* (Nashville, TN: Turner Publishing Co., 2018).

30. Richard Gunderman, "How Smallpox Devastated the Aztecs— and Helped Spain Conquer an American Civilization 500 Years Ago," *The Conversation*, February 19, 2019, https://theconversation.com/how-smallpox-devastated-the-aztecs-and-helped-spain-conquer-an-american-civilization-500-years-ago-111579; Heather Pringle, "How Europeans Brought Sickness to the New World," *Science*, June 4, 2015, https://www.sciencemag.org/news/2015/06/how-europeans-brought-sickness-new-world.

31. Loomis, *Epidemics*.

32. Loomis, *Epidemics*.

33. Loomis, *Epidemics*.

34. Alfred W. Crosby, "Virgin Soil Epidemics as a Factor in the Aboriginal Depopulation in America," *William and Mary Quarterly* 33, no. 2 (1976): 289–99, https://doi.org/10.2307/1922166.

35. J. N. Hays, *The Burdens of Disease: Epidemics and Human Response in Western History* (Piscataway, NJ: Rutgers University Press, 2009).

36. These estimates for R were computed by a consortium of public health experts at Yale, Harvard, and Stanford universities; see https://covidestim.org.

37. The CDC still uses antiquated titles such as "non-Hispanic white" and "Hispanic or Latino" as well as a listing that contains various Indigenous groups. In place of these labels I will use the terms "white," "Latinx," and "Indigenous" to replace these CDC labels when discussing CDC and other data using these titles.

38. CDC, "Risk for COVID-19 Infection, Hospitalization, and Death By Race/Ethnicity" (2022), https://www.cdc.gov/coronavirus/2019 -ncov/covid-data/investigations-discovery/hospitalization-death-by -race-ethnicity.html. Last accessed April 30, 2022.

39. Office of National Statistics, "Updating Ethnic Contrasts in Deaths involving the Coronavirus (COVID-19), England: 24 January 2020 to 31 March 2021," https://www.ons.gov.uk /peoplepopulationandcommunity/birthsdeathsandmarriages /deaths/articles/updatingethniccontrastsindeathsinvolvingthecoro naviruscovid19englandandwales/24january2020to31march2021. Last accessed July 8, 2022.

40. Benjamin Seligman, Maddalena Ferranna, and David E. Bloom, "Social Determinants of Mortality from COVID-19: A Simulation Study using NHANES," *PLOS Medicine* 18, no. 1 (2021): e1003490, https://doi.org/10.1371/journal.pmed.1003490.

41. Richard Rothstein, *The Color of Law* (New York, NY: Liveright Publishing Corp., 2018).

42. Tanzina Vega, "Where's the Empathy for Black Poverty and Pain?," *CNN.com*, May 5, 2017, https://www.cnn.com/2017/05 /05/opinions/empathy-gap-in-viewing-black-poverty-and-pain -tanzina-vega/index.html.

Chapter 2. Differences of Density

1. Patrick Brennan, "Getting Out of the Crescent City: Irish Immigration and the Yellow Fever Epidemic of 1853," *Louisiana History: The Journal of the Louisiana Historical Association* 52, no. 2 (2011): 189–205, http://www.jstor.org/stable/23074685.

2. Robert C. Reinders, *End of an Era: New Orleans, 1850–1860* (New Orleans: Pelican Publishing, 1964), 73. Quoted from Brennan (2001).

3. Richard Campanella, "Before I-10, the New Basin Canal Flowed through New Orleans," *Preservation in Print*, November 1, 2019, https://prcno.org/before-i-10-the-new-basin-canal-flowed-through-new-orleans/.
4. "Report of the Sanitary Commission of New Orleans on the Epidemic Yellow Fever of 1853," published by the Authority of the City Council of New Orleans, 1854, https://archive.org/stream/65030340R.nlm.nih.gov/65030340R_djvu.txt.
5. "Report of the Sanitary Commission of New Orleans," City Council of New Orleans; Brennan, "Getting Out of the Crescent City," 189–205; Katherine Vest, "La Fièvre Jaune: An Exhibition Plan on St. Patrick's Cemetery, Irish Immigrants, and the Role of the Catholic Church during the 1853 Yellow Fever Epidemic in New Orleans" (master's thesis, University of New Orleans, 2019), https://scholarworks.uno.edu/td/2651. The description of the events surrounding the demise of Mr. McGuigan was primarily taken from testimony given in the report. I also relied on the research of Patrick Brennan and Katherine Vest.
6. Jonathan B. Pritchett and Insan Tunali, "Strangers' Disease: Determinants of Yellow Fever Mortality during the New Orleans Epidemic of 1853," *Explorations in Economic History* 32, no. 4 (1995): 517–39, https://doi.org/10.1006/exeh.1995.1022.
7. Jo Ann Carrigan, "Yellow Fever in New Orleans, 1853: Abstractions and Realities," *Journal of Southern History* 25, no. 3 (1959): 339–55, https://doi.org/10.2307/2954767. Quotes and descriptions cited from Carrigan are taken from Erasmus Darwin Fenner, *History of the Epidemic Yellow Fever, at New Orleans, Louisiana, in 1853* (New York: Clayton & Co., 1854), 25.
8. Brennan, "Getting Out of the Crescent City," 189–205.
9. Carrigan, "Yellow Fever in New Orleans, 1853," 339–55.
10. Carrigan, "Yellow Fever in New Orleans, 1853," 339–55.
11. Laura D. Kelley, "Yellow Fever in New Orleans," *64 Parishes*, January 16, 2001 (updated February 9, 2021), https://64parishes.org/entry/yellow-fever-in-louisiana; Anna Faherty, "The Stranger Who Started an Epidemic," *Welcome Collection*, June 15, 2017, https://wellcomecollection.org/articles/WsT4Ex8AAHruGfXH.

12. Pritchett and Tunali, "Strangers' Disease," 517–39.

13. Brennan, "Getting Out of the Crescent City," 189–205.

14. "Coronavirus: First Death Confirmed in Europe," *BBC News,* February 15, 2020, https://www.bbc.com/news/world-europe-51514837.

15. Kate Eby, "Coronavirus Timeline: Tracking Major Moments of COVID-19 Pandemic in San Francisco Bay Area," *ABC7 Bay Area,* July 6, 2022, https://abc7news.com/timeline-of-coronavirus-us-covid-19-bay-area-sf/6047519/.

16. Joseph Goldstein and Andrea Salcedo, "For 4 Days, the Hospital Thought He Had Just Pneumonia. It Was Coronavirus," *New York Times,* March 10, 2020, https://www.nytimes.com/2020/03/10/nyregion/coronavirus-new-rochelle-pneumonia.html.

17. Lateshia Beachum, "New York's 'Patient Zero' Breaks His Silence after Surviving Covid-19," *Washington Post,* May 11, 2020, https://www.washingtonpost.com/nation/2020/05/11/patient-zero-new-york-coronavirus/.

18. Goldstein and Salcedo, "For 4 Days, The Hospital Thought."

19. Daniel Wolfe and Daniel Dale, "It's Going to Disappear: A Timeline of Trump's Comments that Covid-19 will Vanish," *CNN,* October 31, 2020, https://www.cnn.com/interactive/2020/10/politics/covid-disappearing-trump-comment-tracker.

20. Laura Wamsley, "March 11, 2020: The Day Everything Changed," *NPR.org,* March 11, 2021, https://www.npr.org/2021/03/11/975663437/march-11-2020-the-day-everything-changed.

21. Unless otherwise noted, data for this chapter comes from the Johns Hopkins Coronavirus website: https://coronavirus.jhu.edu.

22. Brian Rosenthal, "Density Is New York City's Big 'Enemy' in the Coronavirus Fight," *New York Times,* March 23, 2020, https://www.nytimes.com/2020/03/23/nyregion/coronavirus-nyc-crowds-density.html.

23. LaGuardia Airport provides mostly domestic service other than a small number of flights to Canadian and Caribbean locations.

24. Bureau of Transportation Statistics, "Top 10 U.S. Airports, Ranked by 2018 International Scheduled Enplanements on U.S. and Foreign Airlines," table 12, https://www.bts.dot.gov/table-12

-top-10-us-airports-ranked-2018-international-scheduled
-enplanements-us-and-foreign-airlines.

25. Jason Barr and Troy Tassier, "Are Crowded Cities the Reason for the COVID-19 Pandemic?," *Observations* (blog), *Scientific American*, April 17, 2020, https://blogs.scientificamerican.com /observations/are-crowded-cities-the-reason-for-the-covid-19 -pandemic/; Jason Barr and Troy Tassier, "Escape from New York?: Density and the Coronavirus Trajectory," *Building the Skyline*, April 20, 2020, https://buildingtheskyline.org/covid19 -and-density. Research summarized from both blogs.

26. Barr and Tassier, "Are Crowded Cities the Reason?"

27. Barr and Tassier, "Are Crowded Cities the Reason?"

28. Shima Hamidi, Sadegh Sabouri, and Reid Ewing, "Does Density Aggravate the COVID-19 Pandemic?," *Journal of the American Planning Association* 86, no. 4 (2020): 495–509, http://doi.org/10.1080/01944363.2020.1777891. A comprehensive study of over 900 metropolitan areas by researchers at the Johns Hopkins Bloomberg School of Public Health found that city size was more important than density in the spring 2020 wave.

29. Deneb Cesana, Ole Benedictow, and Raffaella Bianucci, "The Origin and Early Spread of the Black Death in Italy: First Evidence of Plague Victims from 14th-Century Liguia," *Anthropological Science* 125, no. 1 (2017): 15–24, https://www.jstage .jst.go.jp/article/ase/125/1/125_161011/_html/-char/en.

30. Marc Morillon, Bertrand Mafart, and Thierry Matton, "Yellow Fever in Europe during the 19th Century," last accessed July 9, 2022, preprint available at http://bertrand.mafart.free.fr /paleoanthropology_paleopathology_full_text_mafart /Yellowfever_history_europe_mafart.pdf; C. La Chastel, "The 'Plague' of Barcelona. Yellow Fever Epidemic of 1821," *Bulletin de la Societe de pathologie exotique* 92, no. 5 (1999): 405–7. French. PMID: 11000949.

31. Peter McCandless, "History: Yellow Fever," *Charleston Currents,* April 25, 2016, https://charlestoncurrents.com/2016/04 /history-yellow-fever.

32. Jerrold M. Michael, "The National Board of Health: 1879–1883," *Public Health Reports* 126, no. 1 (2011): 123–29, http://doi.org/10.1177/003335491112600117.

33. Molly Caldwell Crosby, *The American Plague: The Untold Story of Yellow Fever, the Epidemic that Shaped Our History* (New York: Berkley Books, 2006).

34. "The Great Fever: 1878 Epidemic," *American Experience*, PBS, https://www.pbs.org/wgbh/americanexperience/features/fever-1878-epidemic.

35. Thomas H. Baker, "YELLOWJACK: The Yellow Fever Epidemic of 1878 in Memphis, Tennessee," *Bulletin of the History of Medicine* 42, no. 3 (1968): 241–64, http://www.jstor.org/stable/44450733.

36. Baker, "YELLOWJACK," 241–64.

37. Baker, "YELLOWJACK," 241–64.

38. "The Great Fever: 1878 Epidemic," PBS.

39. Baker, "YELLOWJACK," 241–64.

40. Baker, "YELLOWJACK," 241–64.

41. Baker, "YELLOWJACK," 241–64.

42. Baker, "YELLOWJACK," 241–64.

43. Baker, "YELLOWJACK," 241–64.

44. Baker, "YELLOWJACK," 241–64.

45. Crosby, *The American Plague*.

46. Baker, "YELLOWJACK," 241–64.

47. The United States Census Bureau divides up the geography of the United States into areas of different resolution. One of the units of area is called the Zip Code Tabulation Areas, or ZCTAs. With some variation, these correspond roughly to zip codes of the United States Postal Service. New York City has 177 ZCTAs. I use these ZCTAs as the neighborhood boundaries in the discussion below.

48. Real estate advertisement for 200 East 59th St. condominiums, last accessed July 8, 2022, https://200east59.com.

49. Jay Pitter, "Urban Density: Confronting the Distance Between Desire and Disparity," *Azure*, April 17, 2020, https://www.azuremagazine.com/article/urban-density-confronting-the-distance-between-desire-and-disparity.

50. Some studies use persons per bedroom, but both measures identify the same neighborhoods as most overcrowded in New York City.

51. The difference grows to 33 percent larger if one considers neighborhoods with income in the top and bottom 10 percent.

52. Raw data provided by urban economist Jason Barr at Rutgers University–Newark. Calculations by the author.

53. Raw data provided by urban economist Jason Barr at Rutgers University–Newark. Calculations by the author.

54. Mitchell L. Moss and Carson Qing, "The Dynamic Population of Manhattan," March 2012, preprint available at https://wagner.nyu.edu/files/rudincenter/dynamic_pop_manhattan.pdf.

55. Joseph Goldstein, Luis Ferré-Sadurni, and Aaron Randle, "Coronavirus in NY: Desperate for a Test, They Couldn't Get One," *New York Times,* March 11, 2020, https://www.nytimes.com/2020/03/11/nyregion/coronavirus-testing-newyork.html.

56. Erin Schumaker, "Frustration and Confusion Mounts among Some Doctors and Patients Who Can't Get Coronavirus Tests," *ABCnews.com*, March 17, 2020, https://abcnews.go.com/Health/frustration-confusion-mounts-doctors-patients-coronavirus-tests/story?id=69555689.

57. Schumaker, "Frustration and Confusion Mounts."

58. Joshua Gans, *The Pandemic Information Gap: The Brutal Economics of COVID-19* (Cambridge, MA: MIT Press, 2020).

59. Goldstein, Ferré-Sadurni, and Randle, "Coronavirus in NY."

60. As a threshold, I consider the zip code tabulation areas that rank in the tenth and ninetieth percentiles as the least and most impoverished.

61. Divya Siddarth et al., "Evidence Roundup: Why Positive Test Rates Need to Fall Below 3%," Harvard Global Health Institute, May 29, 2020. Last accessed July 9, 2022. https://globalhealth.harvard.edu/evidence-roundup-why-positive-test-rates-need-to-fall-below-3/.

62. Siddarth et al., "Evidence Roundup."

63. George Borjas, "Demographic Determinants of Testing Incidence and COVID-19 Infections in New York City Neighborhoods," National Bureau of Economic Research, Working Paper 26952,

April 2020, https://www.nber.org/papers/w26952. Economist George Borjas also analyzed this data using levels of income across neighborhoods and found similar patterns using income to sort neighborhoods.

64. New York City Planning, "Immigrant Settlement Patterns in New York City," *The Newest New Yorkers*, 2013 ed., 23–94, https://www1.nyc.gov/assets/planning/download/pdf/data-maps /nyc-population/nny2013/chapter3.pdf.

65. Institute for Children, Poverty, and Homelessness, "Overcrowd-ing in New York City Community Districts," *On the Map: The Dynamics of Family Homelessness in New York City*, 2016, https://www.icphusa.org/wp-content/uploads/2016/04 /Overcrowding.pdf.

66. New York City Health, "Age Adjusted Rate of Fatal Lab Confirmed COVID-19 Cases per 100,000 by Race/Ethnicity Group," 2020, https://www1.nyc.gov/assets/doh/downloads/pdf /imm/covid-19-deaths-race-ethnicity-04082020-1.pdf.

67. Jarvis Chen and Nancy Krieger, "Revealing the Unequal Burden of COVID-19 by Income, Race/Ethnicity, and Household Crowding: US County versus Zip Code Analyses," *Journal of Public Health Management and Practice* 27 (2021): S43–S56, https://doi.org/10.1097/PHH.0000000000001263.

68. Leah Donnella, "How Yellow Fever Turned New Orleans into the 'City of the Dead,'" *NPR.org*, October 31, 2018, https:// www.npr.org/sections/codeswitch/2018/10/31/415535913/how -yellow-fever-turned-new-orleans-into-the-city-of-the-dead.

69. Jo Ann Carrigan, "Yellow Fever in New Orleans, 1853."

70. Donnella, "How Yellow Fever Turned New Orleans."

71. Donnella, "How Yellow Fever Turned New Orleans."

72. Edward R. Sullivan, *Rambles and Scrambles in North and South America* (London: R. Bentley, 1852), 216. Quoted from Brennan, "Getting Out of the Crescent City," 189–205.

73. Richard Campanella, "Before I-10, the New Basin Canal Flowed through New Orleans," Preservation Resource Center of New Orleans, November 1, 2019, https://prcno.org/before-i-10-the -new-basin-canal-flowed-through-new-orleans/.

74. Haidee Chu et al., "One in 10 Local COVID Victims Destined for Hart Island, NYC's Potter's Field," *TheCity.com,* March 24, 2021, https://www.thecity.nyc/missing-them/2021/3/24 /22349311/nyc-covid-victims-destined-for-hart-island-potters -field.

Chapter 3. One (Unlucky) Spark

1. Details of Mary Mallon's life are taken from Filio Marineli et al., "Mary Mallon (1869–1938) and the History of Typhoid Fever," *Annals of Gastroenterology* 26, no. 2 (2013): 132–34; Judith Walzer Leavitt, *Typhoid Mary: Captive to the Public's Health* (Boston: Beacon Press, 1996); John Fabian Witt, *American Contagions: Epidemics and the Law from Smallpox to COVID-19* (New Haven: Yale UP, 2020); George Soper, "Typhoid Mary," *The Military Surgeon* 45, no. 1 (1919), 1–15.

2. Subsequent research has shown that this role as an asymptomatic carrier is not unusual. Between 1 and 6 percent of those infected with the bacteria causing typhoid fever remain asymptomatic. There were likely many others like Mary in her time, especially in New York City. See also https://med.stanford.edu/news/all -news/2013/08/scientists-get-a-handle-on-what-made-typhoid -marys-infectious-microbes-tick.html.

3. Marineli et al., "Mary Mallon (1869–1938)," 132–34.

4. Virginia Pitzer, Cayley C. Bowles, and Stephen Baker, "Predicting the Impact of Vaccination on the Transmission Dynamics of Typhoid in South Asia: A Mathematical Modeling Study," *PLOS Neglected Tropical Diseases* 8, no. 1 (2014): e2642, https://doi .org/10.1371/journal.pntd.0002642.

5. Luigi Amoroso, "Vilfredo Pareto," *Econometrica* 6, no. 1 (1938): 1–21, https://doi.org/10.2307/1910081.

6. Kevin Kruse, "The 80/20 Rule and How It Can Change Your Life," *Forbes*, May 7, 2016, https://www.forbes.com/sites /kevinkruse/2016/03/07/80-20-rule/?sh=6c6756853814.

7. Paula Rooney, "Microsoft's CEO: 80-20 Rule Applies to Bugs, Not Just Features," *CRN*, October 3, 2002, https://www.crn

.com/news/security/18821726/microsofts-ceo-80-20-rule-applies
-to-bugs-not-just-features.htm.

8. Alison P. Galvani and Robert M. May, "Dimensions of Super-spreading," *Nature* 438, no. 7066 (2005): 293–95, https://doi
.org/10.1038/438293a.

9. Carl Zimmer, "Most People with Coronavirus Won't Spread It.
Why Do a Few Infect Many?," *New York Times,* June 30, 2020,
https://www.nytimes.com/2020/06/30/science/how-coronavirus
-spreads.html; James O. Lloyd-Smith et al., "Superspreading and
the Effect of Individual Variation on Disease Emergence," *Nature*
438, no. 7066 (2005): 355–59.

10. Becky Little, "SARS Pandemic: How the Virus Spread Around
the World in 2003," *History,* March 17, 2020, https://www
.history.com/news/sars-outbreak-china-lessons.

11. Cathy Goudie, "SARS Timeline," *New Scientist*, May 14, 2003,
https://www.newscientist.com/article/dn3732-sars-timeline.

12. Carrie Arnold, "Modern-Day Typhoid Marys: Superspreaders
Can Turn a Minor Outbreak into a Pandemic," *Slate,* December 27, 2012, https://slate.com/technology/2012/12/superspreaders
-of-disease-sars-and-other-pandemics-are-spread-by-modern-day
-typhoid-marys.html.

13. Akira Endo, Adam J. Kucharski, and Sebastion Funk, "Estimat-
ing the Overdispersion in COVID-19 Transmission Using
Outbreak Sizes outside China," *Wellcome Open Research 5*
(2020): 67, https://doi.org/10.12688/wellcomeopenres.15842.3.

14. Max S. Y. Yau et al., "Characterizing Superspreading Events and
Age-Specific Infectiousness of SARS-CoV-2 Transmission in
Georgia, USA," *Proceedings of the National Academy of
Sciences* 117, no. 36 (2020): 22430–35, https://doi.org/10.1073
/pnas.2011802117.

15. Adam Dillon et al., "Clustering and Superspreading Potential of
Severe Acute Respiratory Syndrome Coronavirus 2 (SARS-
CoV-2) Infections in Hong Kong," *Nature Medicine* 26 (2020):
1714–19, https://doi.org/10.21203/rs.3.rs-29548/v1.

16. Kai Kupferschmidt, "Why Do Some COVID-19 Patients Infect
Many Others whereas Most Don't Spread the Virus at All?,"

Science, May 19, 2020, https://www.science.org/news/2020/05
/why-do-some-covid-19-patients-infect-many-others-whereas
-most-don-t-spread-virus-all?_ga=2.195263855.277584553
.1631051028-302294344.1631051028.

17. "Andrew Jerome Mitchell—1956–2020—Obituary," M. L. King
Funeral Directors, https://www.mlkmemorialchapels.com/index
.cfm/obituary/andrew-mitchell.

18. "Andrew Jerome Mitchell," M. L. King Funeral Directors.

19. Ellen Barry, "Days After a Funeral in a Georgia Town, Coronavirus 'Hit Like a Bomb,'" *New York Times*, March 30, 2020,
https://www.nytimes.com/2020/03/30/us/coronavirus-funeral
-albany-georgia.html.

20. "Johnny B. Carter—1949–2020—Obituary," M. L. King
Funeral Directors, https://www.mlkmemorialchapels.com
/obituary/johnny-carter.

21. "Johnny B. Carter," M. L. King Funeral Directors.

22. Barry, "Days After a Funeral."

23. "QuickFacts: New York City, New York; Albany City, Georgia," United States Census Bureau, accessed May 5, 2022,
https://www.census.gov/quickfacts/fact/table/newyorkcitynewyork,
albanycitygeorgia/PST045221.

24. For example, 12 percent of Albany residents have a disability
compared to 7 percent of New York City residents; 75 percent of
Albany residents are Black compared to 24 percent of New York
City residents; and college completion rates of New York City
residents are twice as great as those of Albany residents.

25. Carl Zimmer, "Most People with Coronavirus Won't Spread It.
Why Do a Few Infect Many?," *New York Times,* June 30, 2020,
https://www.nytimes.com/2020/06/30/science/how-coronavirus
-spreads.html.

26. Aimee Groth, "Bill Clinton Was a Ridiculously Good Networker
at Age 22," *Business Insider*, May 5, 2011, https://www.business
insider.com/bill-clinton-networking-2011-5.

27. Maddy Osman, "Wild and Interesting Facebook Statistics and
Facts," *Kinsta*, January 3, 2021, https://kinsta.com/blog/facebook
-statistics.

28. Sara Del Valle et al., "Mixing Patterns between Age Groups in Social Networks," *Social Networks* 29 (2007): 544.

29. "Passenger Boarding (Enplanement) and All-Cargo Data for US Airports," Federal Aviation Administration, accessed June 25, 2022, https://www.faa.gov/airports/planning_capacity/passenger_allcargo_stats/passenger.

30. I thank Pam Papish for the example of a child traveling throughout a school day.

31. Mark E. J. Newman, "Assortative Mixing in Networks," *Physical Review Letters* 89, no. 20 (2002): 208701, https://doi.org/10.1103/PhysRevLett.89.208701.

32. Marc Fortier, "What We Know About the 70+ Coronavirus Cases Linked to Biogen's Boston Meeting," *NBC Boston*, March 6, 2020, https://www.nbcboston.com/news/coronavirus/what-we-know-about-the-coronavirus-cases-linked-to-biogens-boston-meeting/2086974.

33. Jacob E. Lemieux et al., "Phylogenetic Analysis of SARS-CoV-2 in the Boston Area Highlights the Role of Recurrent Importation and Superspreading Events," *Science* 371, no. 6529 (2020), https://doi.org/10.1126/science.abe3261.

34. Lemieux et al., "Phylogenetic Analysis."

35. Angus Chen, "Genetic Fingerprints Suggest Superspreader Biogen Conference Seeded 40% of Boston Coronavirus Cases," *WBUR*, August 25, 2020, https://www.wbur.org/news/2020/08/25/genetic-fingerprints-biogen-superspreader-boston.

36. Jim O'Connell, "COVID-19 and Homelessness in Boston: Thoughts from the Initial Surge," *Harvard Medical School Primary Care Review*, June 30, 2020, https://info.primarycare.hms.harvard.edu/review/covid-homelessness-boston.

37. Taylor Romine, "'We Need to Fix It Quickly.' Asymptomatic Coronavirus Cases at Boston Homeless Shelter Raise Red Flag," *CNN.com*, April 17, 2020, https://www.cnn.com/2020/04/17/us/boston-homeless-coronavirus-outbreak/index.html.

38. Meghan Henry et al., "The 2019 Annual Homeless Assessment Report (AHAR) to Congress, Part 1: Point-In-Time Estimates of Homelessness," US Department of Housing and Urban

Development, January 2020, https://www.huduser.gov/portal
/sites/default/files/pdf/2019-AHAR-Part-1.pdf.

39. "Veteran Homelessness: Overview of State and Federal Resources," National Conference of State Legislatures, May 22,
2020, https://www.ncsl.org/research/military-and-veterans-affairs
/veteran-homelessness-an-overview-of-state-and-federal-resources
.aspx.

40. "Mental Illness and Homelessness," National Coalition for the
Homeless, July 2009, https://www.nationalhomeless.org
/factsheets/Mental_Illness.pdf.

41. O'Connell, "COVID-19 and Homelessness in Boston."

42. "Here's Everyone at the White House Rose Garden SCOTUS
Event Now Called a Likely 'Superspreader.' Help Us ID Them
All," USA Today, October 7, 2020, https://www.usatoday.com
/in-depth/news/investigations/2020/10/07/likely-rose-garden
-covid-superspreader-white-house-drew-hundreds/3636925001.

43. Larry Buchanan et al., "Inside the White House Event Now
Under Covid-19 Scrutiny," New York Times, October 5, 2020,
https://www.nytimes.com/interactive/2020/10/03/us/rose-garden
-event-covid.html.

44. Larry Buchanan et al., "Tracking the White House Coronavirus
Outbreak," New York Times, October 14, 2020, https://www
.nytimes.com/interactive/2020/10/02/us/politics/trump-contact
-tracing-covid.html.

45. Richard J. Baron, Marianne M. Green, and Yul D. Ejnes,
"Seeing the Rose Garden Superspreader Convocation as a 'Never
Event,'" STAT News, October 19, 2020, https://www.statnews
.com/2020/10/19/seeing-rose-garden-superspreader-convocation
-as-a-never-event.

46. In the early days of the internet, Réka Albert, Hawoong Jeong,
and Albert-László Barabási were the first to discover this
property of robustness and fragility in networks. Their work
examined robustness and fragility on hub-and-spoke–based
internet connections. See their article "Error and Attack Toler-
ance of Complex Networks," Nature 406, no. 6794 (2000):
378–82, https://doi: 10.1038/35019019.

47. This strategy came about while seeking a solution to a vaccine-allocation problem and is termed *acquaintance vaccination*. However, I cast this notion in terms of the airport metaphor that I have been using throughout. The original research can be found in Reuven Cohen, Shlomo Havlin, and Daniel ben-Avraham, "Efficient Immunization Strategies for Computer Networks and Populations," *Physical Review Letters* 91 (2003): 24, https://doi.org/0.1103/PhysRevLett.91.247901.

48. Akira Endo et al., "Implication of Backward Contact Tracing in the Presence of Overdispersed Transmission in COVID-19 Outbreaks," *Wellcome Open Research* 5 (2020): 239, https://doi.org/10.12688/wellcomeopenres.16344.1; Sadamori Kojaku et al., "The Effectiveness of Backward Contact Tracing in Networks," *Nature Physics* 17 (2021): 652–58, https://doi.org/10.1038/s41567-021-01187-2.

49. Tim Loh, "Contact Tracers Eye Cluster-Busting to Tackle Covid's New Surge," *Bloomberg*, November 3, 2020, https://www.bloomberg.com/news/articles/2020-11-03/contact-tracers-eye-cluster-busting-to-tackle-covid-s-new-surge.

50. Christie Aschwanden, "Contact Tracing, a Key Way to Slow COVID-19, Is Badly Underused by the US," *Scientific American*, July 21, 2020, https://www.scientificamerican.com/article/contact-tracing-a-key-way-to-slow-covid-19-is-badly-underused-by-the-u-s.

51. Dyani Lewis, "Why Many Countries Failed at COVID Contact-Tracing—But Some Got It Right," *Nature* 588, no. 7838 (2020): 384–387, https://doi: 10.1038/d41586-020-03518-4, https://www.nature.com/articles/d41586-020-03518-4.

52. Loh, "Contact Tracers Eye Cluster-Busting."

53. Lewis, "Why Many Countries Failed."

Chapter 4. Bridges of Disease

1. Patrick Wallis, "A Dreadful Heritage: Interpreting Epidemic Disease at Eyam, 1666–2000," *History Workshop Journal* 61, no. 1 (2006): 31–56, https://www.jstor.org/stable/25472836?seq=1.

2. For background reading, see David McKenna, "Eyam Plague: The Village of the Damned," *BBCnews.com*, November 5, 2016, https://www.bbc.com/news/uk-england-35064071; Victoria Mason, "Why Is Eyam Significant?," *Historic UK,* https://www.historic-uk.com/HistoryUK/HistoryofEngland/Why-Is-Eyam-Significant/; and Wallis, "A Dreadful Heritage," 31–56.

3. Jeffrey Travers and Stanley Milgram, "An Experimental Study of the Small World Problem," *Sociometry* 32, no. 4 (1969): 425–443, https://doi.org/10.2307/2786545.

4. Bruce Schechter, *My Brain Is Open: The Mathematical Journeys of Paul Erdős* (New York: Simon and Schuster, 1998).

5. Schechter, *My Brain Is Open.*

6. The search tool is available at https://mathscinet.ams.org/mathscinet/freeTools.html?version=2.

7. The website is located at https://oracleofbacon.org.

8. The website is located at https://www.imdb.com.

9. Information about the charity is available at https://www.sixdegrees.org/about.

10. Ronald S. Burt, *Structural Holes: The Social Structure of Competition* (Cambridge: Harvard University Press, 1995).

11. I. O. Orubuloye, Pat Caldwell, and John C. Caldwell, "The Role of High-Risk Occupations in the Spread of AIDS: Truck Drivers and Itinerant Market Women in Nigeria," *International Family Planning Perspectives* 19, no. 2 (1993): 43–71, https://doi.org/10.2307/2133418; Nosipho Faith Makhakhe et al., "Sexual Transactions between Long Distance Truck Drivers and Female Sex Workers in South Africa," *Global Health Action* 10, no. 1 (2017), https://doi.org/10.1080/16549716.2017.1346164.

12. Artis Curiskis et al., "Federal COVID Data 101: Working with CMS Nursing Home Data," The COVID Tracking Project, March 4, 2021, https://covidtracking.com/analysis-updates/federal-covid-data-101-working-with-cms-nursing-home-data.

13. Artis Curiskis et al., "What We Know—and What We Don't Know—about the Impact of the Pandemic on Our Most Vulnerable Community," The COVID Tracking Project, March 31, 2021, https://covidtracking.com/nursing-homes-long-term-care-facilities.

14. M. Keith Chen, Judith A. Chevalier, and Elisa F. Long, "Nursing Home Staff Networks and COVID-19," *Proceedings of the National Academy of Sciences* 118, no. 1 (2021): e2015455118, https://doi.org/10.1073/pnas.2015455118.

15. Shamez N. Ladhani et al., "Increased Risk of SARS-CoV-2 Infection in Staff Working across Different Care Homes: Enhanced COVID-19 Outbreak Investigations in London Care Homes," *Journal of Infection* 81, no. 4 (2020): 621–624, https://doi.10.1016/j.jinf.2020.07.027.org.

16. Courtney Harold Van Houtven, Nicole DePasquale, and Norma B. Coe, "Essential Long-Term Care Workers Commonly Hold Second Jobs and Double- or Triple-Duty Caregiving Roles," *Journal of American Geriatrics Society* 68, no. 8 (2020): 1657–1660, https://doi.10.1111/jgs.16509.org.

17. Will Englund, "In a Relentless Pandemic, Nursing-Home Workers Are Worn Down and Stressed Out," *Washington Post*, December 3, 2020, https://www.washingtonpost.com/business/2020/12/03/nursing-home-burnout/.

18. Paraprofessional Healthcare Institute, *Direct Care Workers in the United States: Key Facts* (September 8, 2020), https://phinational.org/resource/direct-care-workers-in-the-united-states-key-facts/.

19. Jose F. Figueroa et al., "Community-Level Factors Associated with Racial and Ethnic Disparities in COVID-19 Rates in Massachusetts," *Health Affairs* 39, no. 11 (2020), https://doi.org/10.1377/hlthaff.2020.01040.

20. Diego A. Martinez et al., "Latino Household Transmission of Severe Acute Respiratory Syndrome Coronavirus 2," *Clinical Infectious Diseases* 74, no. 9 (2022): 1675–1677, https://doi.org/10.1093/cid/ciab753.

21. Anabel Munoz, "Multigenerational Households Wait for Vaccine as California Releases Demographics of Distribution," *ABC7.com*, February 18, 2021, https://abc7.com/ca-mulgenerational-households-vaccine-distribution-latino-covid-statistics-california-update/10349282/.

22. April Simpson et al., "One Home, Many Generations: States Addressing Covid Risk among Families," *NBCnews.com*,

March 27, 2021, https://www.nbcnews.com/news/latino/latino -multigenerational-households-risk-covid-states-address-vaccine -rcna511.

23. Tim Arango, "'We Are Forced to Live in These Conditions': In Los Angeles, Virus Ravages Overcrowded Homes," *New York Times,* January 23, 2021, https://www.nytimes.com/2021/01/23 /us/los-angeles-crowded-covid.html.

24. Arango, "We Are Forced."

25. Marjolein Schat, "Justinian's Foreign Policy and the Plague: Did Justinian Create the First Pandemic?," https://www.montana.edu /historybug/yersiniaessays/schat.html. Last accessed July 11, 2022.

26. John Kelly, *The Great Mortality: An Intimate History of the Black Death, The Most Devastating Plague of All Time* (New York: Harper Collins, 2005), 8.

27. Mark Wheelis, "Biological Warfare at the 1346 Siege of Caffa," *Emerging Infectious Diseases* 8, no. 9 (2002): 971–975, https:// wwwnc.cdc.gov/eid/article/8/9/01-0536_article.

28. Wheelis, "Biological Warfare."

29. Wheelis, "Biological Warfare."

30. Wheelis, "Biological Warfare."

31. John Seven, "The Black Death: A Timeline of the Gruesome Pandemic," *History.com*, April 16, 2020, https://www.history .com/news/black-death-timeline.

32. Ricci P. H. Yue, Harry F. Lee, and Connor Y. H. Wu, "Trade Routes and Plague Transmission in Pre-Industrial Europe," *Scientific Reports* 7, no. 1 (2017), https://doi.org/10.1038 /s41598-017-13481-2.

33. Geoff Manaugh and Nicola Twilley, *Until Proven Safe: The History and Future of Quarantine* (New York: Farrar, Straus, and Giroux, 2021).

34. Francesca Bezzone, "Venetian Quarantine: The History of the Lazzaretto Vecchio and Lazzaretto Nuovo Islands," *L'Italo Americano,* August 24, 2020, https://italoamericano.org/venetian -quarantine-the-history-of-the-lazzaretto-vecchio-and-lazaretto -nuovo-islands/.

35. Frank M. Snowden, *Epidemics and Society: From the Black Death to the Present* (New Haven: Yale University Press, 2019).

36. Snowden, *Epidemics and Society*.

37. Joshua S. Loomis, *Epidemics: The Impacts of Germs and Their Power over Humanity* (Nashville: Turner Publishing, 2018).

38. J. C. McDonald, "The History of Quarantine in Britain during the 19th Century," *Bulletin of the History of Medicine* 25, no. 1 (1951): 22–44, http://www.jstor.org/stable/44443588.

39. Norman Howard-Jones, *The Scientific Background of the International Sanitary Conferences 1851–1938* (Geneva: World Health Organization, 1975), https://apps.who.int/iris/bitstream /handle/10665/62873/14549_eng.pdf.

40. Howard-Jones, *The Scientific Background*.

41. Michael Christopher Low, "Empire and the Hajj: Pilgrims, Plagues, and Pan-Islam under British Surveillance, 1865–1908," *International Journal of Middle East Studies* 40, no. 2 (2008): 269–90, http://www.jstor.org/stable/30069613.

42. Howard-Jones, *The Scientific Background*.

43. Manaugh and Twilley, *Until Proven Safe*.

44. Scott E. Page, "Reopening the Office? Here's How to Stymie Transmission of Covid," *Harvard Business Review,* July 28, 2020, https://hbr.org/2020/07/reopening-the-office-heres-how-to -stymie-transmission-of-covid-19.

Chapter 5. Safer than the City

1. George Blecher, "I Left My Troubled City Behind. Now I Feel Guilty," *New York Times*, May 16, 2020, https://www.nytimes .com/2020/05/16/nyregion/coronavirus-leaving-nyc.html.

2. Billy G. Smith, *Ship of Death: A Voyage That Changed the Atlantic World* (New Haven: Yale University Press, 2013).

3. Thomas Jefferson, "To James Madison from Thomas Jefferson, 1 September 1793," *United States National Archives Founders Online*, https://founders.archives.gov/documents/Madison/01-15 -02-0063.

4. William Kashatus, "Plagued! Philadelphia's Yellow Fever Epidemic of 1793," *Pennsylvania Heritage*, Spring 1993, http://paheritage.wpengine.com/article/plagued-philadelphias -yellow-fever-epidemic-1793/.

5. John Fabian Witt, *American Contagions: Epidemics and the Law from Smallpox to COVID-19* (New Haven: Yale University Press, 2020).

6. Charles E. Rosenberg, *The Cholera Years: The United States in 1832, 1849, and 1866* (Chicago and London: University of Chicago Press, 1987).

7. Rosenberg, *The Cholera Years*, 3.

8. Quoted in Rosenburg, *The Cholera Years*, from "Diary of a Young Man in Albany, July 18, 1832," Manuscript Division, New York Historical Society.

9. Charles Rosenberg, "The Cholera Epidemic of 1832 in New York City," *Bulletin of the History of Medicine* 33, no. 1 (1959): 37–49.

10. Rosenberg, "The Cholera Epidemic."

11. Helen Ouyang, "I'm an E.R. Doctor in New York. None of Us Will Ever Be the Same," *New York Times,* May 27, 2020, https://www.nytimes.com/2020/04/14/magazine/coronavirus-er -doctor-diary-new-york-city.html.

12. Ouyang, "I'm an E.R. Doctor."

13. Terry Nguyen, "How to Get Groceries when Delivery Services Are Slammed," *Vox.com,* April 8, 2020, https://www.vox.com /the-goods/2020/4/8/21213919/grocery-delivery-slammed -coronavirus-freshdirect-instacart.

14. Pew Research Center, *Mobile Fact Sheet* (April 7, 2021), https://www.pewresearch.org/internet/fact-sheet/mobile/.

15. Sam Blum, "Popular Apps Are Tracking and Selling Your Location Data to an Alarming Degree," *Popular Mechanics*, December 10, 2018, https://www.popularmechanics.com /technology/security/a25459046/apps-selling-location-data/.

16. Jennifer Valentino-DeVries et al., "Your Apps Know Where You Were Last Night, and They're Not Keeping It Secret," *New York Times,* December 10, 2018, https://www.nytimes.com/interactive /2018/12/10/business/location-data-privacy-apps.html.

17. Kevin Quealy, "The Richest Neighborhoods Emptied Out Most as Coronavirus Hit New York City," *New York Times,* May 15, 2020, https://www.nytimes.com/interactive/2020/05/15/upshot/who-left-new-york-coronavirus.html.

18. Quealy, "The Richest Neighborhoods Emptied Out."

19. Joshua David Stein, "The City's One-Percenters Flee the Rest of Us to the Hamptons," *New York Magazine,* March 20, 2020, https://nymag.com/intelligencer/2020/03/coronavirus-nyc-one-percenters-flee-to-the-hamptons.html.

20. Stein, "The City's One-Percenters Flee."

21. Anita DeClue and Billy G. Smith, "Wrestling the 'Pale Faced Messenger': The Diary of Edward Garrigues during the 1798 Philadelphia Yellow Fever Epidemic," *Pennsylvania History: A Journal of Mid-Atlantic Studies* 65 (1998): 243–268, http://www.jstor.org/stable/27774168.

22. Giovanni Boccaccio, *The Decameron*, trans. G.H. McWilliam, 2nd ed. (London: Penguin Books, 2003).

23. Erin Blakemore, "The Mysterious Epidemic That Terrified Henry VIII," *History.com*, March 19, 2020, https://www.history.com/news/the-mysterious-epidemic-that-terrified-henry-viii.

24. John L. Flood, "'Safer on the Battlefield Than in the City': England, the 'Sweating Sickness' and the Continent," *Renaissance Studies* 17, no. 2 (June 2003): 147–176, https://www.jstor.org/stable/24413344?seq=1.

25. Alfredo Morabia, "Epidemiology's 350th Anniversary: 1662–2012," *Epidemiology* 24, no. 2 (2013): 179–183, http://www.jstor.org/stable/23487815.

26. Kira L.S. Newman, "Shutt Up: Bubonic Plague and Quarantine in Early Modern England," *Journal of Social History* 45, no. 3 (2012): 809–834, http://www.jstor.org/stable/41678910.

27. Newman, "Shutt Up: Bubonic Plague."

28. Newman, "Shutt Up: Bubonic Plague."

29. Blakemore, "The Mysterious Epidemic That Terrified Henry VIII."

30. Becky Little, "When London Faced a Pandemic—And a Devastating Fire," *History.com*, March 25, 2020, https://www.history.com/news/plague-pandemic-great-fire.

31. "The Second Parliament of Charles II: Sixth Session (Oxford)—Begins 9/10/1665," in *The History and Proceedings of the House of Commons: Volume 1 1660–1680* (London: Chandler, 1742), 85–92. Found on *British History Online*, http://www.british-history.ac.uk/commons-hist-proceedings/vol1/pp85-92.

32. Mary Elizabeth Wilson, "The Power of Plague," *Epidemiology* 6, no. 4 (1995): 458–60, http://www.jstor.org/stable/3702102.

33. Erin Shaw, "The Origins of Banking in Greenwich Village: Yellow Fever and the Establishment of Bank Street," *Researching Greenwich Village History* (blog), October 1, 2013, https://greenwichvillagehistory.wordpress.com/2013/10/01/3660/.

34. Shaw, "The Origins of Banking."

35. William Gribbin, "Divine Providence or Miasma? The Yellow Fever Epidemic of 1822," *New York History* 53, no. 3 (1972): 282–98, http://www.jstor.org/stable/23164699.

36. The data that I discuss below is downloaded from the Opportunity Insights web page, found at https://opportunityinsights.org. It is based on mobility data from Google and aggregated by a team of academic researchers at Brown University and Harvard University. More information about their methods and research team are available at https://tracktherecovery.org. Analysis of the data is my own.

37. Matthew Ormseth, "The Line at This Costco Begins at 2:55 a.m. as Coronavirus Spooks Shoppers," *Los Angeles Times*, March 18, 2020, https://www.latimes.com/california/story/2020-03-18/coronavirus-pandemic-shopping-lines-costco-anxiety.

38. Greater London Authority, "Coronavirus (COVID-19) Mobility Report," London Datastore, last accessed July 13, 2022, https://data.london.gov.uk/dataset/coronavirus-covid-19-mobility-report.

39. Abha Bhattarai, "'If Coronavirus Doesn't Get Us, Starvation Will': A Growing Number of Americans Say They Can't Afford to Stock up on Groceries," *Washington Post*, March 20, 2020, https://www.washingtonpost.com/business/2020/03/20/if-coronavirus-doesnt-get-us-starvation-will-growing-number-americans-say-they-cant-afford-stock-up-groceries.

40. Bhattarai, "'If Coronavirus Doesn't Get Us.'"

41. Bhattarai, "'If Coronavirus Doesn't Get Us.'"

42. J. C. McDonald, "The History of Quarantine in Britain during the 19th Century." *Bulletin of the History of Medicine* 25, no. 1 (1951): 22–44. http://www.jstor.org/stable/44443588.

43. Jim Tankersley, Maggie Haberman, and Roni Caryn Rabin, "Trump Considers Reopening Economy, over Health Experts' Objections," *New York Times*, March 24, 2020, https://www.nytimes.com/2020/03/23/business/trump-coronavirus-economy.html.

44. Heather Long, "Over 10 Million Americans Applied for Unemployment Benefits in March as Economy Collapsed," *Washington Post*, April 3, 2020, https://www.washingtonpost.com/business/2020/04/02/jobless-march-coronavirus.

45. Hamada S. Badr et al., "Association between Mobility Patterns and COVID-19 Transmission in the USA: A Mathematical Modelling Study," *The Lancet* 20, no. 11 (2020): 1247–1254, https://doi.org/10.1016/S1473-3099(20)30553-3; Xiaojiang Li, Abby E. Rudolph, Jeremy Mennis, "Association between Population Mobility Reductions and New COVID-19 Diagnoses in the United States Along the Urban–Rural Gradient, February–April, 2020," *Preventing Chronic Disease* 17 (October 2020), https://www.cdc.gov/pcd/issues/2020/20_0241.html; Edward L. Glaeser, Caitlin Gorback, and Stephen J. Redding, "How Much Does COVID-19 Increase with Mobility? Evidence from New York and Four Other U.S. Cities" (working paper, National Bureau of Economic Research, October 2020), https://www.nber.org/papers/w27519.

46. Caroline Modarressy-Tehrani and Louise McLoughlin, "They Thought COVID-19 Was a Hoax, until They Fell Ill," *NBCnews online*, August 8, 2020, https://www.nbcnews.com/news/us-news/they-thought-covid-was-hoax-until-they-fell-ill-n1236183.

47. Janelle Griffith, "14 in Texas Family Test Positive for Coronavirus after Small Gathering, 1 Dies," *NBCnews online*, July 27, 2020, https://www.nbcnews.com/news/us-news/14-texas-family-test-positive-coronavirus-after-small-gathering-1-n1234980.

48. Tony Green, "A Harsh Lesson in the Reality of COVID-19," *Dallas Voice*, July 24, 2020, https://dallasvoice.com/a-harsh-lesson-in-the-reality-of-covid-19/.

49. Heejung Chung et al., *Working from Home during the COVID-19 Lockdown: Changing Preferences and the Future of Work* (Birmingham: University of Birmingham, 2020), https://www.birmingham.ac.uk/Documents/college-social-sciences/business/research/wirc/epp-working-from-home-COVID-19-lockdown.pdf.

50. Kim Parker, Juliani Menasce Horowitz, and Rachel Minkin, "How the Coronavirus Outbreak Has—and Hasn't—Changed the Way Americans Work," Pew Research Center, December 9, 2020, https://www.pewresearch.org/social-trends/2020/12/09/how-the-coronavirus-outbreak-has-and-hasnt-changed-the-way-americans-work/.

51. Parker, Horowitz, and Minkin, "How the Coronavirus Outbreak."

52. Jesse Matheson, Gianni De Fraja, and James Rockey, "Five Charts That Reveal How Remote Working Could Change the UK," *The Conversation*, February 3, 2021, https://theconversation.com/five-charts-that-reveal-how-remote-working-could-change-the-uk-154418.

53. Matheson, Fraja, and Rockey, "Five Charts."

54. USAFacts, *Monthly Public Transit Ridership Is 65% Lower Than before the Pandemic*, October 13, 2020, https://usafacts.org/articles/covid-public-transit-decline/.

55. Scott Calvert, "COVID-19 Pandemic Likely Improved Your Commute to Work," *Wall Street Journal*, January 3, 2021, https://www.wsj.com/articles/covid-19-pandemic-likely-improved-your-commute-to-work-11609669801.

56. Tom Krisher, "Used Vehicle Prices Up as Supply Sinks, but Relief Is Coming," *Associated Press*, October 14, 2020, https://apnews.com/article/virus-outbreak-prices-e329d1f56e879360939736fab27189dd.

57. Madelaine Criden, *The Stranded Poor: Recognizing the Importance of Public Transportation for Low-Income Households*

(Washington, DC: National Association for State Community Service Programs, 2008), https://nascsp.org/wp-content/uploads/2018/02/issuebrief-benefitsofruralpublictransportation.pdf.

58. Cathy Bussewitz, "Fears and Tension Mount for Commuters Still Heading to Work," *Associated Press,* December 10, 2020, https://apnews.com/article/new-york-health-transportation-coronavirus-pandemic-98c309f705004e22a6d1832e96a1014d.

59. Bussewitz, "Fears and Tension Mount."

60. "Rush Hour Commuters 'Nervous' After PM Eases Lockdown Measures," *NewsChain*, May 11, 2020, https://www.newschainonline.com/news/rush-hour-commuters-nervous-after-pm-eases-lockdown-measures-7626.

61. David Wickert, "Have MARTA Bus Cuts Affected You? Talk to Us," *Atlanta Journal-Constitution*, September 2, 2020, https://www.ajc.com/news/commuting-blog/have-marta-bus-cuts-affected-you-talk-to-us/FT3RDRSBHRBZTCYFUTCOHCGD24/.

62. Liz Ohanesian, "How Public Transit Riders Are Managing Their Metro Commutes during the Pandemic," *Los Angeles Magazine*, August 5, 2020, https://www.lamag.com/citythinkblog/public-transit-pandemic/.

63. For this section, I define *an impoverished county* to be one with more than 25 percent of residents in poverty. I define an *affluent county* as one with less than 5 percent of residents in poverty.

64. Jonathan Steinberg et al., "COVID-19 Outbreak among Employees at a Meat Processing Facility—South Dakota, March–April 2020," *Morbidity and Mortality Weekly Report* 69, no. 31 (August 7, 2020): 1015–1019, https://www.cdc.gov/mmwr/volumes/69/wr/mm6931a2.htm.

65. Steinberg et al., "COVID-19 Outbreak."

66. Jessica Lussenhop, "Coronavirus at Smithfield Pork Plant: The Untold Story of America's Biggest Outbreak," *BBC News*, April 17, 2020, https://www.bbc.com/news/world-us-canada-52311877.

67. Lussenhop, "Coronavirus at Smithfield."

68. Mia Jankowicz, "The South Dakota Slaughterhouse Linked to More than Half the State's Coronavirus Cases Had Offered

Employees a $500 'Responsibility Bonus' to Come to Work in April," *Business Insider*, April 16, 2020, https://www .businessinsider.com/south-dakota-slaughterhouse-coronavirus -responsibility-bonus-2020-4.

69. Nathaniel Meyersohn, "Groceries Were Hard to Find for Millions. Now It's Getting Even Worse," *CNN*, June 9, 2020, https://www.cnn.com/2020/06/09/business/food-deserts -coronavirus-grocery-stores/index.html.

70. Rachel Siegel, "For the Unemployed, Rising Grocery Prices Strain Budgets Even More," *Washington Post*, August 6, 2020, https://www.washingtonpost.com/business/2020/08/04/grocery -prices-unemployed/.

71. U.S. Bureau of Labor Statistics, *Consumer Price Index: 2020 in Review*, January 15, 2021, https://www.bls.gov/opub/ted/2021 /consumer-price-index-2020-in-review.htm.

72. Rachel Siegel, "For the Unemployed, Rising Grocery Prices Strain Budgets Even More," *Washington Post*, August 6, 2020, https://www.washingtonpost.com/business/2020/08/04/grocery -prices-unemployed/.

73. Stephen Fried, *Rush: Revolution, Madness, and the Visionary Doctor Who Became a Founding Father* (New York: Crown, 2018).

74. Sarah Pruitt, "When the Yellow Fever Outbreak of 1793 Sent the Wealthy Fleeing Philadelphia," *History.com*, June 11, 2020, https://www.history.com/news/yellow-fever-outbreak -philadelphia.

75. William Kashatus, "Plagued! Philadelphia's Yellow Fever Epidemic of 1793," *Pennsylvania Heritage*, Spring 1993, http://paheritage.wpengine.com/article/plagued-philadelphias -yellow-fever-epidemic-1793/.

76. Pruitt, "When the Yellow Fever Outbreak."

77. Absalom Jones and Richard Allen, *A Narrative of the Proceedings of the Black People, during the Late Awful Calamity in Philadelphia, in the Year 1793: And a Refutation of Some Censures, Thrown Upon Them in Some Late Publications* (Philadelphia: William W. Woodward, 1794), https://collections

.nlm.nih.gov/bookviewer?PID=nlm:nlmuid-2559020R-bk#page
/1/mode/2up.

78. Allen and Jones, *A Narrative of the Proceedings*, 18.

79. Allen and Jones, *A Narrative of the Proceedings*, 16.

80. Sandy Hingston, "What Two Centuries of Census Records
    Taught Us about Philadelphia," *Philadelphia Magazine*, January 18, 2020, https://www.phillymag.com/news/2020/01/18
    /philadelphia-census-records/.

81. "COVID: Bus Drivers 'Three Times More Likely to Die' than
    Other Workers," *BBC News*, March 19, 2021, https://www.bbc
    .com/news/uk-england-london-56455845.

82. Louis Beckett, "Revealed: Nearly 100 US Transit Workers Have
    Died of COVID-19 amid Lack of Basic Protections," *The
    Guardian*, April 20, 2020, https://www.theguardian.com/world
    /2020/apr/20/us-bus-drivers-lack-life-saving-basic-protections
    -transit-worker-deaths-coronavirus.

83. Louis Beckett, "Detroit Bus Driver Dies of Coronavirus after
    Posting Video about Passenger Coughing," *The Guardian*, April 3,
    2020, https://www.theguardian.com/us-news/2020/apr/03/detroit
    -bus-driver-dies-coronavirus-video-passenger-coughing.

84. Jennifer Hassan, "Tributes Pour In for British Rail Worker
    Who Died after Being Spat At by Man Who Said He Had the
    Coronavirus," *Washington Post*, May 13, 2020, https://www
    .washingtonpost.com/world/2020/05/13/tributes-pour-british
    -rail-worker-who-died-after-being-spat-by-man-who-said-he-had
    -coronavirus/.

85. Cory Stieg, "Line Cooks Have the Highest Risk of Dying during
    Pandemic, plus Other Riskiest Jobs: Study," *CNBC*, February 3,
    2021, https://www.cnbc.com/2021/02/02/jobs-where-workers
    -have-the-highest-risk-of-dying-from-covid-study.html.

86. Yea-Hung Chen et al., "Excess Mortality Associated with the
    COVID-19 Pandemic among Californians 18–65 Years of Age,
    by Occupational Sector and Occupation: March through
    October 2020," *PLOS ONE*, June 4, 2021, https://doi.org/10
    .1371/journal.pone.0252454.

87. Chen et al., "Excess Mortality."

Chapter 6. Below the Margin

1. Maria Hernandez, "Op-Ed: I Got COVID-19 While Working at Ralphs. People Like Me Need a Voice in Workplace Safety," *Los Angeles Times*, September 14, 2020, https://www.latimes.com/opinion/story/2020-09-14/ralphs-worker-covid-safetly-workplace.
2. Hernandez, "Op-Ed: I Got COVID-19."
3. Hye Jin Rho, Hayley Brown, and Shawn Fremstad, *A Basic Demographic Profile of Workers in Frontline Industries* (Washington, DC: Center for Economic Policy Research, April 2020), https://cepr.net/wp-content/uploads/2020/04/2020-04-Frontline-Workers.pdf.
4. Rho, Brown, and Fremstad, *A Basic Demographic Profile.*
5. Jim Zarroli and Avie Schneider, "3.3 Million File Unemployment Claims, Shattering Records," NPR, March 26, 2020, https://www.npr.org/2020/03/26/821580191/unemployment-claims-expected-to-shatter-records.
6. This data is available at https://tracktherecovery.org/.
7. Elise Gould and Jori Kandra, *Wages Grew in 2020 Because the Bottom Fell Out of the Low-Wage Labor Market* (Washington, DC: Economic Policy Institute, February 24, 2021), https://www.epi.org/publication/state-of-working-america-wages-in-2020/.
8. Gould and Kandra, *Wages Grew in 2020.*
9. Congressional Research Service, *Unemployment Rates during the COVID-19 Pandemic*, August 20, 2021, https://sgp.fas.org/crs/misc/R46554.pdf.
10. Ella Koeze, "A Year Later, Who Is Back to Work and Who Is Not?," *New York Times*, March 9, 2021, https://www.nytimes.com/interactive/2021/03/09/business/economy/covid-employment-demographics.html.
11. Alaa Elassar, "She Lost Her Business Due to Coronavirus. Now She's Supporting Her Four Children by Running Their Lemonade Stand," CNN, September 19, 2020, https://www.cnn.com/2020/09/19/us/lemonade-stand-family-coronavirus-trnd/index.html.
12. Elassar, "She Lost Her Business."

13. "Food Insecurity in the U.S.," U.S. Department of Agriculture Economic Research Service, updated October 17, 2022, https://www.ers.usda.gov/topics/food-nutrition-assistance/food-security-in-the-u-s/measurement/#insecurity.

14. Diane Schanzenbach and Abigail Pitts, *How Much Has Food Insecurity Risen? Evidence from the Census Household Pulse Survey* (Evanston, IL: Institute for Policy Research, June 10, 2020), https://www.ipr.northwestern.edu/documents/reports/ipr-rapid-research-reports-pulse-hh-data-10-june-2020.pdf.

15. Schanzenbach and Pitts, *How Much Has Food Insecurity Risen?*

16. Kimi Ceridon, "I Grew Up with the Shame of Food Insecurity. Decades Later, I Still Obsess over What I Eat," *Bon Appétit*, June 23, 2021, https://www.bonappetit.com/story/childhood-food-insecurity.

17. Ceridon, "I Grew Up with the Shame."

18. Ceridon, "I Grew Up with the Shame."

19. Ceridon, "I Grew Up with the Shame."

20. Ceridon, "I Grew Up with the Shame."

21. Ceridon, "I Grew Up with the Shame."

22. Mimi Whitefield, "Cars Line up for Hours at the Food Pantry. How the Pandemic Ravaged South Florida," Feeding South Florida, November 2, 2020, https://feedingsouthflorida.org/cars-line-up-for-hours-at-the-food-pantry-how-the-pandemic-ravaged-south-florida/.

23. Megan Sheets, "Startling Drone Footage Shows 1.5 Mile-Long Line of Cars Waiting Outside a Drive-thru Food Bank in Miami That Gives Out 2.5 Million Meals per Week as Coronavirus Effects Leave Millions Hungry," Feeding South Florida, August 9, 2021, https://feedingsouthflorida.org/1-5-mile-long-line-of-cars-waits-outside/.

24. Alaa Elassar, "She Lost Her Job in the Pandemic. She Can't Even Afford the Dollar Store to Feed Her Kids," CNN, September 28, 2020, https://www.cnn.com/2020/09/24/us/child-hunger-family-food-insecurity-coronavirus-trnd/index.html.

25. Carmen Sesin, "'In Triage Mode': South Florida Food Banks Worry about Dwindling Supplies," *NBC News*, December 1,

2020, https://www.nbcnews.com/news/latino/triage-mode-south
-florida-food-banks-worry-about-dwindling-supplies-n1249550.

26. Sharen Cohen, "Millions of Hungry Americans Turn to Food
Banks for 1st Time," *Associated Press*, December 7, 2020,
https://apnews.com/article/race-and-ethnicity-hunger-coronavirus
-pandemic-4c7f1705c6d8ef5bac241e6cc8e331bb.

27. Cohen, "Millions of Hungry Americans."

28. Cohen, "Millions of Hungry Americans."

29. Kim Parker, Rachel Minkin, and Jesse Bennett, *Economic Fallout
from COVID-19 Continues to Hit Lower-Income Americans the
Hardest* (Washington, DC: Pew Research Center, May 28, 2021),
https://www.pewresearch.org/social-trends/2020/09/24/economic
-fallout-from-covid-19-continues-to-hit-lower-income-americans
-the-hardest/.

30. Parker, Minkin, and Bennett, *Economic Fallout*.

31. "Coal in the United States," Indiana Geological and Water
Survey, Indiana University, https://igws.indiana.edu/Coal/.

32. Frank Parker Stockbridge, "Health at Home to Help the Army:
Improving the Sanitary Conditions in the United States in Order
to Help the Army Win the War," *The World's Work*, April 1918,
608. Quoted from Nancy Bristow, *American Pandemic: The
Lost Worlds of the 1918 Influenza Epidemic* (New York: Oxford
University Press, 2012).

33. John M. Barry, "How the Horrific 1918 Flu Spread across
America," *Smithsonian Magazine*, November 1, 2017, https://www
.smithsonianmag.com/history/journal-plague-year-180965222/.

34. Teamus Bartley, "'There Wasn't a Mine Runnin' a Lump O' Coal':
A Kentucky Coal Miner Remembers the Influenza Pandemic of
1918–1919," University of Kentucky, Library Oral History
Project, http://historymatters.gmu.edu/d/107/.

35. Barry, "How the Horrific 1918 Flu Spread across America."

36. Barry, "How the Horrific 1918 Flu Spread across America."

37. Barry, "How the Horrific 1918 Flu Spread across America."

38. Rev. John McDowell, "Life of a Coal Miner," *The World's Work*
1902, 2659–60, https://energyhistory.yale.edu/library-item/rev
-john-mcdowell-life-coal-miner-1902.

39. Karen Clay, "Pandemics and the Labor Market—Then and Now," *IZA World of Labor*, March 25, 2020, https://www.heinz.cmu.edu/media/2020/March/karen-clay-iza-pandemics-and-the-labor-market.

40. Simon Heffer, "What the Spanish Flu Pandemic Teaches Us Today," *New Statesman*, May 6, 2020, https://www.newstatesman.com/politics/health/2020/05/what-spanish-flu-pandemic-teaches-us-today.

41. Heffer, "What the Spanish Flu Pandemic."

42. Heffer, "What the Spanish Flu Pandemic."

43. Rachel King, "More than 110,000 Eating and Drinking Establishments Closed in 2020," *Fortune*, January 26, 2021, https://fortune.com/2021/01/26/restaurants-bars-closed-2020-jobs-lost-how-many-have-closed-us-covid-pandemic-stimulus-unemployment/.

44. King, "More than 110,000."

45. Andy Kiersz, "Alexandria Ocasio-Cortez Defended Being 'Just a Waitress' in Latest Twitter Spat. There Are 10.7 Million Americans Employed in Food Service, Though What They Earn Depends on the Role," *Business Insider*, May 6, 2019, https://www.businessinsider.com/how-much-are-restaurant-workers-paid-2019-5#8-cooks-make-a-median-of-26230-a-year-and-there-are-1137590-employed-in-the-restaurant-industry-15.

46. Katie Okamoto, "'Challenging Is Not Nearly a Strong Enough Word,'" *Eater*, February 18, 2021, https://www.eater.com/22288274/high-risk-restaurant-workers-navigating-pandemic-covid-19.

47. Okamoto, "'Challenging is Not Nearly.'"

48. Nina Friend, "What Restaurant Workers Wish You Knew," *Food & Wine*, January 14, 2021, https://www.foodandwine.com/fwpro/what-restaurant-workers-wish-you-knew.

49. Friend, "What Restaurant Workers."

50. Friend, "What Restaurant Workers."

51. Eli Rosenberg, "'The Final Straw': How the Pandemic Pushed Restaurant Workers over the Edge," *Washington Post*, September 7, 2021, https://www.washingtonpost.com/business/2021/05/24/restaurant-workers-shortage-pay/.

52. Rosenberg, "'The Final Straw.'"

53. Rosenberg, "'The Final Straw.'"

54. Sophia Chang, "Report: Being a Restaurant Worker during a Pandemic Is Even Worse Than You Think," *Gothamist*, December 2, 2020, https://gothamist.com/food/report-being-restaurant -worker-during-pandemic-even-worse-you-think.

55. Chang, "Report."

56. Chang, "Report."

57. Chang, "Report."

58. Courtney Vinopal, "The Pandemic Forced Millions Out of a Job. Some Say They Can't Return to the Way Things Were," PBS, June 17, 2021, https://www.pbs.org/newshour/economy/the -pandemic-forced-millions-out-of-a-job-some-say-they-cant -return-to-the-way-things-were.

59. Will Englund, "In a Relentless Pandemic, Nursing-Home Workers Are Worn Down and Stressed Out," *Washington Post*, December 4, 2020, https://www.washingtonpost.com/business /2020/12/03/nursing-home-burnout/.

60. Englund, "In a Relentless Pandemic."

61. Englund, "In a Relentless Pandemic."

62. Englund, "In a Relentless Pandemic."

63. Bryce Covert, "'They Just Feel That They've Been Violated,'" *Atlantic*, April 16, 2021, https://www.theatlantic.com/health /archive/2021/04/the-pandemic-broke-americas-health-care -workers/618600/.

64. Data available at "Long-Term-Care COVID Tracker," The COVID Tracking Project, https://covidtracking.com/nursing -homes-long-term-care-facilities.

65. Conan Brady et al., "Nursing Home Staff Mental Health during the Covid-19 Pandemic in the Republic of Ireland," *International Journal of Geriatric Psychiatry* 37, no. 1 (2021): 1–10, https://doi.org/10.1002/gps.5648.

66. Mo Shenjiang and Junqi Shi, "The Psychological Consequences of the COVID-19 on Residents and Staff in Nursing Homes," *Work, Aging and Retirement* 6, no. 4 (2020): 254–259. https:// doi.org/10.1093/workar/waaa021.

67. Shenjiang and Shi, "The Psychological Consequences."
68. Yinfei Duan et al., "Care Aides Working Multiple Jobs: Considerations for Staffing Policies in Long-Term Care Homes during and after the COVID-19 Pandemic," *Journal of Post-Acute and Long-Term Care Medicine* 21, no. 10 (2020), https://doi.org/10.1016/j.jamda.2020.07.036.
69. PHI National, *Direct Care Workers in the United States: Key Facts*, 2020, https://phinational.org/resource/direct-care-workers-in-the-united-states-key-facts/.
70. Matt Sedensky, "Ghost Towns: Nursing Home Staffing Falls amid Pandemic," *Associated Press*, October 7, 2021, https://apnews.com/article/coronavirus-pandemic-nursing-homes-d1befe76a3a0680b57defb6d9f1cfb66.
71. Sedensky, "Ghost Towns."
72. Sedensky, "Ghost Towns."
73. William Wan, "Burned Out by the Pandemic, 3 in 10 Health-Care Workers Consider Leaving the Profession," *Washington Post*, April 23, 2021, https://www.washingtonpost.com/health/2021/04/22/health-workers-covid-quit/.
74. Allan Kulikoff, *From British Peasants to Colonial American Farmers* (Chapel Hill: University of North Carolina Press, 2000).
75. L. R. Poos, "The Social Context of Statute of Labourers Enforcement," *Law and History Review* 1, no. 1 (1983): 27–52, https://doi.org/10.2307/744001. Last accessed June 16, 2022.
76. Dan Jones, *Power and Thrones: A New History of the Middle Ages* (New York: Viking, 2021).
77. Heather Long, Alyssa Fowers, and Andrew Van Dam, "Why America Has 8.4 Million Unemployed When There Are 10 Million Job Openings," *Washington Post*, September 8, 2021, https://www.washingtonpost.com/business/2021/09/04/ten-million-job-openings-labor-shortage/.
78. "The COVID-19 Labor Shortage: Exploring the Disconnect between Business and Unemployed Americans," Society for Human Resources Management, 2021, https://advocacy.shrm.org/wp-content/uploads/2021/07/SHRM-Research_The_Employment_Picture_Comes_Into_Focus.pdf.

79. Claire Cain Miller, "Return to Work? Not with Child Care Still in Limbo, Some Parents Say," *New York Times*, August 5, 2021, https://www.nytimes.com/2021/08/05/upshot/covid-child-care -schools.html?referringSource=articleShare.

80. Miller, "Return to Work?"

81. Rakesh Kochhar, *Two Years of Economics Recovery: Women Lose Jobs, Men Find Them* (Washington, DC: Pew Research Center, July 6, 2011), https://www.pewresearch.org/social-trends /2011/07/06/two-years-of-economic-recovery-women-lose-jobs -men-find-them/.

82. Claire Ewing-Nelson and Jasmine Tucker, *A Year into the Pandemic, Women Are Still Short Nearly 5.1 Million Jobs* (Washington, DC: National Women's Law Center, March 2021), https:// nwlc.org/wp-content/uploads/2021/03/Feb-Jobs-Day-v2.pdf.

83. St. Louis Federal Reserve Bank data available at https://fred .stlouisfed.org/series/LNS11300002.

84. Jessica Bennett, "'I Feel Like I Have Five Jobs': Moms Navigate the Pandemic," *New York Times*, March 20, 2020, https://www .nytimes.com/2020/03/20/parenting/childcare-coronavirus-moms .html.

85. Bennett, "'I Feel Like I Have Five Jobs.'"

86. Ruth Igielnik, *A Rising Share of Working Parents in the U.S. Say It's Been Difficult to Handle Child Care during the Pandemic* (Washington, DC: Pew Research Center, January 26, 2021), https://www.pewresearch.org/fact-tank/2021/01/26/a-rising-share -of-working-parents-in-the-u-s-say-its-been-difficult-to-handle -child-care-during-the-pandemic/.

87. Jessica Grose, "America's Mothers Are in Crisis," *New York Times*, February 4, 2021, https://www.nytimes.com/2021/02/04 /parenting/working-moms-mental-health-coronavirus.html.

88. Grose, "America's Mothers."

89. Grose, "America's Mothers."

90. Amanda Holpuch, "How the 'Shecession' Will Cause Long-Term Harm for Women in the US," *Guardian*, January 4, 2021, https://www.theguardian.com/business/2021/jan/04/shecession -women-economy-c-nicole-mason-interview.

91. Jasmine Tucker and Julie Vogtman, *When Hard Work Is Not Enough: Women in Low-Paid Jobs* (Washington, DC: National Women's Law Center, April 2020), https://nwlc.org/wp-content/uploads/2020/04/Women-in-Low-Paid-Jobs-report_pp04-FINAL-4.2.pdf.

92. This is defined as earnings less than 200 percent of the federal poverty level. This is the standard definition for *the working poor.*

93. Samantha Schmidt, "Women Have Been Hit Hardest by Job Losses in the Pandemic. And It May Only Get Worse," *Washington Post*, May 11, 2020, https://www.washingtonpost.com/dc-md-va/2020/05/09/women-unemployment-jobless-coronavirus/.

94. Schmidt, "Women Have Been Hit Hardest."

95. Claire Ewing-Nelson, *After a Full Month of Business Closures, Women Were Hit Hardest by April's Job Losses* (Washington, DC: National Women's Law Center, May 2020), https://nwlc.org/wp-content/uploads/2020/05/Jobs-Day-April-Factsheet.pdf.

96. Ewing-Nelson, "After a Full Month."

97. Titan Alon et al., "The Impact of COVID-19 on Gender Equality" (working paper, National Bureau of Economic Research, April 2020), https://www.nber.org/system/files/working_papers/w26947/w26947.pdf.

98. Alon et al., "The Impact of COVID-19."

99. Megan Leonhardt, "9.8 Million Working Mothers in the U.S. Are Suffering from Burnout," CNBC, December 3, 2020, https://www.cnbc.com/2020/12/03/millions-of-working-mothers-in-the-us-are-suffering-from-burnout.html.

100. Titan Alon et al., "From Mancession to Shecession: Women's Employment in Regular and Pandemic Recessions" (working paper, National Bureau of Economics Research, April 2021), https://doi.org/10.3386/w28632.

101. Schmidt, "Women Have Been Hit Hardest."

Chapter 7. The Pandemic Dilemma

1. J. Alexander Navarro, "Mask Resistance during a Pandemic Isn't New—in 1918 Many Americans Were 'Slackers,'" *Discover Magazine*, November 3, 2020, https://www.discovermagazine.com/health/mask-resistance-during-a-pandemic-isnt-new-in-1918-many-americans-were.

2. "Wear a Mask and Save Your Life!" *Oakland Tribune*, October 23, 1918, 2, https://quod.lib.umich.edu/f/flu/1440flu.0007.441/1/--wear-a-mask-and-save-your-life?rgn=full+text;view=image;q1=wear+a+mask.

3. Navarro, "Mask Resistance during a Pandemic Isn't New."

4. Christine Hauser, "The Mask Slackers of 1918," *New York Times*, August 3, 2020, https://www.nytimes.com/2020/08/03/us/mask-protests-1918.html.

5. Hauser, "The Mask Slackers of 1918."

6. Hauser, "The Mask Slackers of 1918."

7. Navarro, "Mask Resistance during a Pandemic Isn't New."

8. Navarro, "Mask Resistance during a Pandemic Isn't New."

9. "Three Shot in Struggle with Mask Slacker, Blacksmith Strikes Health Inspector Striving to Enforce Order," *San Francisco Chronicle*, October 29, 1918, https://www.newspapers.com/image/?clipping_id=47945955&fcfToken=eyJhbGciOiJIUzI1NiIsInR5cCI6IkpXVCJ9.eyJmcmVlLXZpZXctaWQiOjI3NTY2MDcxLCJpYXQiOjE2NTc4MTQwMDcsImV4cCI6MTY1NzkwMDQwN30.sbXMgwpWOM5t-7oE0IUPk9mhEebkRhjqvI5bwg4V6u8.

10. "Three Shot in Struggle with Mask Slacker," *San Francisco Chronicle*.

11. Details and quotes taken from "Three Shot in Struggle with Mask Slacker," *San Francisco Chronicle*; Hauser, "The Mask Slackers of 1918"; and Polly J. Price, "How a Fragmented Country Fights a Pandemic," *The Atlantic*, March 19, 2020, https://www.theatlantic.com/ideas/archive/2020/03/how-fragmented-country-fights-pandemic/608284/.

12. Brian Dolan, "Unmasking History: Who Was Behind the Anti-Mask League Protests During the 1918 Influenza Epidemic in San

Francisco?," *eScholarship University of California* (2020), https://doi.org/10.34947/M7QP4M.

13. Brian Dolan, "Unmasking History."

14. Brian Dolan, "Unmasking History."

15. Katie Canales, "Photos Show How San Francisco Had to Convince Its 'Mask Slackers' to Wear Masks after Many Defied the Law While the 1918 Spanish Flu Pandemic Seized the City," *Business Insider,* June 3, 2020, https://www.businessinsider.com /san-francisco-anti-mask-league-1918-spanish-flu-pandemic -2020-5.

16. A historical timeline of the rally can be found on the event web page at https://sturgismotorcyclerally.com/index.php?page =timeline.

17. Mark Walker and Jack Healy, "A Motorcycle Rally in a Pandemic? 'We Kind of Knew What Was Going to Happen,'" *New York Times*, November 6, 2020, https://www.nytimes.com /2020/11/06/us/sturgis-coronavirus-cases.html.

18. Walker and Healy, "A Motorcycle Rally in a Pandemic?"

19. Stephen Groves, "Harleys Everywhere, Masks Nowhere: Sturgis Draws Thousands," *AP News*, August 7, 2020, https://apnews .com/article/virus-outbreak-ap-top-news-nd-state-wire-sd-state -wire-south-dakota-fa074079157ad9a3683445b291daaf39.

20. Brittany Shammas and Lena H. Sun, "How the Sturgis Motor-cycle Rally May Have Spread Coronavirus across the Upper Midwest," *Washington Post*, December 12, 2020, https://www .washingtonpost.com/health/2020/10/17/sturgis-rally-spread/.

21. Frank H. Knight, *Risk, Uncertainty, and Profit* (Boston, New York: Houghton Mifflin, 1921).

22. Peter Dizikes, "Explained: Knightian Uncertainty," MIT News Office, June 2, 2010, https://news.mit.edu/2010/explained -knightian-0602.

23. Nassim Nicholas Taleb, *The Black Swan: The Impact of the Highly Improbable* (New York: Random House, 2007).

24. Michael Baily et al., "Social Networks Shape Beliefs and Behavior: Evidence from Social Distancing during the COVID-19 Pandemic" (working paper, National Bureau of

Economic Research, January 2021), https://doi.org/10.3386 /w28234.

25. Francesco Pierri et al., "Online Misinformation Is Linked to Early COVID-19 Vaccination Hesitancy and Refusal," *Scientific Reports* 12, no. 1 (April 2022), https://doi.org/10.1038/s41598 -022-10070-w.

26. Kellyanne Conway, "Conway: Press Secretary Gave 'Alternative Facts,'" interview by Chuck Todd, *NBCNews.com*, May 25, 2021, https://www.nbcnews.com/meet-the-press/video/conway -press-secretary-gave-alternative-facts-860142147643.

27. Josh Dawsey, Felicia Sonmez, and Paul Kane, "Trump Acknowl- edges He Intentionally Downplayed Deadly Coronavirus, Says Effort Was to Reduce Panic," *Washington Post*, September 10, 2020, https://www.washingtonpost.com/politics/trump-reaction -woodward-interview-coronavirus/2020/09/09/fc21e67e-f2ca -11ea-b796-2dd09962649c_story.html.

28. Laurel Wamsley, "Fired Florida Data Scientist Launches a Coronavirus Dashboard of Her Own," NPR, June 14, 2020, https://www.npr.org/2020/06/14/876584284/fired-florida-data -scientist-launches-a-coronavirus-dashboard-of-her-own.

29. Leonardo Bursztyn et al., "Misinformation during a Pandemic" (working paper, Becker Friedman Institute, 2020), https://bfi .uchicago.edu/working-paper/2020-44/.

30. "Historian John Barry Compares COVID-19 to the 1918 Flu Pandemic," University of Rochester Newscenter, October 6, 2020, https://www.rochester.edu/newscenter/historian-john-barry -compares-covid-19-to-1918-flu-pandemic-454732/.

31. Ben Verde, "Frozen in Time: Bay Ridge Bar Owner Joe Joyce Remembered as Local Legend," *Brooklyn Paper*, April 17, 2020, https://www.brooklynpaper.com/frozen-in-time-bay-ridge-bar -owner-joe-joyce-remembered-as-local-legend/.

32. Ginia Bellafante, "A Beloved Bar Owner Was Skeptical about the Virus. Then He Took a Cruise," *New York Times*, April 18, 2020, https://www.nytimes.com/2020/04/18/nyregion/coronavirus -jjbubbles-joe-joyce.html.

33. Bellafante, "A Beloved Bar Owner Was Skeptical."

34. Bellafante, "A Beloved Bar Owner Was Skeptical."
35. Bellafante, "A Beloved Bar Owner Was Skeptical."
36. Bellafante, "A Beloved Bar Owner Was Skeptical."
37. Bellafante, "A Beloved Bar Owner Was Skeptical."
38. Bellafante, "A Beloved Bar Owner Was Skeptical."
39. Bellafante, "A Beloved Bar Owner Was Skeptical."
40. Bursztyn et al., "Misinformation during a Pandemic."
41. Meghan Glova, "Locals Excited for Famed Sturgis Motorcycle Rally despite COVID Risks," *Central Oregon Daily News*, June 3, 2021, https://centraloregondaily.com/%E2%96%B6%EF%B8%8F -locals-excited-for-famed-sturgis-motorcycle-rally-despite-covid -risks/.
42. Shammas and Sun, "How the Sturgis Motorcycle Rally May Have Spread Coronavirus."
43. Megan Raposa, "SD Governor Criticizes Study Suggesting Sturgis Bike Rally Led to 260,000 Covid-19 Cases," *USA Today*, September 9, 2020, https://www.usatoday.com/story/news/nation /2020/09/08/study-260-000-coronavirus-cases-likely-tied-sturgis -rally/5750587002/.
44. Shammas and Sun, "How the Sturgis Motorcycle Rally May Have Spread Coronavirus."
45. Rosalind J. Carter et al., "Widespread Severe Acute Respiratory Syndrome Coronavirus 2 Transmission among Attendees at a Large Motorcycle Rally and Their Contacts, 30 US Jurisdictions August–September, 2020," *Clinical Infectious Diseases* 73, no. 1 (July 2021): S106–S109, https://doi.org/10.1093/cid/ciab321.
46. Dhaval Dave, Drew McNichols, and Joseph J. Sabia, "The Contagion Externality of a Superspreading Event: The Sturgis Motorcycle Rally and COVID-19," *Southern Economic Journal* 87, no. 3 (2020): 769–807, https://doi.org/10.1002/soej.12475.
47. When an early, non-peer-reviewed draft of their study was made available in September 2020, it created a firestorm of commentary. Newspapers emphasized the upper bound of 260,000. Some researchers claimed the results were too large when matched against case data. Others thought the numbers more plausible. Researchers at the Johns Hopkins University Bloomberg School of

Public Health issued a note of caution, particularly with respect to the uncertainty of the national estimates. That commentary can be found at https://ncrc.jhsph.edu/research/the-contagion-externality -of-a-superspreading-event-the-sturgis-motorcycle-rally-and-covid -19/. Following peer-review, a revised version of the study was published in the *Southern Economic Journal* in December 2020. This version emphasized the lower bound in the discussion of the results more than the previous version.

48. Nir Shafir, "In an Ottoman Holy Land: The Hajj and the Road from Damascus, 1500–1800," *History of Religions* 60, no. 1 (2020): 1–36.

49. Michael Christopher Low, "Empire and the Hajj: Pilgrims, Plagues, and Pan-Islam under British Surveillance, 1865–1908," *International Journal of Middle East Studies* 40, no. 2 (2008): 269–90, http://www.jstor.org/stable/30069613.

50. Eileen Kane, "The Hajj and Europe," *Origins: Current Events in Historical Perspective*, July 2016, https://origins.osu.edu/article /hajj-and-europe.

51. Low, "Empire and the Hajj."

52. Joshua S. Loomis, *Epidemics: The Impact of Germs and Their Power over Humanity* (Nashville: Turner Publishing, 2018).

53. William H. McNeill, *Plagues and Peoples* (New York: Anchor Books, 1998).

54. Loomis, *Epidemics: The Impact of Germs.*

55. Low, "Empire and the Hajj."

56. Loomis, *Epidemics: The Impact of Germs.*

57. Loomis, *Epidemics: The Impact of Germs.*

58. Loomis, *Epidemics: The Impact of Germs.*

59. Harriet Sherwood, "'Let Us Disobey': Churches Defy Lockdown with Secret Meetings," *Guardian*, November 22, 2020, https:// www.theguardian.com/world/2020/nov/22/let-us-disobey -churches-defy-lockdown-with-secret-meetings.

60. Low, "Empire and the Hajj."

61. Low, "Empire and the Hajj."

62. Ed Yong, "The Pandemic's Legacy Is Already Clear: All of This Will Happen Again," *Atlantic*, September 30, 2022, https://www

.theatlantic.com/health/archive/2022/09/covid-pandemic-exposes
-americas-failing-systems-future-epidemics/671608/.

63. H. Holden Thorp, "It Ain't Over 'Til It's Over," *Science* 376,
no. 6594 (2022): 675, https://doi.org/10.1126/science.abq8460.

64. Fenit Nirappil, "The Bar for Reimposing Mask Mandates Is
Getting Higher and Higher," *Washington Post*, May 14, 2022,
https://www.washingtonpost.com/health/2022/05/09/mask
-mandate-covid-cases/.

65. F. Scott Fitzgerald, *The Great Gatsby* (New York: Charles
Scribner's Sons, 1925).

66. John Stuart Mill, *On Liberty* (London: John W. Parker and Son,
1859).

67. Sirin Kale, "Off Their Heads: The Shocking Return of the Rave,"
Guardian, June 30, 2020, https://www.theguardian.com/music
/2020/jun/30/off-their-heads-the-shocking-return-of-the-rave.

68. Mill, *On Liberty*.

69. Brit Dawson, "Inside the UK's Illegal Rave Scene, Flourishing in
Lockdown," *Dazed Digital*, November 20, 2020, https://www
.dazeddigital.com/life-culture/article/51143/1/inside-the-uk-illegal
-rave-scene-flourishing-in-lockdown-coronavirus.

70. Shawn Hubler and Anemona Hartocollis, "Stop Campus
Partying to Slow the Virus? Colleges Try but Often Fail," *New
York Times*, August 22, 2020, https://www.nytimes.com/2020/08
/22/us/college-campus-covid.html.

71. Kevin Stankiewicz and Will Feuer, "Students Are Heading Back
to Campus and So Is the Coronavirus as Colleges Scramble to
Cancel In-Person Classes," CNBC, August 20, 2020, https://www
.cnbc.com/2020/08/19/students-are-heading-back-to-campus-and
-so-is-the-coronavirus-as-colleges-scramble-to-cancel-in-person
-classes.html.

72. Danielle Ivory, Robert Gebeloff, and Sarah Mervosh, "Young
People Have Less Covid-19 Risk, but in College Towns, Deaths
Rose Fast," *New York Times*, December 12, 2020, https://www
.nytimes.com/2020/12/12/us/covid-colleges-nursing-homes.html.

73. Ivory, Gebeloff, and Mervosh, "Young People Have Less
Covid-19 Risk."

74. Ivory, Gebeloff, and Mervosh, "Young People Have Less Covid-19 Risk."
75. Ivory, Gebeloff, and Mervosh, "Young People Have Less Covid-19 Risk."
76. Ivory, Gebeloff, and Mervosh, "Young People Have Less Covid-19 Risk."
77. Ivan Specht et al., "The Case for Altruism in Institutional Diagnostic Testing," *Scientific Reports* 12, no. 1857 (2022), https://doi.org/10.1038/s41598-021-02605-4.
78. Emily Anthes, "Why It Pays to Think Outside the Box on Coronavirus Tests," *New York Times*, March 24, 2021, https://www.nytimes.com/2021/03/24/health/coronavirus-testing-universities-sabeti.html?referringSource=articleShare.
79. Shawn Hubler, "A California University Tries to Shield an Entire City from Coronavirus," *New York Times*, January 30, 2021, https://www.nytimes.com/2021/01/30/us/college-coronavirus-california.html.
80. Hubler, "A California University Tries."
81. Antoine de Bengy Puyvallée and Sonja Kittelsen, "'Disease Knows No Borders': Pandemics and the Politics of Global Health Security," in *Pandemics, Publics, and Politics*, eds. K. Bjørkdahl and B. Carlsen (Singapore: Palgrave Pivot, 2019), https://doi.org/10.1007/978-981-13-2802-2_5.
82. Garrett Hardin, "The Tragedy of the Commons," *Science* 162, no. 3859 (1968): 1243–1248, https://www.science.org/doi/10.1126/science.162.3859.1243.
83. Michael Errigo, "Mets' Chris Bassitt Wants to Halt MLB Covid Testing: 'There's No Reason,'" *Washington Post*, July 7, 2022, https://www.washingtonpost.com/sports/2022/07/07/mets-chris-bassitt-covid/.

Chapter 8. Rogue Waves

1. Nellie Bristol, "Obituary: William H. Stewart," *The Lancet* 372, no. 9633 (2008), https://doi.org/10.1016/S0140-6736(08)61022-3.

2. Brad Spellberg and Bonnie Taylor-Blake, "On the Exoneration of Dr. William H. Stewart: Debunking an Urban Legend," *Infectious Diseases of Poverty* 2, no. 3 (2013), https://doi.org/10.1186/2049-9957-2-3.

3. Katie Kalvaitis, "Penicillin: An Accidental Discovery Changed the Course of Medicine," *Healio News*, August 2008, https://www.healio.com/news/endocrinology/20120325/penicillin-an-accidental-discovery-changed-the-course-of-medicine.

4. T. Butler, "Plague History: Yersin's Discovery of the Causative Bacterium in 1894 Enabled, in the Subsequent Century, Scientific Progress in Understanding the Disease and the Development of Treatments and Vaccines," *Clinical Microbiology and Infection* 20, no. 3 (2014): 202–209, https://doi.org/10.1111/1469-0691.12540.

5. *Use of Vital and Health Records in Epidemiological Research*, Vital and Health Statistics: Documents and Committee Reports (Washington, DC: DHEW Publication, March 1968), https://www.cdc.gov/nchs/data/series/sr_04/sr04_007.pdf.

6. Donald A. Henderson, "The Eradication of Smallpox—An Overview of the Past, Present, and Future," *Vaccine* 29 (2011): D7–D9, https://doi.org/10.1016/j.vaccine.2011.06.080.

7. This data was generously made available from urban economist Jason Barr. He discusses this data in more detail in his blog, *Building the Skyline*, at https://buildingtheskyline.org/mortality-nyc-1/. Beyond the raw data, all calculations are my own.

8. Jacob A. Riis, *How the Other Half Lives: Studies among the Tenements of New York* (New York: Charles Scribner's Sons, 1890).

9. Riis, *How the Other Half Lives*, 46.

10. John W. Sterling, "Part First. Original Communications.: Art. I.—History of the Asiatic Cholera at Quarantine, Staten Island, New-York, in December, 1848, and January, 1849. 2d and 3d January," *New York Journal of Medicine and Collateral Sciences (1843–1856)* 3, no. 1 (1849): 9, https://www.proquest.com/scholarly-journals/part-first-original-communications/docview/136118792.

11. Sterling, "Part First."

12. "Disasters: New York City Cholera Outbreak of 1849," NYC
     Data, last accessed May 2, 2023, https://www.baruch.cuny.edu
     /nycdata/disasters/cholera-1849.html.

13. Jeremy Faust, "Data Snapshot: Are We Overcounting Covid-19
     Deaths? No.," *Inside Medicine* (blog), January 16, 2023,
     https://insidemedicine.substack.com/p/data-snapshot-are-we
     -overcounting.

14. Jeffrey Gettleman and Kai Schultz, "Modi Orders 3-Week Total
     Lockdown for All 1.3 Billion Indians," *New York Times*,
     March 24, 2020, https://www.nytimes.com/2020/03/24/world
     /asia/india-coronavirus-lockdown.html.

15. Gettleman and Schultz, "Modi Orders."

16. Gettleman and Schultz, "Modi Orders."

17. Gettleman and Schultz, "Modi Orders."

18. Sushmita Pathak, "Whatever Happened to . . . the Teen Hailed
     for Cycling 700 Miles with Her Injured Dad?," NPR, Septem-
     ber 7, 2021, https://www.npr.org/sections/goatsandsoda/2021/09
     /07/1033652752/whatever-happened-to-the-teen-hailed-for
     -cycling-700-miles-with-her-injured-dad.

19. Avishek G. Dastidar, "Shramik Specials: 'When the Train Left,
     We Broke into an Applause . . . It Was Spontaneous,'" *Indian
     Express*, January 1, 2021, https://indianexpress.com/article/india
     /shramik-trains-covid-19-india-lockdown-7128238/.

20. Jeffrey Gettleman et al., "The Virus Trains: How Lockdown
     Chaos Spread Covid-19 across India," *New York Times*, Decem-
     ber 15, 2020, https://www.nytimes.com/2020/12/15/world/asia
     /india-coronavirus-shramik-specials.html.

21. Gettleman et al., "The Virus Trains."

22. Dastidar, "Shramik Specials."

23. Dastidar, "Shramik Specials."

24. Gettleman et al., "The Virus Trains."

25. Yashwant Deshmukh et al., "Excess Mortality in India from
     June 2020 to June 2021 during the COVID Pandemic: Death
     Registration, Health Facility Deaths, and Survey Data," med-
     Rxiv preprint, posted July 23, 2021, https://www.medrxiv.org

/content/10.1101/2021.07.20.21260872v1; Abhishek Anand, Justin Sandefur, and Arvind Subramanian, "Three New Estimates of India's All-Cause Excess Mortality during the COVID-19 Pandemic" (working paper, Washington, DC: Center for Global Development, 2021), https://cgdev.org/publication/three-new -estimates-indias-all-cause-excess-mortality-during-covid-19 -pandemic. These two studies counted the excess deaths at the midpoint of 2021 and found similar magnitudes.

26. "The Last Journey of the München," Hapag-Lloyd, November 3, 2018, https://www.hapag-lloyd.com/en/news-insights /insights/2018/11/the-last-journey-of-the--muenchen-.html.

27. Centers for Disease Control and Prevention, *Excess Deaths Associated with Covid-19*, last accessed March 10, 2022, https://www.cdc.gov/nchs/nvss/vsrr/covid19/excess_deaths.htm.

28. Chana Joffe-Walt, "Essential: The Pandemic Forced Jobs to Change, but Then the Workers Changed, Too," *This American Life Podcast*, August 13, 2021, https://www.thisamericanlife.org /744/essential.

29. Paul Berger, "NYC Dead Stay in Freezer Trucks Set Up during Spring Covid-19 Surge," *Wall Street Journal*, November 22, 2020, https://www.wsj.com/articles/nyc-dead-stay-in-freezer -trucks-set-up-during-spring-covid-19-surge-11606050000.

30. David Roos, "How Many Were Killed on D-Day?," *History .com*, June 5, 2019, https://www.history.com/news/d-day -casualties-deaths-allies.

31. Jeremy Samuel Faust, Zhenqiu Lin, and Carlos Del Rio, "Comparison of Estimated Excess Deaths in New York City during the COVID-19 and 1918 Influenza Pandemics," *JAMA Network Open* 3, no. 8 (2020), http://doi.org/10.1001/jamanetworkopen .2020.17527. This study found that while the excess mortality in terms of the number of deaths was slightly higher in the 1918 influenza epidemic in New York City than the pandemic of 2020, the pandemic of 2020 had a larger relative increase in mortality.

32. Riis, *How the Other Half Lives*, 35.

33. Riis, *How the Other Half Lives*, 10.

34. Riis, *How the Other Half Lives*, 36.
35. Archibald Robertson, *Collect Pond, New York City,* 1798, on virtual display, Metropolitan Museum of Art, New York, https://www.metmuseum.org/art/collection/search/11925.
36. Harry Schenawolf, "New York City's Pristine Collect Pond Was a Fresh Water Source for New Yorkers for Nearly Two Hundred Years. What Happened to It?," *Revolutionary War Journal*, July 22, 2019, http://www.revolutionarywarjournal.com/new -york-citys-pristine-collect-pond-was-a-fresh-water-source-for -new-yorkers-for-nearly-two-hundred-years-what-happened -to-it/.
37. Schenawolf, "New York City's Pristine Collect Pond."
38. Schenawolf, "New York City's Pristine Collect Pond."
39. Tricia Kang, "What Lies Beneath: A History of Collect Pond," New York City Tenement Museum (blog), https://www.tenement .org/blog/what-lies-beneath-a-history-of-collect-pond/.
40. Riis, *How the Other Half Lives*, 8.
41. Riis, *How the Other Half Lives*, 8.
42. Charles Dickens, *American Notes for General Circulation* (London: Chapman and Hall, 1842), https://archive.org/details /americannotes00dick/page/588/mode/2up.
43. Dickens, *American Notes*.
44. Tyler Anbinder, *Five Points: The 19th-Century New York City Neighborhood that Invented Tap Dance, Stole Elections, and Became the World's Most Notorious Slum* (New York: Free Press, 2010), 43.
45. Anbinder, *Five Points*, 88.
46. Anbinder, *Five Points*, 74.
47. Alternatively spelled Coulter's Brewery in some accounts and descriptions.
48. Neil Pentecost, "The Old Brewery," *New York City Looking Back* (blog), April 21, 2011, http://newyorklookingback .blogspot.com/2011/04/old-brewery.html.
49. Pentecost, "The Old Brewery."
50. Anbinder, *Five Points*, 69.
51. Anbinder, *Five Points*, 67.

52. John Noble Wilford, "How Epidemics Helped Shape the Modern Metropolis," *New York Times*, April 15, 2008, https://www.nytimes.com/2008/04/15/science/15chol.html.
53. Anbinder, *Five Points*, 23.
54. Wilford, "How Epidemics."
55. Riis, *How the Other Half Lives*, 21.
56. Riis, *How the Other Half Lives*, 21.
57. For a description of the term *othering*, see Edward W. Said, *Orientalism* (New York: Pantheon Books, 1978).
58. Rosemary Horrox, ed., *The Black Death* (Manchester: Manchester University Press, 1994).
59. Horrox, *The Black Death*.
60. Nicholas A. Christakis, *Apollo's Arrow: The Profound and Enduring Impact of Coronavirus on the Way We Live* (New York: Little, Brown Spark, 2020).
61. "The Second Parliament of Charles II: Sixth Session (Oxford)," *The History and Proceedings of the House of Commons: Volume 1, 1660–1680* (London: Chandler, 1742), https://www.british-history.ac.uk/commons-hist-proceedings/vol1/pp85-92.
62. Reuters Staff, "Italian Regional Chief Sorry for Saying Chinese Eat 'Live Mice,'" *Reuters*, February 29, 2020, https://www.reuters.com/article/china-health-italy/italian-regional-chief-sorry-for-saying-chinese-eat-live-mice-idUSL8N2AT0G3.
63. Reuters Staff, "Italian Regional Chef."
64. "COVID-19 Fueling Anti-Asian Racism and Xenophobia Worldwide," *Human Rights Watch*, May 12, 2020, https://www.hrw.org/news/2020/05/12/covid-19-fueling-anti-asian-racism-and-xenophobia-worldwide.
65. Wendy Grossman Kantor, "Filipino American Man Recounts Brutal Attack with Box Cutter on N.Y.C. Subway: 'Nobody Helped,'" *PEOPLE.com*, February 18, 2021, https://people.com/crime/filipino-american-man-recounts-brutal-attack-with-box-cutter-on-n-y-c-subway-nobody-helped/.
66. "Exclusive: 89-Year-Old Woman Who Was Attacked, Set on Fire in Brooklyn Speaks Out," interview by CeFann Kim, *ABC7 New York*, July 25, 2020, https://abc7ny.com/woman-set-on-fire

-elderly-attack-89-year-old-attacked-bensonhurst-crime
/6333749/.

67. Sakshi Venkatraman, "Anti-Asian Hate Crimes Rose 73% Last
Year, Updated FBI Data Says," *NBCNews.com*, October 25,
2021, https://www.nbcnews.com/news/asian-america/anti-asian
-hate-crimes-rose-73-last-year-updated-fbi-data-says-rcna3741.

68. Paul Sakkal, "'Go Back to Your Country': Chinese International
Students Bashed in CBD," *The Age*, April 17, 2020, https://
www.theage.com.au/national/victoria/go-back-to-your-country
-chinese-international-students-bashed-in-cbd-20200417-p54kyh
.html; "COVID-19 Fueling Anti-Asian Racism," *Human Rights
Watch*.

69. Trip Gabriel, "Ohio Lawmaker Asks Racist Question about
Black People and Hand-Washing," *New York Times*, June 11,
2020, https://www.nytimes.com/2020/06/11/us/politics/steve
-huffman-african-americans-coronavirus.html.

70. "Tapper to Azar: This Is Nothing to Celebrate," interview by
Jake Tapper, CNN, May 15, 2020, https://www.cnn.com/videos
/politics/2020/05/17/alex-azar-coronavirus-pandemic-death-toll
-tapper-sot-sotu-vpx.cnn. Full transcript available at https://
transcripts.cnn.com/show/sotu/date/2020-05-17/segment/01.

71. Tomi Akinyemiju et al., "Disparities on the Prevalence of
Comorbidities among US Adults by State Medicaid Expansion
Status," *Preventative Medicine* 88 (2016): 196–202, https://doi
.org/10.1016/j.ypmed.2016.04.009.

72. Jason M. Barr and Troy Tassier, "The Pandemic Tsunami: How
COVID-19 Swept Across America," *Building the Skyline* (blog),
February 25, 2021, https://buildingtheskyline.org/covid-waves/.

73. Dana Ullman, "After a Farmworker in Rural Texas Died of
Complications from COVID-19, His Family and Federal
Investigators Want Answers," *The Fern*, September 16, 2020,
https://thefern.org/2020/09/after-a-farmworker-in-rural-texas
-died-of-complications-from-covid-19-his-family-and-federal
-investigators-want-answers/. The account of Mr. Gomez collects
details from this source.

74. Ullman, "After a Farmworker."

75. Ullman, "After a Farmworker."

76. Ullman, "After a Farmworker."

77. Ullman, "After a Farmworker."

78. Ullman, "After a Farmworker."

79. Vania Patino, "Dalhart Community Leaders Step Up as Hospital Overflows with COVID-19 Cases," *Newschannel0.com*, October 22, 2020, https://www.newschannel10.com/2020/10/22 /dalhart-community-leaders-step-up-hospital-overflows-with -covid-cases/.

80. Navajo Housing Authority, *Phase II Housing Needs Assessment and Demographic Analysis*, August 2011, https://www.navajo housingauthority.org/images/2022/Housing%20Needs%20 Assessment/Navajo_Nation_Housing_Needs_Assessment _091311.pdf.

81. Federal Reserve Bank of Minneapolis, *Navajo Nation Reservation Demographics*, last accessed July 14, 2022, https://www .minneapolisfed.org/indiancountry/resources/reservation-profiles /navajo-nation-reservation.

82. Max Ufberg, "The Navajo Nation Is Being Decimated by This Virus," *Medium*, May 13, 2020, https://mronline.org/2020/05 /20/the-navajo-nation-is-being-decimated-by-this-virus/.

83. Benjamin R. Brady and Howard M. Bahr, "The Influenza Epidemic of 1918–1920 among the Navajos: Marginality, Mortality, and the Implications of Some Neglected Eyewitness Accounts," *American Indian Quarterly* 38, no. 4 (2014): 459–91, https://doi.org/10.5250/amerindiquar.38.4.0459.

84. Hollie Silverman, Konstantin Toropin, and Sara Snider, "Navajo Nation Surpasses New York State for the Highest Covid-19 Infection Rate in the US," CNN, May 18, 2020, https://www .cnn.com/2020/05/18/us/navajo-nation-infection-rate-trnd/index .html.

85. Dennis Wagner and Wyatte Grantham-Philips, "'Still Killing Us': The Federal Government Underfunded Health Care for Indigenous People for Centuries. Now They're Dying of Covid-19," *USA Today*, October 26, 2020, https://www.usatoday .com/in-depth/news/nation/2020/10/20/native-american-navajo

-nation-coronavirus-deaths-underfunded-health-care
/5883514002/.

86. Wagner and Grantham-Philips, "'Still Killing Us.'"

87. Jonathan Nez (@NNPrezNez), "177 New Cases, 9,833 Recoveries, and No Recent Deaths Related to COVID-19," Twitter, December 6, 2020, 7:02 p.m., https://twitter.com/NNPrezNez /status/1335736416488210432/photo/2.

88. "Indian Health Service Profile Fact Sheets," IHS, last accessed July 14, 2022, https://www.ihs.gov/newsroom/factsheets /ihsprofile/.

89. Joshua Cheetham, "Navajo Nation: The People Battling America's Worst Coronavirus Outbreak," *BBC News*, June 15, 2020, https://www.bbc.com/news/world-us-canada-52941984.

90. Wagner and Grantham-Philips, "'Still Killing Us.'"

91. "Dikos Ntsaaígíí-19," Navajo Department of Health, accessed July 1, 2022, https://www.ndoh.navajo-nsn.gov/covid-19.

92. The World Health Organization estimates are slightly larger. Data available from the WHO does not sort deaths by ethnicity and race.

93. Calculations from the author using socioeconomic data from the US Census Bureau and the US Bureau of Labor Statistics in conjunction with pandemic data from USAfacts.org.

94. Jennifer Tolbert, Kendal Orgera, and Anthony Damico, *Key Facts about the Uninsured Population* (San Francisco: Kaiser Family Foundation, November 6, 2020).

95. Samantha Artiga et al., *Health Coverage by Race and Ethnicity, 2010–2019* (San Francisco: Kaiser Family Foundation, July 15, 2021), https://www.kff.org/racial-equity-and-health-policy/issue -brief/health-coverage-by-race-and-ethnicity/.

96. Artiga et al., *Health Coverage.*

97. Tolbert, Orgera, and Damico, *Key Facts.*

98. Data calculations in this paragraph performed by the author using county level death data available at USA Facts, https:// usafacts.org/visualizations/coronavirus-covid-19-spread-map/, and demographic data from the US Census Bureau, https://www .census.gov/data.html.

99. Tolbert, Orgera, and Damico, *Key Facts.*

100. Tolbert, Orgera, and Damico, *Key Facts,* Appendix Table B.

101. Jennifer Tolbert, Kendal Orgera, and Anthony Damico, *Key Facts about the Uninsured Population: Supplemental Tables* (San Francisco: Kaiser Family Foundation, November 6, 2020), https://files.kff.org/attachment/Key-Facts-about-the-Uninsured -Population-Supplemental-Tables.pdf.

102. Tolbert, Orgera, and Damico, *Key Facts.*

103. Davalon, "How Much Does Health Insurance Cost without A Subsidy?," *eHealth,* January 21, 2022, https://www.ehealth insurance.com/resources/affordable-care-act/much-health-insurance -cost-without-subsidy.

104. Jeanine Skowronski, "A State-by-State Guide to Medicaid: Do I Qualify?," PolicyGenius.com, December 8, 2021, https://www .policygenius.com/health-insurance/a-state-by-state-guide-to -medicaid/.

105. John Tozzi, "Why Some Americans Are Risking It and Skipping Health Insurance," *Bloomberg News*, March 26, 2018, https://www.bloomberg.com/news/features/2018-03-26 /why-some-americans-are-risking-it-and-skipping-health -insurance.

106. Tozzi, "Why Some Americans."

107. Tolbert, Orgera, Damico, *Key Facts*, Supplemental Tables.

108. Rachel Garfield, Kendal Orgera, and Anthony Damico, *The Uninsured and the ACA: A Primer—Key Facts about Health Insurance and the Uninsured Amidst Changes to the Affordable Care Act* (San Francisco: Kaiser Family Foundation, January 25, 2019), https://www.kff.org/report-section/the-uninsured-and -the-aca-a-primer-key-facts-about-health-insurance-and-the -uninsured-amidst-changes-to-the-affordable-care-act-how-does -lack-of-insurance-affect-access-to-care/.

Chapter 9. A Curious Practice

1. Stefan Riedel, "Edward Jenner and the History of Smallpox and Vaccination," *Baylor University Medical Center Proceedings* 18,

no. 1 (2005): 21–25, http://doi.org/10.1080/08998280.2005
.11928028.

2. A minority believe this plague to have been caused by measles.

3. Isobel Grundy, *Lady Mary Wortley Montagu: Comet of the Enlightenment* (New York: Oxford University Press, 2001).

4. Lady Mary Wortley Montagu, *Turkish Embassy Letters*, ed. Malcolm Jack (London: William Pickering 1993), available at "Modern History Sourcebook: Lady Mary Wortley Montagu (1689–1762): Smallpox Vaccination in Turkey," Fordham University, https://sourcebooks.fordham.edu/mod/montagu -smallpox.asp.

5. A. Boylston, "The Origins of Inoculation," *Journal of the Royal Society of Medicine* 105, no.7 (2012): 309–313, https://doi.org /10.1258/jrsm.2012.12k044.

6. Ben Franklin, *Autobiography* (New York: Modern Library, 1950), 113–114.

7. Reidel, "Edward Jenner and the History of Smallpox."

8. Reidel, "Edward Jenner and the History of Smallpox."

9. History.com Editors, "Battle of Quebec (1775)," *history.com*, August 21, 2018, https://www.history.com/topics/american -revolution/battle-of-quebec-1775.

10. Philip J. Smith, David Wood, and Paul M. Darden, "Highlights of Historical Events Leading to National Surveillance of Vaccination Coverage in the United States," *Public Health Reports* 126, no. 2 (2011): 3–12, https://doi.org/10.1177 /00333549111260S202.

11. History.com Editors, "Battle of Quebec (1775)."

12. Ian Glynn and Jenifer Glynn, *The Life and Death of Smallpox* (Cambridge: Cambridge University Press, 2004).

13. "From George Washington to William Shippen, Jr. 6 February 1777," *Founders Online*, National Archives, https://founders .archives.gov/documents/Washington/03-08-02-0281.

14. Frank M. Snowden, *Epidemics and Society: From the Black Death to Present* (New Haven: Yale University Press, 2019).

15. Riedel, "Edward Jenner and the History of Smallpox."

16. Riedel, "Edward Jenner and the History of Smallpox."

17. Snowden, *Epidemics and Society.*
18. Snowden, *Epidemics and Society.*
19. Snowden, *Epidemics and Society.*
20. Snowden, *Epidemics and Society.*
21. P. Berche, "Louis Pasteur, from Crystals of Life to Vaccination," *Clinical Microbiology and Infection* 18, no. 5 (2012): 1–6, https://doi.org/10.1111/j.1469-0691.2012.03945.x.
22. Snowden, *Epidemics and Society.*
23. Snowden, *Epidemics and Society.*
24. Michael Underwood, *Debility of the Lower Extremities. In: Treatise on the Diseases of Children* (London: J. Mathews, 1789), 53–57.
25. Snowden, *Epidemics and Society.*
26. Snowden, *Epidemics and Society.*
27. Anda Baicus, "History of Polio Vaccination," *World Journal of Virology* 1, no. 4 (2012): 108–14, https://doi.org/10.5501/wjv.v1.i4.108.
28. Joshua S. Loomis, *Epidemics: The Impact of Germs and Their Power over Humanity* (Nashville: Turner Publishing, 2018).
29. Naomi Rogers, "Race and the Politics of Polio: Warm Springs, Tuskegee, and the March of Dimes," *American Journal of Public Health* 97, no. 5 (2007): 784–95, https://doi.org/10.2105/AJPH.2006.095406.
30. Paul Harmon, "The Racial Incidence of Poliomyelitis in the United States with Special Reference to the Negro," *Journal of Infectious Diseases* 58, no. 3 (1936): 331–336, https://doi.org/10.1093/infdis/58.3.331; quoted by Rogers, "Race and the Politics of Polio," 784–95.
31. Rogers, "Race and Politics," 784–95.
32. Rogers, "Race and Politics," 784–95.
33. Rogers, "Race and Politics," 784–95.
34. Baicus, "History of Polio Vaccination," 108–14.
35. Baicus, "History of Polio Vaccination," 108–14.
36. Baicus, "History of Polio Vaccination," 108–14.
37. Snowden, *Epidemics and Society.*
38. Snowden, *Epidemics and Society.*

39. Snowden, *Epidemics and Society*.
40. Tom D. Y. Chin and William M. Marine, "The Changing Pattern of Poliomyelitis Observed in Two Urban Epidemics: Kansas City and Des Moines, 1959," *Public Health Reports* 76, no. 7 (1961): 553–563.
41. Chin and Marine, "The Changing Pattern," 553–563.
42. Chin and Marine, "The Changing Pattern," 553–563.
43. Neal Nathanson et al., "Epidemic Poliomyelitis during 1956 in Chicago and Cook County, Illinois," *American Journal of Hygiene* 70, no. 2 (1959): 107–168.
44. Howard D. Siedler et al., "Outbreak of Type 3 Paralytic Poliomyelitis in Washington, D.C., in 1957," *American Journal of Hygiene* 71, no. 1 (1959): 29–44.
45. Joseph G. Molner, Jacob A. Brody, and George H. Agate, "Detroit Poliomyelitis Epidemic, 1958. Preliminary Report," *Journal of the American Medical Association* 169, no. 16 (1959): 1838–1842.
46. Snowden, *Epidemics and Society*.
47. Rogers, "Race and the Politics of Polio," 784–95.
48. Snowden, *Epidemics and Society*.
49. Snowden, *Epidemics and Society*.
50. Richard B. Johns et al., "Two Voluntary Mass Immunization Programs Using Sabin Oral Vaccine," *Journal of the American Medical Association* 183, no. 3 (1963): 171–175, https://doi.org/10.1001/jama.1963.03700030047010.
51. "Polio Once Caused Widespread Panic," Centers for Disease Control and Prevention, last accessed July 15, 2022, https://www.cdc.gov/polio/what-is-polio/polio-us.html.
52. "Past Seasons Vaccine Effectiveness," Centers for Disease Control and Prevention, last accessed July 15, 2022, https://www.cdc.gov/flu/vaccines-work/past-seasons-estimates.html.
53. Amy McKeever, "Why Even Fully Vaccinated Older People Are at High Risk for Severe COVID-19," *National Geographic*, October 19, 2021, https://www.nationalgeographic.com/science/article/why-older-vaccinated-people-face-higher-risks-for-severe-covid-19.

54. James Skipper and George P. Landow, "Wages and Cost of Living in the Victorian Era," Victorian Web, July 16, 2003, https://victorianweb.org/economics/wages2.html.

55. Philip J. Smith, David Wood, and Paul M. Darden, "Highlights of Historical Events Leading to National Surveillance of Vaccination Coverage in the United States," *Public Health Reports* 126, no. 2 (2011): 3–12, https://doi.org/10.1177/00333549111260S202.

56. Elena Conis, "The History of the Personal Belief Exemption," *Pediatrics* 145, no. 4 (2020), https://doi.org/10.1542/peds.2019-2551.

57. Conis, "The History of the Personal Belief Exemption."

58. Conis, "The History of the Personal Belief Exemption."

59. Myong-Hun Chang and Troy Tassier, "Socio-Economic and Spatial Patterns of Vaccine Refusal" (paper, Eastern Economic Association Meetings, Boston, MA, 2019).

60. Chang and Tassier, "Socio-Economic and Spatial Patterns."

61. Chang and Tassier, "Socio-Economic and Spatial Patterns."

62. World Health Organization, "Measles Vaccination Has Saved an Estimated 17.1 Million Lives since 2000," news release, November 12, 2015, https://www.who.int/news/item/12-11-2015-measles-vaccination-has-saved-an-estimated-17-1-million-lives-since-2000.

63. Makia S. Clemmons et al., "Incidence of Measles in the United States, 2001–2015," *Journal of the American Medical Association* 318, no. 13 (2017): 1279–1281, https://doi.org/10.1001/jama.2017.9984.

64. New York City Department of Health and Mental Hygiene, *Alert # 10: Update on Measles Outbreak in New York City and Citywide Recommendations*, May 24, 2019, https://www1.nyc.gov/assets/doh/downloads/pdf/han/alert/2019/update-measles-outbreak.pdf.

65. "Measles" Vaccine Knowledge Project, June 9, 2022, https://vk.ovg.ox.ac.uk/vk/measles, last accessed July 15, 2022.

66. *Confirmed Cases of Measles Mumps and Rubella in England and Wales: 1996 to 2021*, UK Health Security Agency, Immunisation

and Vaccine Preventable Diseases Division, February 1, 2022, https://www.gov.uk/government/publications/measles-confirmed -cases/confirmed-cases-of-measles-mumps-and-rubella-in-england -and-wales-2012-to-2013.

67. Stephanie Soucheray, "US Measles Cases Top 1,200 as UK Loses 'Measles Free' Status," *Center for Infectious Disease Research and Policy News*, August 19, 2019, https://www.cidrap.umn.edu /news-perspective/2019/08/us-measles-cases-top-1200-uk-loses -measles-free-status.

68. Gary Finnegan, "France Measles Outbreak: Babies Hit Hardest," *Vaccines Today*, November 7, 2018, https://www.vaccinestoday .eu/stories/france-measles-outbreak-babies-hit-hardest/.

69. Finnegan, "France Measles Outbreak."

70. Data from The World Bank can be found at https://data.worldbank .org/indicator/SH.IMM.MEAS?locations=UA.

71. Tim Whewell, Kateryna Shypko, and Diana Kuryshko, "The Budding Doctor Who Died of Measles," *BBC News*, June 22, 2019, https://www.bbc.com/news/stories-48668841.

72. Meredith Wadman, "Measles Cases Have Tripled in Europe, Fueled by Ukrainian Outbreak," *Science*, February 12, 2019, https://www.science.org/content/article/measles-cases-have -tripled-europe-fueled-ukrainian-outbreak.

73. Data from The World Bank can be found at https://data.worldbank .org/indicator/SH.IMM.MEAS?locations=UA.

74. Roman Rodyna, "Measles Situation in Ukraine during the Period 2017–2019," *European Journal of Public Health* 29, no. 4 (2019), https://doi.org/10.1093/eurpub/ckz186.496; World Health Organization, "Strengthening Response to Measles Outbreak in Ukraine," news release, January 22, 2020, https:// www.who.int/europe/news/item/22-01-2020-strengthening -response-to-measles-outbreak-in-ukraine.

75. Whewell, Shypko, and Kuryshko, "The Budding Doctor."

76. Jacqui Thornton, "Measles Cases in Europe Tripled from 2017 to 2018," *British Medical Journal* 364 (2019), https://doi.org/10 .1136/bmj.l634.

77. Thornton, "Measles Cases in Europe."

78. Active management of forests does exactly this spacing of trees and brush to try to limit the risk of forest fires. See Beth Rands, "Making Forests Stronger through Active Management," *Forestry* (blog), US Department of Agriculture, July 29, 2021, https://www.usda.gov/media/blog/2019/03/01/making-forests -stronger-through-active-management.

79. Myong-Hun Chang and Troy Tassier, "Spatially Heterogeneous Vaccine Coverage and Externalities in a Computational Model of Epidemics," *Computational Economics* 58 (2021): 27–55, https://doi.org/10.1007/s10614-019-09918-7.

80. Mallory Locklear, "'Not a Zero-Sum Game': Sharing Vaccines Is in Countries' Best Interests," *Yale News,* September 21, 2021, https://news.yale.edu/2021/09/21/not-zero-sum-game-sharing -vaccines-countries-best-interests.

81. Peter J. Hotez, *Preventing the Next Pandemic: Vaccine Diplomacy in a Time of Anti-Science* (Baltimore: Johns Hopkins University Press, 2021).

82. "Vaccine Tracker," European Centre for Disease Prevention and Control, last accessed July 15, 2022, https://vaccinetracker .ecdc.europa.eu/public/extensions/COVID-19/vaccine-tracker .html#uptake-tab.

83. Josh Holder, "Tracking Coronavirus Vaccinations around the World," *New York Times*, January 29, 2021, https://www.nytimes .com/interactive/2021/world/covid-vaccinations-tracker.html.

84. Holder, "Tracking Coronavirus Vaccinations."

85. Seth Berkley, "COVAX Explained," *Vaccines Work* (blog), Gavi, September 3, 2020, https://www.gavi.org/vaccineswork/covax -explained.

86. Benjamin Mueller and Rebecca Robbins, "Where a Vast Global Vaccination Program Went Wrong," *New York Times*, August 2, 2021, https://www.nytimes.com/2021/08/02/world/europe/covax -covid-vaccine-problems-africa.html.

87. Keith Collins and Josh Holder, "What Data Shows about Vaccine Supply and Demand in the Most Vulnerable Places,"

New York Times, December 9, 2021, https://www.nytimes.com
/interactive/2021/12/09/world/vaccine-inequity-supply.html.

88. Collins and Holder, "What Data Shows."
89. Mueller and Robbins, "Where a Vast Global Vaccination."
90. Mueller and Robbins, "Where a Vast Global Vaccination"; Staff,
   "Pfizer: Nigeria Drug Trial Victims Get Compensation," *BBC
   News*, August 11, 2011, https://www.bbc.com/news/world-africa
   -14493277.
91. Mueller and Robbins, "Where a Vast Global Vaccination."
92. Jason Law, "What Is a 'Vaccine Desert' and How Do We Avoid
   Them?," *Boston 25 News*, February 11, 2021, https://www
   .boston25news.com/news/health/what-is-vaccine-desert-how-do
   -we-avoid-them/SKLDQBGGFVCKFJJR2C3H54CZDI/.
93. Paola Rosa-Aquino, "America's Next Covid Obstacle: Vaccine
   Deserts," *NY Magazine: Intelligencer*, March 11, 2021, https://
   nymag.com/intelligencer/2021/03/americas-next-covid-obstacle
   -vaccine-deserts.html.
94. Jacey Fortin, "Woman, 90, Walked Six Miles in the Snow for a
   Vaccine," *New York Times*, February 18, 2021, https://www
   .nytimes.com/2021/02/18/us/fran-goldman-covid-vaccine-seattle
   .html.
95. Tori Marsh, "'Vaccine Deserts' Threaten to Prolong COVID-19
   Vaccine Rollout and Widen Disparities," *GoodRx Health*,
   January 14, 2021, https://www.goodrx.com/blog/covid-19-vaccine
   -deserts-threaten-rollout/.
96. Benjamin Rader et al., "Spatial Accessibility Modeling of
   Vaccine Deserts as Barriers to Controlling SARS-CoV-2,"
   medRxiv preprint, posted June 12, 2021, https://www.medrxiv
   .org/content/10.1101/2021.06.09.21252858v1.full.pdf.
97. Rader et al., "Spatial Accessibility."
98. Rader et al., "Spatial Accessibility."
99. Rader et al., "Spatial Accessibility."
100. Kellen Browning, "Seniors Seeking Vaccines Have a Problem:
   They Can't Use the Internet," *New York Times*, February 28,
   2021, https://www.nytimes.com/2021/02/28/technology/seniors
   -vaccines-technology.html.

101. Browning, "Seniors Seeking Vaccines."
102. Browning, "Seniors Seeking Vaccines."
103. Browning, "Seniors Seeking Vaccines."
104. Nambi Ndugga et al., *Latest Data on COVID-19 Vaccinations by Race/Ethnicity* (San Francisco: Kaiser Family Foundation, July 14, 2022), https://www.kff.org/coronavirus-covid-19/issue-brief/latest-data-on-covid-19-vaccinations-race-ethnicity/.
105. Ndugga et al., *Latest Data on COVID-19.*
106. Ndugga et al., *Latest Data on COVID-19.*
107. Natasha Williams et al., "Assessment of Racial and Ethnic Disparities in Access to COVID-19 Vaccination Sites in Brooklyn, New York," *JAMA Network Open* 4, no. 6 (2021), http://doi.org/10.1001/jamanetworkopen.2021.13937.
108. Data collected from "Vaccinations in the United States," Centers for Disease Control and Prevention, https://www.cdc.gov/coronavirus/2019-ncov/vaccines/distributing/reporting-counties.html. A few states had to be excluded from this data analysis due to inconsistencies in reporting methods or lack of data provided at the county level. These included AK, CO, GA, HI, TX, VA and some counties in a few other states that did not report vaccine statistics due to the small population of the county. In total, 2,489 counties out of 3,143 counties in the country are included in the analysis.
109. "Household Pulse Survey COVID-19 Vaccination Tracker," United States Census Bureau, December 22, 2021, https://www.census.gov/library/visualizations/interactive/household-pulse-survey-covid-19-vaccination-tracker.html.
110. Elizabeth A. Dobis and David McGranahan, "Rural Residents Appear to be More Vulnerable to Serious Infection or Death from Coronavirus COVID-19," US Department of Agriculture Economic Research Service, February 1, 2021, https://www.ers.usda.gov/amber-waves/2021/february/rural-residents-appear-to-be-more-vulnerable-to-serious-infection-or-death-from-coronavirus-covid-19/.
111. Dobis and McGranahan, "Rural Residents."

Chapter 10. Compassion, Not Tools

1. John Snow, *On the Mode of Communication of Cholera* (London: John Churchill, 1855).
2. Snow, *On the Mode.*
3. Snow, *On the Mode.*
4. Henry Whitehead, "Special Investigation of Broad Street," June 5, 1855, https://kora.matrix.msu.edu/files/21/120/15-78-7D -22-1855-07-CIC-Whitehead.pdf.
5. The child was not named by Snow or Whitehead. However, a genealogist named Dave Boylan uncovered Frances's name. Dave Boylan, "Finding Baby Lewis," available at https://kora.matrix.msu .edu/files/21/120/15-78-AD-22-johnsnow-a0a1f7-a_11479.pdf.
6. Whitehead, "Special Investigation," 159.
7. Whitehead, "Special Investigation," 160.
8. Frank M. Snowden, *Epidemics and Society: From the Black Death to the Present* (New Haven: Yale University Press, 2019).
9. Charles Dickens, *Oliver Twist* (London: Penguin Books, 2002).
10. Snowden, *Epidemics and Society.*
11. Snowden, *Epidemics and Society.*
12. Rudolf Carl Virchow, "Report on the Typhus Epidemic in Upper Silesia," *American Journal of Public Health* 96, no. 12 (2006): 2102–2105, https://doi.org/10.2105/ajph.96.12.2102.
13. Virchow, "Report on the Typhus Epidemic," 2102–5.
14. Virchow, "Report on the Typhus Epidemic," 2102–5.
15. Virchow, "Report on the Typhus Epidemic," 2102–5.
16. Virchow, "Report on the Typhus Epidemic," 2102–5.
17. Virchow, "Report on the Typhus Epidemic," 2102–5.
18. Klaus W. Lange, "Rudolf Virchow, Poverty and Global Health: From 'Politics as Medicine on a Grand Scale' to 'Health in All Policies,'" *Global Health Journal* 5, no. 3 (2021): 149–154, https://doi.org/10.1016/j.glohj.2021.07.003.
19. Lange, "Rudolf Virchow," 149–154.
20. Lange, "Rudolf Virchow," 149–154.
21. Amy L. Fairchild et al., "The Exodus of Public Health: What History Can Tell Us About the Future," *American Journal of*

Public Health 100, no. 1 (2010): 54–63, https://doi.org/10.2105/AJPH.2009.163956.

22. Allan M. Brandt and Martha Gardner, "Antagonism and Accommodation: Interpreting the Relationship between Public Health and Medicine in the United States during the 20th Century," *American Journal of Public Health* 90, no. 5 (2000): 707–715, https://doi.org/10.2105/ajph.90.5.707.

23. Fairchild et al., "The Exodus of Public Health," 54–63.

24. Paul Starr, *The Social Transformation of American Medicine: The Rise of a Sovereign Profession and the Making of a Vast Industry* (New York: Basic Books, 1982).

25. Brandt and Gardner, "Antagonism and Accommodation," 707–715.

26. Ed Yong, "How Public Health Took Part in Its Own Downfall," *Atlantic*, October 23, 2021, https://www.theatlantic.com/health/archive/2021/10/how-public-health-took-part-its-own-downfall/620457/. Quote given to Ed Yong by Amy Fairchild.

27. Fairchild et al., "The Exodus of Public Health," 54–63.

28. Brandt and Gardner, "Antagonism and Accommodation," 707–715.

29. Brandt and Gardner, "Antagonism and Accommodation," 707–715.

30. Brandt and Gardner, "Antagonism and Accommodation," 707–715.

31. H. Holden Thorp, "It Ain't Over 'til It's Over," *Science* 376, no. 6594 (2022): 675, https://doi.org/10.1126/science.abq8460.

32. For examples see Thomas McKeown, *The Modern Rise of Population* (New York: Academic Press, 1976) and Thomas McKeown, R. G. Record, and R. D. Turner, "An Interpretation of the Decline of Mortality in England and Wales during the Twentieth Century," *Population Studies* 29, no. 3 (1975): 391–422.

33. James Colgrove, "The McKeown Thesis: A Historical Controversy and Its Enduring Influence," *American Journal of Public Health* 92, no. 5 (2002): 725–729.

34. For examples, see Donald A. Barr, *Health Disparities in the United States: Social Class, Race, Ethnicity, and the Social*

Determinants of Health (Baltimore: Johns Hopkins University Press, 2008) and Daniel E. Dawes, *The Political Determinants of Health* (Baltimore: Johns Hopkins University Press, 2020).

35. James Reason, *Human Error* (Cambridge, MA: Cambridge University Press, 1990).

36. James Reason, "Human Error: Models and Management," *British Medical Journal* 320 (2000): 768–770, https://doi.org/10 .1136/bmj.320.7237.768.

37. Justin Larouzee and Jean-Christophe Le Coze, "Good and Bad Reasons: The Swiss Cheese Model and Its Critics," *Safety Science* 126 (2020), https://doi.org/10.1016/j.ssci.2020.104660.

38. Siobhan Roberts, "The Swiss Cheese Model of Pandemic Defense," *New York Times*, December 5, 2020, https://www .nytimes.com/2020/12/05/health/coronavirus-swiss-cheese -infection-mackay.html.

39. Details of Mr. Contreras taken from Kate Cimini and Jackie Botts, "Close Quarters: California's Overcrowded Homes Fuel Spread of Coronavirus among Workers," *Cal Matters*, June 12, 2020, updated December 10, 2020, https://calmatters.org/projects /overcrowded-housing-california-coronavirus-essential-worker/.

40. Matteo Forgiarini, Marcello Gallucci, and Angelo Maravita, "Racism and the Empathy for Pain on our Skin," *Frontiers in Psychology* 23 (2011), https://doi.org/10.3389/fpsyg.2011 .00108.

41. W. E. B. Du Bois, *The Philadelphia Negro: A Social Study* (Philadelphia: University of Pennsylvania Press, 1899, reprinted 1996).

42. David R. Williams and Michelle Sternthal, "Understanding Racial-Ethnic Disparities in Health: Sociological Contributions," *Journal of Health and Social Behavior* 51 (2010): S15–S27, http://doi.org/10.1177/0022146510383838.

43. I thank Pam Papish for the genesis of this comment.

44. Mike Dorning, "Getting Covid Gets You Fired When You're a Food Worker on a Visa," *Bloomberg News*, July 31, 2020, https://news.bloomberglaw.com/coronavirus/u-s-visa-rules-trap -migrant-workers-in-virus-infested-dorms.

45. Corina Knoll, "'What Do I Do Next?': Orphaned by Covid, Two Teens Find Their Way," *New York Times*, May 29, 2021, https://www.nytimes.com/2021/05/29/nyregion/covid-death-mom-teens.html.

46. Knoll, "'What Do I Do Next?'"

47. Knoll, "'What Do I Do Next?'"

48. Dan Treglia et al., "Hidden Pain: Children Who Lost a Parent or Caregiver to COVID-19 and What the Nation Can Do to Help Them," COVID Collaborative, December 2021, https://www.covidcollaborative.us/assets/uploads/pdf/HIDDEN-PAIN.Report.Final.pdf.

49. Susan D. Hillis et al., "COVID-19-Associated Orphanhood and Caregiver Death in the United States," *Pediatrics* 148, no. 6 (2021), https://doi.10.1542/peds.2021-053760.org.

50. H. Juliette T. Unwin et al., "Global, Regional, and National Minimum Estimates of Children Affected by COVID-19-Associated Orphanhood and Caregiver Death, by Age and Family Circumstance up to Oct. 21, 2021: An Updated Modelling Study," *The Lancet* 6, no. 4 (2022): 249–259, https://www.thelancet.com/journals/lanchi/article/PIIS2352-4642(22)00005-0/fulltext.

51. Ed Yong, "How the Pandemic Defeated America," *Atlantic*, July 30, 2021, https://www.theatlantic.com/magazine/archive/2020/09/coronavirus-american-failure/614191/.

52. Liz Ford, "'Covid Has Magnified Every Existing Inequality'—Melinda Gates," *Guardian*, September 15, 2020, https://www.theguardian.com/global-development/2020/sep/15/covid-has-magnified-every-existing-inequality-melinda-gates.

53. Philip Blumenshine et al., "Pandemic Influenza Planning in the United States from a Health Disparities Perspective," *Emerging Infectious Disease* 14, no. 5 (2008): 709–715, https://doi.org/10.3201/eid1405.071301.

54. Alison P. Galvani et al., "Universal Healthcare as Pandemic Preparedness: The Lives and Costs That Could Have Been Saved during the COVID-19 Pandemic," *Proceedings of the National Academy of Sciences* 199, no. 25 (2022), https://doi.org10.1073/pnas.2200536119.

55. Paul Starr, *The Social Transformation of American Medicine: The Rise of a Sovereign Profession and the Making of a Vast Industry* (New York: Basic Books, 1982).

56. Martin Luther King Jr., "Beyond Vietnam—A Time to Break the Silence," speech at Riverside Church, New York City, April 4, 1967, https://www.americanrhetoric.com/speeches /mlkatimetobreaksilence.htm.

INDEX

Page numbers in *italics* indicate illustrations.

291, 322–24; focus on individual risk, 16–17; food shortages, 139–40; as great equalizer, idea of, 4–5, 162; grocery delivery during, 131; health risk of, 23, 24–25, 29, 200; hospitalization rates, 26, 266; housing insecurity and, 82, 83, 131; ICU care, 130, 308–9; impact on children, 188, 335–36; labor market and, 144, 146–47, 170, 185–87, 190–91; layers of protection from, 326–27; less-cautious groups, 205–7; in long-term care facilities, 107–8; mathematical models, 224–25; migrant workers and, 263–65; minority communities and, 5, 26, 250–51, 261–63, 262; misinformation about, 202–3, 204; mobility patterns during, 139, *140*; number of cases, 39–40, 209–10, 309–10; origin of, 3, 139; popular views of, 143–45; preventive measures against, 16, 23, 87–88, 112, 113, 145–46, 233–34, 322; protests against restrictions, 197–98, 214; public health social programs, 95–96; religion and, 211, 214; reproduction number, 23–24, 55; retreat from, 125–26, 131–35; risk aversion and, 199, 205–6; in rural areas, 74, 308–10; shopping experience, 139–43, 144–45; social impact of, 122, 145–46, 165–67, 330–31, 334–36; spread of, 37, 55, 71–72, 106, 118, 205, 261, 356n28; stay-at-home orders, 39, 112, 120, 129–30, 141; super-spreading events, 71–76, 81–87, 113–14, 197–98, 216–17, 220–22; Swiss cheese model, 325–26; time spent outside homes during, 142–44; treatment of, 130, 215–16, 340; Trump's policy on, 204; undetected infections, 57–58; variants and strains, 82, 306, 307–8, 324; waves of, 246–47, 248, 263, 307–8

COVID-19 mortality: of ethnic and racial minorities, 336, 400n92; per capita, 74; versus 1918 influenza mortality, 395n31; poverty and, 271; statistics on, 16, 26–27, 43, 65, 107–8, 245, 248, 340–41; of uninsured population, 272–73; white population and, 262

polio (*cont.*)
deaths from, 248; outbreaks,
283–84, 286–87; race and,
287; severe cases, 284;
socioeconomic aspect, 287,
339; symptoms, 284;
treatment of, 285
polio vaccination: attenuated
vaccine, 285; criticism of,
286; Cuban program, 289;
development of, 283,
285–86, 288; distribution
of, 287–88, 306; mandate,
291; opposition to, 291–92;
rates of, 287; Sabin vaccine,
288, 289, 300; Salk vaccine,
286, 288, 323–24
Pollock, Brad, 225
Pompeo, Mike, 259
poorhouses, 315, 332
population density: epidemic
risk and, 40–41, 43; in
high-income and impover-
ished neighborhoods,
49–50, 51, 52–53; infectious
diseases and, 14, 52, 54,
59–60, 64; types of, 50;
of urban environment,
12–13. *See also* dominant
density; forgotten density;
inward density; upward
density
Portland, Oregon: influenza
epidemic of 1918, 195
Portugal: COVID-19 vaccination rates, 300–301

preventative medicine, 322,
327, 340
Prince of Wales Hospital, 71
prisoner's dilemma, 227
Pritchett, Jonathan, 36–37
Procopius, 115
public health: emergencies,
231–32; evolution of, 320,
321–22; versus medicine,
320–21; necessity of pro-
grams, 95; nutrition and,
341–42; origin of field of,
319; reform of, 316, 317;
social factors in, 320
public health interest versus
commercial interests
debates, 120–22
public transit ridership:
COVID-19 pandemic and,
140, 141, 147–49

quarantines, 97–98, 99,
118–19, 120, 121, 129
Quebec City: siege of,
280–81
Quintana, Noel, 260

R (reproduction number):
definition of, 8; DOTS factors
of, 9–10, 23; exposure risk
and, 23; of infectious disease,
8–11
rabies vaccine, 283
Ralphs (supermarket chain),
163–64
Ramos, Sidney, 178

Reason, James, 325; *Human Error*, 324
Redfield, Robert, 39
Reinders, Robert, 30
restaurant workers: COVID-19 impact on, 161, 174–75, 178–79, 191; exposure risk, 175–76, 178; layoffs, 174, 192; sexual harassment of, 178; treatment from patrons, 176, 177; wages, 175, 176–77
retail stores: closure of, 191; COVID-19 infections, 163; time spent in, 140, 142, 145
"return to normal," 276, 304, 332, 335
Riis, Jacob, 251, 253; *How the Other Half Lives*, 238, 253, 257–58
risk: uncertainty and, 199–200, 201, 203
risk acceptance, 232, 233, 234
risk aversion, 198–99, 205, 216
Rivera, Betty, 112
Robertson, Archibald, 251
Robert Wood Johnson Foundation, 83
Rogers, Naomi, 284, 285
rogue waves of epidemics, 246, 249
Rolph, James, 194, 196
Romania: COVID-19 vaccination rates, 301
Roosevelt, Franklin, 285

Roosevelt Warm Springs Institute for Rehabilitation, 285
Rose Garden reception: as super-spreader event, 85–86, 87, 205
Rosenberg, Charles, 128, 129
Ross, Ronald, 7–8, 24
Rush, Benjamin, 127, 128, 157–58
Rush, Julia, 158
Russia: cholera outbreaks, 213
Ryder, Kate, 191

Sabin, Albert Bruce, 288, 289, 324
Sabin polio vaccine, 236, 288, 289, 300, 324
Salk, Jonas, 285–86, 288, 323
Salk polio vaccine, 236, 286, 288, 306, 323–24
Salmonella typhi, 67
Salomon, Adriana, 334, 335, 336
Salomon, Magalie, 334
Salomon, Xavier, 334–35, 336–37, 341
Sand City, CA, 328
San Francisco, CA: influenza epidemic of 1918, 195–96
sanitation, 316, 319
SARS (severe acute respiratory syndrome), 38, 69, 70–71, 80, 113
Sault Ste. Marie airport, 78–79, 88, 92

typhoid fever: asymptomatic carriers, 70, 360n2; outbreaks of, 67–68; reproduction number of, 68, 70; spread of, 68–69; symptoms, 66

Typhoid Mary, 66, 67, 68

typhus, 21, 317–19

Uganda: COVID-19 vaccination rates, 302

Ukraine: measles outbreaks, 295–97, 298

Ullman, Dana, 265

Underwood, Michael, 283

unemployment: COVID-19 and, 144, 146–47, 165–66; decline of, 165; gender and, 166; government benefits, 173; Great Recession and, 187; racial and ethnic factor, 166; single parenting and, 166–67; statistics, 165–66; of women, 187–88

uninsured population, 261, 271–73, 274–75, 304, 308, 310

United Kingdom: COVID-19 contact tracing, 95; excess deaths, 246; household income, 149–50; industrial revolution, 12; influenza epidemic of 1918, 173–74; measles vaccination, 295; mobility patterns, 142–43;

New Poor Laws, 315–16; Ordinance of Labourers of 1349, 184; Peasants' Revolt of 1381, 185; public works program, 316; sanitation system, 316; smallpox vaccination, 279, 280, 291; Statute of Labourers of 1351, 185; stay-at-home order, 141; urban population of, 12

United States: coal production, 171; excess mortality, 246, 247, *262, 263*; heavy industry, 171; household income, 149–50; urban population of, 12

universal health care, xii, 339, 341–42

upward density, 52–53, 59

urgent care system, 275

vaccination: discovery of, 282–83; effectiveness of, 289–91; herd immunity and, 299; hesitancy, 295; invention of, 281; mandates, 216, 291, 292; misinformation about, 202; personal belief exemption, 292, 293, 294; religious exemption from, 291–92; spoiled doses, 302. *See also* COVID-19 vaccination; influenza vaccination; polio vaccination

vaccine-allocation problem, 365n47